Certified Hospice and Palliative Nurse (CHPN®) Exam Review

A Study Guide With Review Questions

Patricia Moyle Wright, PhD, CRNP, ACNS-BC, CHPN, CNE

SPRINGER PUBLISHING COMPANY

Springer Publishing Company, LLC
11 West 42nd Street
New York, NY 10036
www.springerpub.com
http://connect.springerpub.com

Acquisitions Editor: Elizabeth Nieginski
Compositor: diacriTech

ISBN: 978-0-8261-1969-8
ebook ISBN: 978-0-8261-1974-2
DOI: 10.1891/9780826119742

19 20 21 22 / 5 4 3 2 1

The author and the publisher of this Work have made every effort to use sources believed to be reliable to provide information that is accurate and compatible with the standards generally accepted at the time of publication. Because medical science is continually advancing, our knowledge base continues to expand. Therefore, as new information becomes available, changes in procedures become necessary. We recommend that the reader always consult current research and specific institutional policies before performing any clinical procedure. The author and publisher shall not be liable for any special, consequential, or exemplary damages resulting, in whole or in part, from the readers' use of, or reliance on, the information contained in this book. The publisher has no responsibility for the persistence or accuracy of URLs for external or third-party Internet websites referred to in this publication and does not guarantee that any content on such websites is, or will remain, accurate or appropriate.

The Hospice and Palliative Credentialing Center (HPCC®) is the sole owner of the Certified Hospice and Palliative Nurse (CHPN®) certification program. HPCC does not endorse any CHPN certification exam review resources or have a proprietary relationship with Springer Publishing Company. Direct permission requests to LeonardM@hpna.org.

Library of Congress Cataloging-in-Publication Data
Names: Wright, Patricia Moyle, author.
Title: Certified hospice and palliative nurse (CHPN®) exam review : a study guide with review
    questions / Patricia Moyle Wright, PhD, CRNP, ACNS-BC, CHPN, CNE.
Description: New York, NY : Springer Publishing Company, LLC, [2020] | Includes bibliographical
    references and index.
Identifiers: LCCN 2019015623 | ISBN 9780826119698 | ISBN 9780826119742 (e-book)
Subjects: LCSH: Hospice nurses–Examinations, questions, etc. | Palliative treatment–Examinations,
    questions, etc. | Nursing–Examinations, questions, etc.
Classification: LCC RT87.T45 W74 2020 | DDC 616.02/9076–dc23
LC record available at https://lccn.loc.gov/2019015623

Contact us to receive discount rates on bulk purchases.
We can also customize our books to meet your needs.
For more information please contact: sales@springerpub.com

Patricia Moyle Wright: https://orcid.org/0000-0002-0005-0759

Publisher's Note: New and used products purchased from third-party sellers are not guaranteed for quality, authenticity, or access to any included digital components.

Printed in the United States of America.

Register Now for Online Access to Your Book!

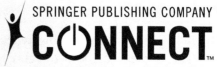

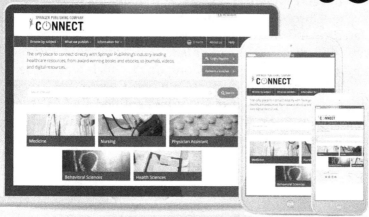

Your print purchase of *Certified Hospice and Palliative Nurse (CHPN®) Exam Review* **includes online access to the contents of your book**—increasing accessibility, portability, and searchability!

Access today at:

http://connect.springerpub.com/content/book/978-0-8261-1974-2
or scan the QR code at the right with your smartphone
and enter the access code below.

H5KHMAF4

Scan here for quick access.

SPRINGER PUBLISHING COMPANY
View all our products at springerpub.com

Patricia Moyle Wright, PhD, CRNP, ACNS-BC, CHPN, CNE, is a professor of nursing at the University of Scranton in Scranton, Pennsylvania, where she teaches in the undergraduate and graduate nursing programs. Dr. Wright brings more than 20 years of experience in the field of hospice and palliative care to her teaching and truly loves to inspire students to provide the best possible care to those facing their last moments. She also continues to provide direct care to terminally ill patients through her work as a per diem hospice nurse practitioner.

Outside of the classroom and clinical settings, Dr. Wright shares her love of end-of-life nursing care with others through her writing. She is the author of numerous articles on issues related to end-of-life care, including perinatal loss. She is coeditor of the award-winning text *Perinatal and Pediatric Bereavement in Nursing and Other Health Professions* (Springer Publishing Company), which was chosen as the 2016 AJN Book of the Year in the category of Palliative Care and Hospice. She is also the author of a ready reference text for nurses entitled *Fast Facts for the Hospice Nurse: A Concise Guide to End-of-Life Care*, which was published by Springer Publishing Company, as well as numerous articles and book chapters on end-of-life care.

This book is dedicated to all of the nurses who touch the lives of patients and families facing end-of-life issues each day. You have chosen to work in the most sacred of spaces, the nexus of life and death. May your work be a shining light in the darkest of times, and may you inspire others through your care and professionalism.

Contents

SECTION V: PATIENT AND FAMILY CARE, EDUCATION, AND ADVOCACY

SECTION VI: PRACTICE ISSUES

SECTION VII: PRACTICE TEST

Preface

This book is offered to hospice and palliative care nurses to assist their preparation for taking the Certified Hospice and Palliative Nurse (CHPN®) certification examination. When I prepared to take the hospice certification exam for the first time in 1999, there were no certification preparation texts or courses. Pulling together resources to study was a challenge. Since then, numerous texts have been published on end-of-life care, and the field has grown by leaps and bounds. Interest in demonstrating expertise through certification as a hospice and palliative care nurse has continually grown, as recognition of one's expertise brings not only professional satisfaction but also personal pride.

Since this text is a practice and certification review for hospice and palliative care nurses preparing for the CHPN certification examination, the book follows the test outline offered by the Hospice and Palliative Credentialing Center. In seven sections, this book offers tips on test-taking, an outline of the CHPN certification examination (Section I), a review of life-limiting conditions in adult patients (Section II), a review of pain and symptom management (Sections III and IV), a review of education and advocacy in patient and family care (Section V), a review of practice issues (Section VI), and a full-length practice test with answers and rationales (Section VII). Practice questions are also included at the ends of Chapters 3 through 22.

The content included in this book is one of many resources available. My hope is that it will be a useful tool as it does cover the specific content on the examination outline and offers hundreds of practice questions. Best wishes as you prepare to demonstrate excellence in hospice and palliative care through certification.

Acknowledgments

I gratefully acknowledge my family's unwavering support for my determination to write about, teach, and practice end-of-life nursing. First, I thank my parents for the selfless love you have offered me throughout my life. It has taught me to give unselfishly to others. I am also grateful to my husband, David, for supporting me through every twist and turn of my career. Your love and light saw me through and helped me to continue this work. I also thank my children, Dominic and Vivian, for your patience with me as you often waited for me to finish "just one more sentence." May you also find fulfillment and inspiration in your life's work.

I would also like to gratefully acknowledge the editorial staff of Springer Publishing Company for their outstanding professionalism and dedication to the nursing profession. I am especially grateful to Elizabeth Nieginski and Rachel Landes for their support and assistance through the completion of this book.

Test Preparation

1

The Hospice and Palliative Nursing Examination

*Nursing certifications recognize those individuals who
demonstrate an advanced knowledge base, along with qualifications
and skills within a particular specialty.*
—Fritter and Shimp (2016, p. 8)

LEARNING OBJECTIVES

After completing this section, the nurse will be able to

1. Discuss the importance of earning certification as a Hospice and Palliative Nurse
2. Describe the process of applying for and renewing certification through the Hospice and Palliative Credentialing Center
3. Identify various resources for content review and test preparation
4. Describe the application process for the exam
5. Develop a system for tracking recertification requirements over the 5-year renewal period

Certification as a Hospice and Palliative Nurse demonstrates knowledge and experience in the role of the hospice and palliative nurse. The exam includes material that is important for everyday practice in the specialty field of end-of-life and palliative care. In this chapter, detailed information about the exam is presented. However, the reader is strongly encouraged to read the entire Certified Hospice and Palliative Nurse (CHPN®) Candidate Handbook, which is available at advancingexpertcare.org/chpn.

WHY BECOME CERTIFIED?

Certification in a nursing specialty demonstrates personal and professional commitment to excellence in practice. In today's fast-paced and ever-changing healthcare arena, there is an increased need for professionals to demonstrate knowledge and expertise. Personal benefits of certification include external validation of knowledge and expertise, personal empowerment, and a sense of accomplishment. Certification may also lead to increased marketability, career ladder progression, and peer recognition (Fritter & Shimp, 2016).

Certification in the area of hospice and palliative care is encouraged for nurses as a way of demonstrating competence. According to the Hospice and Palliative Credentialing Center (HPCC, 2019a), "the purpose of certification is to promote delivery of comprehensive palliative care through the certification of qualified hospice and palliative care professionals" (p. 1). Successful completion of the certification exam demonstrates that the certificant has the requisite knowledge for certification in this practice specialty. Further, certification demonstrates a commitment to the specialty (Fritter & Shimp, 2016) and encourages further professional growth in the area of hospice and palliative care (HPCC, 2019a).

▨ ABOUT THE CERTIFIED HOSPICE AND PALLIATIVE NURSE EXAMINATION

In 1994, the first hospice certification exam was offered by the Hospice Nurses Association (HNA), which was renamed the Hospice and Palliative Nurses Association in 2002. The first certificants were awarded the credential CRNH, Certified Registered Nurse Hospice. In 1997, in response to the results of a role delineation study conducted by the HNA, the certification test was renamed the Certified Hospice and Palliative Nurse (CHPN) Examination to recognize that palliative care is a critical part of hospice care. Certificants were then awarded the credential CHPN upon successful completion of the exam.

The Hospice and Palliative Credentialing Center

HPCC is an organization dedicated to advancing expert care for those who are seriously ill. The HPCC offers certification examinations for Advanced Practice Registered Nurses, RNs, Licensed Practical Nurses/Licensed Vocational Nurses, Nursing Assistants, administrators, and perinatal loss professionals such as nurses, social workers, and chaplains. The board of the HPCC is responsible for all aspects of the certification process. The HPCC Board of Directors is responsible for development and maintenance of the CHPN examination and partners with the testing agency, PSI Services, to ensure secure administration of the exam.

Testing Agency: PSI Services

PSI Services is contracted "by the HPCC to assist in the development, administration, scoring, and analysis of the HPCC certification examinations" (Hospice and Palliative Credentialing Center, 2019a, p. 1). In addition to providing the HPCC assistance with development and administration of the exam, PSI processes the exam results and reports them to the examinee and to the HPCC. Paper applications for the exam are also processed by PSI Services.

Applying for the Exam

Prior to applying for the CHPN examination, eligibility should be established. Eligibility for the CHPN examination includes the following:

1. Current and active nursing licensure in the United States or its territories or in Canada
2. 500 hours of practice in the area of hospice and palliative nursing within the most recent 12 months OR 1,000 hours of practice within the most recent 24 months

If eligibility requirements are met, the application process can be undertaken. According to the HPCC (2019a), there are two ways to register for the CHPN exam:

1. Visit advancingexpertcare.org/chpn and choose the test you wish to take under the "Certification" tab. Click "Begin online exam application" under the heading "Online Exam Application." Select the appropriate options in the drop-down menus, which will lead to the PSI website, where you can register for the exam.
2. Instead of completing the application online, you may complete a paper application, which can be found in the Candidate Handbook that is available at documents.goamp.com/Publications/candidateHandbooks/HPCC-CHPN-Handbook.pdf. The completed application and fee (payable by credit card, personal check, cashier's check, or money order) should then be mailed to PSI Services using the address in the Candidate Handbook. It may take up to 2 weeks to process a paper application. The candidate will be contacted by PSI and given a website address and a toll-free phone number that can be used to schedule the exam.

Requests for Special Accommodations

Requests for special accommodations due to disability may be made at the time of application for the examination. The Examination Accommodations form is included in the Candidate Handbook, which can be found at documents.goamp.com/Publications/candidateHandbooks/HPCC-CHPN-Handbook.pdf. All requests must be signed by an appropriate professional and submitted to PSI Services by the application deadline.

Scheduling the Examination

The CHPN examination is administered during specific testing windows. Applications must be received and processed by the application date in order for an applicant to take the examination during the testing window. Applications that are submitted prior to the Application Start Date or after the Application Deadline will not be processed. Applications are processed strictly according to the following schedule:

Testing Window	Application Start Date	Paper Application Deadline	Online Application Deadline
March 1–March 31	December 1	January 15	February 15
June 1–June 30	March 1	April 15	May 15
September 1– September 30	June 1	July 15	August 15
December 1– December 31	September 1	October 15	November 15

The CHPN Examination is administered at PSI Assessment Centers throughout the United States. The examination is administered by appointment at a PSI testing center. Available appointment times may vary from testing center to testing center, with some centers offering evening or Saturday appointments. Testing centers are closed for certain holidays during each testing window. Examination appointments are available on a first-come, first-serve basis (HPCC, 2019a). If a date or time is not available at one testing center, it may be wise to check availability at another nearby testing center.

> **Key Point**
>
> Testing center locations can be found at online.goamp.com/CandidateHome/displayTCList.aspx?pExamID=20735.

The Day of the Examination

On the day of the examination, arrive at the testing center at least 15 minutes prior to the appointment to allow time for verification of the appointment and security procedures. Those arriving more than 15 minutes late for the appointment will not be admitted.

At the center, go to the PSI test center check-in area. Bring two forms of identification. The primary form of identification must be government issued, with a photo. All forms of identification must be current. Expired forms of identification cannot be used. Examples of valid primary forms of identification are as follows:

- Driver's license with photograph
- State identification card with photograph
- Passport with photograph
- Military identification card with photograph

Temporary identification cards, Social Security cards, employment identification cards, and student identification cards may be used as secondary forms of identification if they include a photograph and a signature. However, they may not be used as the primary form of identification.

Once the examinee's identity is verified, the examinee will sign the roster and will be directed to the computer station. A photograph of the examinee will be taken and will remain on-screen during the examination. The score report will also include the photograph. During the examination, no notes, cameras, cell phones, recorders, calculators, or pagers are allowed. Belongings will be secured in a soft locker by the testing center. If a candidate's personal items do not fit in the soft locker, the candidate will not be tested that day. No one may accompany the examinee into the testing area or reception area. Any examinee who is observed with personal or restricted items in the testing room will be dismissed (HPCC, 2019a).

Practice Examination

Prior to beginning the computerized certification examination, the examinee will be offered practice questions on the computer to ensure comfort with the electronic testing process. The questions presented to the examinee during the practice test *do not* count toward the test score. When the examinee quits the practice exam, the timed examination begins.

■ EXAMINATION OUTLINE

The CHPN examination consists of 150 multiple-choice questions. Of those 150 questions, 15 questions are trial questions that are not scored. Thus, a total of 135 questions, which have equal weight, are scored for the examination. The trial questions are interspersed throughout the examination and are indistinguishable from the scored questions. Responses to trial questions do not affect the outcome of the examination. Examinees are allotted a total of 3 hours to complete the examination. Those who pass the examination are awarded the credential CHPN (HPCC, 2019a).

Content

The content that is included on the CHPN certification examination is directly related to work performed by hospice and palliative nurses as identified through a role delineation study that was conducted by the HPCC (2019b). The content is reflective of the knowledge base that a hospice and palliative nurse with 2 years of practice experience in this specialty area should have attained.

A detailed outline is provided in the Candidate Handbook (HPCC, 2019a) and is included in the following table. Questions on the exam correspond to an area that is specified on the outline. Further, the outline provides candidates with the relative importance of each area on the exam by denoting the percentage of the test that is related to that topic.

Topic	Percentage of CHPN Examination
Patient Care: Life-Limiting Conditions in Adult Patients	18
Patient Care: Pain Management	22
Patient Care: Symptom Management	24
Patient and Family Care, Education and Advocacy	24
Practice Issues	12

Note: The Candidate Handbook (HPCC, 2019a) provides a detailed outline of the test. CHPN, Certified Hospice and Palliative Nurse.

To further explicate the examination content, 22% is recall of information, 60% requires the candidate to apply the information to patient situations, and 18% requires the candidate to analyze situations, synthesize information, determine solutions, and/or evaluate the interventions (HPCC, 2019b).

During the Examination

Examinees may comment on individual test questions throughout the examination. This can be done by clicking on the COMMENT button that appears to the left of the TIME button on the screen. To ensure

> **Key Point**
>
> On the CHPN examination, generic drug names are provided. Exceptions may be made in certain cases as deemed necessary by the examination development committee (HPCC, 2019a).

the security of the examination, examinees will not receive feedback regarding their comments. All questions are the copyrighted property of the HPCC. Copying, reproducing, recording, distributing, or sharing any part of the examination is strictly forbidden by law and may incur civil and criminal penalties (HPCC, 2019a).

■ AFTER THE EXAMINATION

Getting the Results

When the examination is over, a brief survey regarding your examination experience appears on the screen. Following this, instructions to report to the examination proctor to obtain a score report will appear. The score report obtained at the testing center will indicate whether the result was "pass" or "fail."

The score report will also indicate the raw scores in each of the content areas. The raw score is the number of questions that were answered correctly. Raw scores help the examinee identify areas of strengths and areas in need of further review. The report will also include the scaled score, which is derived from the raw score and is a score between 0 and 99. The scaled score, rather than the raw score, is used to account for variations in the difficulty of different versions of the examination. A scaled score of 75 is needed to pass the exam (HPCC, 2019a).

I've Passed! Now What?

Those who successfully pass the examination may use the designation CHPN after their name to indicate that they are a CHPN. Within a few weeks of passing the examination, an official certificate will be issued by mail from the HPCC. The certificant's name will also appear in the certification verification online system, which can be accessed via the following link: advancingexpertcare.org/HPNA/HPCC/CertificationWeb/Certification_Verification.aspx. The certification period is 4 years.

Renewal Requirements

Certificants are required to complete the requirements for the Certified Hospice and Palliative Nurse Hospice and Palliative Alternative Recertification (CHPN HPAR). Renewal of certification through this method requires that the CHPN fulfill practice hour requirements and also demonstrate ongoing professional development.

Practice Hour Requirements

In order to renew certification as a CHPN, the nurse must have an unrestricted license to practice as a RN in the United States, its territories, or Canada. The nurse must also have completed 500 practice hours in the specialty in the most recent 12 months or 1,000 hours in the specialty in the most recent 24 months prior to submitting the application for renewal of certification (HPCC, 2018).

Ongoing Professional Development

Professional Development Activities includes four distinct areas: situational judgment exercise (SJE), continuing education, scholarly accomplishments, and/or professional contributions. The certificant accrues points in each of these

Key Point
The LearningBuilder platform may be accessed through advancingexpertcare. org/chpn/. In the LearningBuilder platform, certificants may add their professional accomplishments to their online record at any time during the certification cycle.

areas based on their activity. In total, 100 points must be accrued during the certification period. All certificants must log their accomplishments in the LearningBuilder platform during the certification cycle (see advancingex-pertcare.org/chpn).

A brief summary of the requirements is offered in the following table, but please refer to the Candidate Handbook for the most up-to-date information.

Category	Requirements	Maximum Point Limit
Practice Hours and Licensure	500 practice hours in the specialty in the most recent 12 months or 1,000 hours in the specialty in the most recent 24 months prior to submitting the application for renewal of certification **and** An unrestricted license to practice as a RN in the United States, its territories, or Canada	N/A
Professional Development Activities	A. **SJE:** This is a required online exercise B. **Continuing Education:** 60 minutes = 1 contact hour = 1 HPAR point; 30 minutes = 0.5 contact hour = 0.5 HPAR points C. **Scholarly Accomplishments:** 1 academic credit = 15 HPAR points; 1 HPAR point is awarded for every 10 minutes of a professional presentation starting with 20 minutes; professional publications accrue points depending on the type of publication	**SJE:** 20 points maximum **Continuing Education:** No maximum **Scholarly Accomplishments:** Academic Education: 45 points maximum Professional Presentations: 20 points maximum Professional Publications: 75 points maximum

(continued)

(continued)

Category	Requirements	Maximum Point Limit
	D. **Professional Contributions:** 25 hours of precepting students who are enrolled in an accredited academic healthcare program = 5 HPAR points; 40 hours of orienting staff = 5 HPAR points; 1 year of volunteer service in a healthcare-related organization = 5 HPAR points	**Professional Contributions:** Precepting Students = 20 points maximum; Orienting Staff = 5 points maximum; Volunteer Service = 10 points maximum

CHPN, Certified Hospice and Palliative Nurse; HPAR, Hospice Palliative Alternative Recertification; SJE, Situational Judgment Exercise.

Requirements for Recertification

The CHPN HPAR requirements must be met during the certification period, and the renewal applications must be submitted between January 1 and December 31 in the year that the certification will expire.

Reactivation of an Expired Credential

If a certificant misses the deadline for renewal of recertification, the LearningBuilder platform can be used to submit the materials for reactivation of the credential. The option of reactivation is available for 3 years after the expiration of the credential. In order to meet the criteria for reactivation of the credential, professional development and practice hours are required. All professional development activities must be completed during the reporting period, which is stated in the individual's learning plan in the LearningBuilder platform. In addition to meeting the requirements for recertification, the certificant must also contact HPCC to request reactivation and pay the reactivation fee.

What If I Don't Pass?

If a candidate does not successfully pass the CHPN examination, it can be taken again in a subsequent testing window. The applicant must submit a new application and the testing fee.

Chapter Summary
• Certification as a hospice and palliative nurse demonstrates expertise that is gained with approximately 2 years of clinical experience in the specialty.
• The HPCC offers certification testing during four testing windows in March, June, September, and December.
• An applicant for the CHPN examination may apply online or by mail.
• The complete test outline for the CHPN examination is available online at advancing-expertcare.org/chpn.

▪ REFERENCES

Fritter, E., & Shimp, K. (2016). What does certification in professional nursing practice mean? *Academy of Medical Surgical Nurses, 25*(2), 8–10. Retrieved from https://www.amsn.org/sites/default/files/private/medsurg-matters-newsletterarchives/marapr16.pdf

Hospice and Palliative Credentialing Center. (2018). *Certified hospice and palliative nurse.* Retrieved from https://advancingexpertcare.org/chpn/

Hospice and Palliative Credentialing Center. (2019a). *CHPN® candidate handbook.* Retrieved from http://documents.goamp.com/Publications/candidateHandbooks/HPCC-CHPN-Handbook.pdf

Hospice and Palliative Credentialing Center. (2019b). *Role delineation study.* Retrieved from https://advancingexpertcare.org/role-delineation/

2 Preparing for the Examination

> *In a word, before undertaking any enterprise, careful preparation must be made.*
> —Cicero (1913, p. 73)

LEARNING OBJECTIVES

After completing this section, the nurse will be able to

1. Develop a study plan for the Certified Hospice and Palliative Nurse (CHPN®) examination
2. Identify resources for CHPN examination preparation
3. Utilize appropriate strategies for answering examination questions
4. Choose electronic resources that can be used for test preparation

Certification in any nursing specialty is the mark of excellence and expertise. The goal of taking the examination is to leave the testing center with a new credential, having demonstrated competence in a specific area of practice. The idea of failing the examination is frightening and discouraging, especially considering the cost of the examination. Therefore, although careful preparation does not always ensure a positive outcome, it certainly helps to have the material organized mentally. Further, thorough preparation decreases test anxiety, which can unnerve even the best-prepared examinees.

PREPARATION

Preparation for certification examinations requires careful planning. A study plan that includes 1 to 3 hours per day during the 12-week period in advance of the test date is recommended. The Certified Hospice and Palliative Nurse (CHPN) test outline, available in Chapter 1,

The Hospice and Palliative Nursing Examination, should be used to break down material into small sections. In preparing for the examination, each of the chapters that follows in this book can be used to organize material, to practice questions, and to identify areas that require more focused review. Some sources recommend purchasing at least two different review books (or online reviews) so that the material can be reviewed in different ways (Leik, 2018). In addition to this review book, the Hospice and Palliative Nurses Association (HPNA) also offers an online review course that can be accessed at advancingexpertcare.org/HPNA/Education/Certification_Review_Courses/HPNAweb/Certification_Review.aspx?hkey=c3ad3f93-d90d-4655-b6f2-14c4984a1de5.

HPNA also offers face-to-face review courses at the Annual Clinical Practice Forum. This conference provides a forum for networking among hospice and palliative care nurses and sessions covering topics such as symptom management, hospice leadership, and the importance of self-care. More information can be found at advancingexpertcare .org/ClinicalPracticeForum.

> **Key Point**
>
> The End-of-Life Nursing Education Consortium (ELNEC) curriculum was developed in 2000 to provide end-of-life training for RNs. Today, nearly 24,000 nurses and other healthcare professionals have attended ELNEC courses (American Association of Colleges of Nursing, 2019).

Additional Resources

In addition to this text and the resources offered by the HPNA, reliable information regarding hospice and palliative nursing practice can be accessed by attending the ELNEC courses that are offered throughout the world. Although these courses are not review courses for the CHPN examination, they do include up-to-date information on pain and symptom management, cultural aspects of end-of-life care, communication, loss, grief, and bereavement, and working with patients in their final hours.

Another excellent source of information is the Annual Assembly of the American Academy of Hospice and Palliative Medicine (AAHPM) and HPNA. This conference is offered annually and is attended by over 3,000 hospice and palliative care professionals. Sessions focus on topics such as symptom management, communication with patients and families, spiritual aspects of care, and end-of-life care planning. Conferences such as this can help bring hospice professionals up-to-date with topics that are covered on the CHPN exam.

> **Key Point**
>
> Information about the Annual Assembly can be found at aahpm.org/meetings/assembly.

▪ PREPARATION STRATEGIES

Many nurses who have spent years in practice have not taken tests in some time. Although their skills and judgment in practice are excellent, standardized testing can be a stressful experience due to fear of the unknown or fear of failure. Careful preparation using various study methods and test-taking strategies can be helpful. Also, developing a systematic way of reading and answering each question as it appears on the screen can help improve preparedness. Some of these strategies will be discussed in the following sections.

Use Various Study Methods

Using the chapters that follow, organize the material into small sections that you can study each day. Plan to devote 1 to 3 hours each night for 8 to 12 weeks to properly prepare for the examination. When reviewing the material, develop a strategy for keeping track of material that you want to review. Some find it helpful to highlight key terms in the text with the plan to reread the material at a later time. There are also several other ways to capture material for easy review.

Note cards can be used to write down key concepts that will be reviewed again in the future. When developing note cards, the key is to keep the material simple. On one side of the card, write the concept and on the other side write only two to three key points about the concept that are important to remember. These cards can be used for self-study as often as needed until the material is mastered. Note cards can also be used to write review questions, with the question on one side and the answer on the other. Using a combination of both methods may also be helpful. Color coding note cards and grouping them together by topic is another way to organize material.

Another great way to memorize material is through the use of mnemonic devices. Mnemonic devices are techniques used to help remember concepts more easily, such as images, acronyms, and rhymes that bring information to mind more easily. For example, the acronym PQRST is commonly used to remember aspects of pain assessment:

P: Palliative and provocative factors

Q: Quality of the pain

R: Radiation

S: Severity

T: Timing

Acronyms like these are useful for jarring one's memory and for organizing information in a systematic way. Rhymes also help to put information together, so be creative when organizing materials for study. Imagery may also be a helpful tool when envisioning a patient with symptoms of a specific illness. Drawing images to help remember specific concepts is a great way to call to mind key concepts. One way of organizing material in a visual fashion is through the use of concept mapping. Concept mapping in an active learning strategy that involves constructing a diagram. Within the diagram, key concepts are captured in individual boxes or "nodes" and lines are drawn between and among the nodes to represent the relationships between the concepts (Karpicke & Blunt, 2011) (see Figure 2.1).

Example of a Concept Map

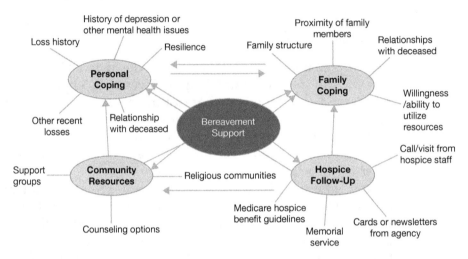

FIGURE 2.1 Concept map of bereavement support.

Developing a Plan

Once the approach to studying is chosen, it is important to follow certain "rules" of studying. First, review the test outline and list the topics according to the content that you find most challenging or least familiar. When you study, focus on unfamiliar things first. Once that material is mastered, more familiar material can be reviewed. This plan is a good way to economize study time.

When focusing on unfamiliar material, plan to devote several hours to learning one or two major concepts. Be sure to allow enough time to do this learning so that the material can be mastered, but do not get lost in rabbit holes. The CHPN examination is designed to test knowledge that is expected of a hospice and palliative care nurse with about 2 years of experience. It will not include in-depth questions on obscure topics.

Use Electronic Resources to Prepare for Electronic Testing

Electronic testing differs from paper and pencil examinations in several ways. The most notable is that the examinee cannot write on the exam during the test. Familiarity with online learning and online review of material may help increase comfort with the online format of the CHPN certification examination. For example, online note card programs are available to help organize material electronically. One advantage of using this type of tool is that the information can be accessed anywhere using a tablet, computer, or phone, which allows for on-the-go studying. Online review courses and online practice tests are also available.

Develop a Method for Answering Questions

The questions on standardized tests are developed by content experts who are also experts in test writing. Therefore, although there is only one correct answer, the other choices, which are called distractors, may seem plausible. The examinee must avoid being pulled toward responses that "seem" like good answers but are not actually the correct answers to the question. Distractors require the examinee to carefully read each question, to develop a plan to break the question down systematically, and then to determine the correct answer.

First, it is critical to read each question carefully. When reading the question, note key words in the stem of the question, paying close attention to important words such as "not"or "except" that direct the question in a specific way.

> **Key Point**
>
> In a well-written exam question, distractors contain familiar words that are not pertinent to the question or concepts that are commonly confused with the correct answer.

The stem will provide all of the information necessary to answer the question. Note important information such as the age of the patient in a scenario, the diagnosis, or the stage of a terminal illness. Sometimes, a scenario will be presented that provides a brief history of an illness and asks the nurse to consider what to expect next. Questions like these require an understanding of the disease process, but are essentially knowledge questions. Twenty-two percent of the CHPN examination is composed of knowledge-based, or recall, questions (Hospice and Palliative Credentialing Center, 2019). Knowledge questions can be recognized by the inclusion of terms like "What would the nurse expect next?" or "The nurse knows that . . . ." Knowledge questions can also appear as simple completion questions, such as in the following example.

Example of a Knowledge-Level Question

Which of the following is not covered by the Hospice Medicare Benefit?

A. Social worker visits

B. Bereavement services

C. Long-term care

D. Medications

Answering this type of question requires the nurse to eliminate three out of four distractors. But doing so requires thorough knowledge of the Hospice Medicare Benefit. Specifically, options A and B can be eliminated because Medical Social Services and Bereavement Services are considered to be core services. To eliminate D, the nurse must be aware that only medications related to the terminal illness are covered by the Hospice Medicare Benefit. So, the term "medications" is too broad to be the correct choice. Respite care can take place in a long-term care facility, but long-term care services are not covered by the Hospice Medicare Benefit. Therefore, C is the correct response.

Other questions require the examinee to demonstrate an understanding of some aspect of clinical practice and exhibit clinical judgment. In such questions, a scenario may be presented and the question may be phrased with a term such as "The best intervention is" or "What should the nurse do first?" Questions that specify "highest priority" test the nurse's ability to not only choose an appropriate intervention but also to determine which intervention is most important at that given time. In this way, the nurse's ability to plan and implement care that ensures the best outcome for the patient and family is assessed. Sixty percent of the CHPN examination questions are application questions (Hospice and Palliative Credentialing Center, 2019).

Example of an Application Question

The family of a patient who is actively dying calls the on-call hospice nurse to report that the patient appears to be in pain. There is an order for subcutaneous morphine sulfate 5 mg PRN q4h for pain, but the family is hesitant to administer it because the patient's respirations are shallow at 30 per minute. The nurse's best response is

A. "In the late stages of a disease process, pain is not a common concern, so there is no need to administer the morphine at this time."

B. "Administer the morphine, but monitor the respirations carefully and give naloxone if respirations become very shallow or fall below 10 per minute."

C. "Administer the morphine now to promote comfort. A nurse is available by phone 24 hours a day and a home visit can be made, if needed."

D. "What I hear you saying is that you are having trouble managing the patient's pain. Let us arrange for a transfer to the inpatient unit."

To correctly answer this question, the nurse must be able to unfold the various aspects of the stem. The most important information is that the patient is actively dying, appears to be in pain, and has an order for pain medication. Knowing that the goal of hospice care is to promote comfort, the best intervention involves administering the pain medication. However, since the family is viewed as the unit of care in hospice, the family's concerns must also be addressed. Therefore, the best response involves both managing the patient's pain and addressing the family's concerns. So, A can be eliminated because it is incorrect—pain is always a concern in hospice care. B can be eliminated because during the course of the dying process, respirations are expected to become shallower; the main concern is the patient's comfort. C addresses both the concerns of the family and the needs of the patient. It is also consistent with hospice philosophy, so it is the correct response. There is no evidence that the family is unable to manage the patient's symptoms or that inpatient care is required; therefore, D is not the correct the answer.

Evaluation questions prompt the candidate to synthesize the information in a patient scenario and determine whether an intervention is required. Further, the nurse must determine whether the steps taken were appropriate or effective, and whether further intervention is necessary. Evaluation questions may require the nurse to consider which symptom has the greatest impact on the choice of interventions. Or a scenario may be given in which a patient is experiencing several symptoms and numerous interventions are being implemented, and then the nurse may be asked to determine which intervention should be stopped due to adverse effects. Evaluation questions are usually complex and require time and higher-level thinking to determine the best response. Eighteen percent of the CHPN examination is composed of evaluation questions (Hospice and Palliative Credentialing Center, 2019).

Example of an Evaluation Question

A patient who has stage IV breast cancer is taking the bisphosphonate, clodronic acid. The treatment can be considered effective if

A. Serum calcium levels decrease

B. Pain level decreases from 9 to 4

C. Appetite increases

D. Fatigue decreases

Answering an evaluation question requires the examinee to synthesize knowledge, apply that knowledge to the scenario, and then draw a conclusion. In the example, the nurse would need to know that stage IV breast cancer involves bone metastases and that bisphosphonates are prescribed to decrease bone pain. The assessment skills needed involve linking the knowledge about the disease process with the treatment and deciding which assessments are key.

The example requires the examinee to choose the exact assessment that reveals whether the intervention is effective in a hospice population. With this in mind, A is a challenging distractor because one might see a decrease in serum calcium levels if bone metastases has slowed. However, the question is not asking for a general effect of the drug, so this response is not correct. Knowing that the bisphosphonate is prescribed for hospice patients to reduce pain, the nurse can most effectively determine that the intervention is effective if pain decreases.

Therefore, B is the correct choice. C and D may occur as pain decreases, but they are not the main goals of the pharmacological intervention stated in the question.

General Test-Taking Strategies

Regardless of the type of question that appears on the screen during the examination, there are several strategies that can be used to eliminate distractors. For example,

> **Key Point**
>
> Be sure to read each question carefully to see whether the answer requires a fact to be identified, an intervention is required, or an intervention must be evaluated. This process will help to eliminate distractors that do not address what is being asked in the question.

- When answering a question, be sure to not read into the information given in the stem of the question. Questions on standardized examinations are based in a perfect world, not in the real clinical practice setting. So, do not make assumptions about what might be implied. Use only the information given in the stem of the question to choose the response.

- When choosing a response, try to narrow down the choices by eliminating as many distractors as possible. Often, distractors that contain words like "never" or "always" can be eliminated since very few things in patient care are absolute. Once two distractors are eliminated, reread the stem of the question to be sure you are focused on what the question is really asking.

- When rereading the stem of the question, pay close attention to key words in the stem to narrow your focus strictly to what is being asked. Review the stem for pertinent information about the patient in the scenario, such as the patient's age, diagnosis, and current symptoms or treatments. Sometimes it is helpful to write this information on the scrap paper provided during the exam and then use the nursing process to determine whether an intervention, assessment, or evaluation is needed.

- Remember that no matter how "good" the distractors seem to be, there is only one correct answer to each question.

In addition to studying and carefully reading each question, it is important to manage test anxiety before and during the examination.

Reducing Test Anxiety

Test anxiety is rooted in feeling out of control about the material on the test, the questions themselves, or the outcome of the examination. Test-takers sometimes feel so overcome with test anxiety that it can inhibit their ability to focus on the test questions and respond accurately, even if they know the material very well. Therefore, it is critical to recognize test anxiety and to take steps to manage it prior to and during the examination.

One helpful strategy for managing test anxiety is to reflect on strategies that have been helpful in the past to manage anxiety related to standardized examinations, such as deep breathing and visualization. There are many guided meditation exercises available online that may help to relieve stress in the weeks leading up to the examination.

On the day of the examination, try to leave anxiety from past tests or disappointment about previous undesirable test results in the past. Stay focused on the present moment throughout the exam. Take one question at a time. If unsure of an answer, mark a response, mark the question for review, and then move on to the next question. When all questions have been completed, go back to double-check any marked questions.

CONCLUSION

Preparation is key to successfully completing the examination and earning certification. Using a study plan to master the material is crucial to organizing the information and feeling confident on the day of the test. But

Key Point
To help alleviate stress, use the 4-7-8 breathing technique. Inhale while slowly counting to 4, hold the breath for 7 seconds, and then exhale slowly while counting to 8.

it is also important to cultivate calm and to overcome test anxiety. On test day, arrive early for the exam and plan to succeed!

Chapter Summary
• Preparation for the CHPN examination should take place over a 12-week period, at least.
• Developing an individualized study guide, starting with the least familiar content, is a good way to organize study material.
• Using several different study strategies may help recall and application of material.
• Using relaxation and stress-reduction strategies can help reduce test anxiety that can interfere with test performance.
• Twenty-two percent of the CHPN examination questions are recall (knowledge based), 60% are application questions, and 18% are evaluation questions.

REFERENCES

American Association of Colleges of Nursing. (2019). *About ELNEC*. Retrieved from https://www.aacnnursing.org/ELNEC/About

Cicero, M. (1913). *De Officiis* (W. Miller, Trans.). Cambridge, MA: Harvard University Press.

Hospice and Palliative Credentialing Center. (2019). *CHPN® candidate handbook.* Retrieved from https://advancingexpertcare.org/HPNA/Certification/Credentials/RN_CHPN/HPCC/Certification Web/CHPN.aspx?hkey=19bf12b2-5123-4ee1-9496-6c8a30dc2c3bCHPN

Karpicke, J. D., & Blunt, J. R. (2011). Retrieval practice produces more learning than elaborative studying with concept mapping. *Science, 331*(6018), 772–775. Retrieved from http://science.sciencemag.org/

Leik, M. T. (2018). *Adult-gerontology nurse practitioner certification intensive review: Fast facts and practice questions* (3rd ed.). New York, NY: Springer Publishing Company.

Life-Limiting Conditions in Adult Patients

3 Disease Progression and Imminent Death

Prediction is very difficult, especially if it's about the future.
—Nils Bohr, Nobel Laureate in Physics

LEARNING OBJECTIVES

After completing this section, the nurse will be able to

1. Identify trajectories for common end-of-life diseases
2. Explain the purpose of using disease trajectory models
3. Apply knowledge of disease trajectories to patient care
4. Identify the signs of impending death
5. Assess and treat symptoms that manifest throughout the dying process
6. Describe family support needs related to the patient's imminent death

DISEASE PROGRESSION

Most diseases progress in a somewhat predictable manner. Knowledge of the expected disease trajectory is essential for prognostication. Illness trajectory models allow clinicians to explain and predict symptoms associated with the patient's overall decline in function. Murray, Kendall, Boyd, and Sheikh (2005) described three common illness trajectories illustrating the process from diagnosis to death in several terminal diseases (see Figure 3.1).

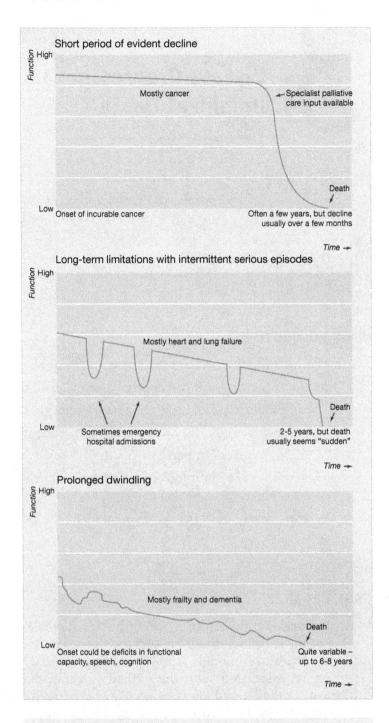

FIGURE 3.1 Disease trajectories.

Source: Murray, S. A., Kendall, M., Boyd, K., & Sheikh, A. (2005). Illness trajectories and palliative care. *BMJ, 330,* 1007–1011. doi:10.1136/bmj.330.7498.1007. Retrieved from www.bmj.com. Reprinted with permission.

Trajectory 1

In the first trajectory depicted, the patient experiences relative wellness followed by a short but predictable period of decline leading to death. Trajectory 1 (Figure 3.1) is typically associated with cancer diagnoses, and the expected time from terminal diagnosis to death is approximately 6 months without intervention. During the period of decline, the patient may experience symptoms of weight loss, gradual decreased ability to engage in activities of daily living, and a progressive decline in overall condition. Such patients are most likely to access palliative care and hospice services because of the predictability of the disease process.

Trajectory 2

The second trajectory, depicted in Figure 3.1, is characterized by periods of relative well-being punctuated by acute exacerbations that may require hospitalization. After each exacerbation, the patient's level of overall health declines somewhat, with a clear declinatory pattern discernable over time. This trajectory is associated with chronic illnesses such as heart failure and chronic obstructive pulmonary disease (COPD). The time from terminal diagnosis to death is longer than the process in the first trajectory and may span a period of 2 to 5 years or more.

Trajectory 3

The third trajectory (Figure 3.1) is associated with chronic conditions such as dementia, frailty, and debility. Such diseases involve a gradual functional decline over a period of 6 to 8 years without acute exacerbation. However, patients may fall subject to acute illnesses, such as pneumonia or cardiac events, that unexpectedly lead to their death.

Prognostication and Disease Trajectories

Knowledge of the expected disease trajectories for common terminal conditions provides the clinician with an important but singular data point. Clinicians must integrate information from several sources to draw reasonable conclusions about life expectancy and the course of the illness. Some tools commonly used to help clinicians prognosticate are:

- The Functional Assessment Staging (FAST) scale (Reisberg, 1987), for patients who have dementia (see Figure 3.2)
- The Karnofsky Scale (Karnofsky & Burchenal, 1949), for measuring patient health status over time (see Figure 3.3)

Functional Assessment Scale (FAST)	
1	No difficulty either subjectively or objectively.
2	Complains of forgetting location of objects. Subjective work difficulties.
3	Decreased job functioning evident to co-workers. Difficulty in travelling to new locations. Decreased organizational capacity.*
4	Decreased ability to perform complex task (e.g., planning dinner for guests, handling personal finances, such as forgetting to pay bills, etc.)
5	Requires assistance in choosing proper clothing to wear for the day, season or occasion (e.g. pt may wear the same clothing repeatedly, unless supervised)*
6	Occasionally or more frequently over the past weeks* for the following **A)** Improperly putting on clothes without assistance or cueing **B)** Unable to bathe properly (not able to choose proper water temp) **C)** Inability to handle mechanics of toileting (e.g., forget to flush the toilet, does not wipe properly or dispose of toilet tissue) **D)** Urinary incontinence **E)** Fecal incontinence
7	**A)** Ability to speak limited to approximately ≤ 6 intelligible different words in the course of an average day or in the course of an intensive interview. **B)** Speech ability is limited to the use of a single intelligible word in an average day or in the course of an intensive interview. **C)** Ambulatory ability is lost (cannot walk without personal assistance). **D)** Cannot sit up without assistance (e.g., the individual will fall over if there are not lateral rests [arms] on the chair). **E)** Loss of ability to smile. **F)** Loss of ability to hold up head independently.
*Scored primarily on information obtained from a knowledgeable informant.	

FIGURE 3.2 FAST Scale.

Source: Reisberg, B. (1987). Functional assessment staging (FAST). Retrieved from https://www .researchgate.net/journal/0048-5764_Psychopharmacology_bulletin. Reprinted with permission.

- The Palliative Performance Scale (PPS; Victoria Hospice Society, 2001), a modified version of the Karnofsky Scale, also used to measure health status over time (see Figure 3.4)
- The Eastern Cooperative Oncology Group Performance Scale (ECOG; Oken et al., 1982), used to measure disease progression, most often for patients who have a cancer diagnosis (see Figure 3.5; Wright, 2017)

Karnofsky Score (KS)	Definition
100	Normal; no complaints; no evidence of disease
90	Able to carry on normal activity; minor signs or symptoms of disease
80	Normal activity with effort; some sign or symptoms of disease
70	Cares for self; unable to carry on normal activity or do active work
60	Requires occasional assistance, but is able to care for most personal needs
50	Requires considerable assistance and frequent medical care
40	Disabled; requires special care and assistance
30	Severely disabled; hospitalization is indicated, although death not imminent
20	Very sick; hospitalization necessary; active support treatment is necessary
10	Moribund; fatal processes progressing rapidly
0	Dead

FIGURE 3.3 Karnofsky Scale.

Source: Karnofsky, D. A., & Burchenal, J. H. (1949). *The clinical evaluation of chemotherapeutic agents.* New York, NY: Columbia University Press. Reprinted with permission.

All prognostication tools are intended to provide evidence of the degree of the patient's functionality. Successive use of a specific tool can indicate a pattern of decline over time. With this information, the interdisciplinary care team can more effectively work with patients and families to develop goals of care during serious illness.

Establishing Goals of Care

Serious illnesses necessitate serious attention to the patient's goals of care and to the patient's comfort. So, when a patient is diagnosed with a chronic, potentially terminal illness, treatment options are reviewed and the patient and family are asked to make decisions about which options they find acceptable. During these serious conversations, the benefits of treatments are weighed against the potential risks. The expected quality of life throughout the disease process, with or without treatment, should be considered when determining which approaches to treatment align with the patient's goals.

The development of a circumscript document that outlines the patient's goals and end-of-life wishes is paramount in the decision-making process. In the event that the patient is not able to make their wishes known, the document provides clinicians and families with a guide for aligning care with the patient's goals. There are several documents that can be used to communicate goals of care and patients' end-of-life wishes.

Version 2

PPS Level	Ambulation	Activity & Evidence of Disease	Self-Care	Intake	Conscious Level
100%	Full	Normal activity & work No evidence of disease	Full	Normal	Full
90%	Full	Normal activity & work Some evidence of disease	Full	Normal	Full
80%	Full	Normal activity *with* Effort Some evidence of disease	Full	Normal or reduced	Full
70%	Reduced	Unable Normal Job/Work Significant disease	Full	Normal or reduced	Full
60%	Reduced	Unable hobby/house work Significant disease	Occasional assistance necessary	Normal or reduced	Full or Confusion
50%	Mainly Sit/Lie	Unable to do any work Extensive disease	Considerable assistance required	Normal or reduced	Full or Confusion
40%	Mainly in Bed	Unable to do most activity Extensive disease	Mainly assistance	Normal or reduced	Full or Drowsy +/– Confusion
30%	Totally Bed Bound	Unable to do any activity Extensive disease	Total Care	Normal or reduced	Full or Drowsy +/– Confusion
20%	Totally Bed Bound	Unable to do any activity Extensive disease	Total Care	Minimal to sips	Full or Drowsy +/– Confusion
10%	Totally Bed Bound	Unable to do any activity Extensive disease	Total Care	Mouth care only	Drowsy or Coma +/– Confusion
0%	Death	-	-	-	-

Instructions for Use of PPS (see also definition of terms)

1. PPS scores are determined by reading horizontally at each level to find a 'best fit' for the patient which is then assigned as the PPS% score.

2. Begin at the left column and read downwards until the appropriate ambulation level is reached, then read across to the next column and downwards again until the activity/evidence of disease is located. These steps are repeated until all five columns are covered before assigning the actual PPS for that patient. In this way, 'leftward' columns (columns to the left of any specific column) are 'stronger' determinants and generally take precedence over others.

FIGURE 3.4 Palliative Performance Scale, version 2.

Source: Victoria Hospice Society. (2001). Palliative Performance Scale (PPSv2). Retrieved from http://www.npcrc.org/files/news/palliative_performance_scale_PPSv2.pdf. Reprinted with permission.

Example 1: A patient who spends the majority of the day sitting or lying down due to fatigue from advanced disease and requires considerable assistance to walk even for short distances but who is otherwise fully conscious level with good intake would be scored at PPS 50%.

Example 2: A patient who has become paralyzed and quadriplegic requiring total care would be PPS 30%. Although this patient may be placed in a wheelchair (and perhaps seem initially to be at 50%). The score is 30% because he or she would be otherwise totally bed bound due to the disease or complication if it were not for caregivers providing total care including lift/transfer. The patient may have normal intake and full conscious level.

Example 3: However, if the patient in example 2 was paraplegic and bed bound but still able to do some self-care such as feed themselves, then the PPS would be higher at 40 or 50% since he or she is not 'total care.

3. PPS scores are in 10% increments only. Sometimes, there are several columns easily placed at one level but one or two which seem better at a higher or lower level. One then needs to make a 'best fit' decision. Choosing a 'half-fit' value of PPS 45%, for example, is not correct. The combination of clinical judgment and 'leftward precedence' is used to determine whether 40% or 50% is the more accurate score for that patient.

4. PPS may be used for several purposes. First, it is an excellent communication tool for quickly describing a patient's current functional level. Second, it may have value in criteria for workload assessment or other measurements and comparisons. Finally, it appears to have prognostic value.

Definition of Terms for PPS

As noted below, some of the terms have similar meanings with the differences being more readily apparent as one reads horizontally across each row to find an overall 'best fit' using all five columns.

1. Ambulation

The items **'mainly sit/lie,' 'mainly in bed,'** and **'totally bed bound'** are clearly similar. The subtle differences are related to items in the self-care column. For example, 'totally bed 'bound' at PPS 30% is due to either profound weakness or paralysis such that the patient not only can't get out of bed but is also unable to do any self-care. The difference between 'sit/lie' and 'bed' is proportionate to the amount of time the patient is able to sit up VS need to lie down.

'Reduced ambulation' is located at the PPS 70% and PPS 60% level. By using the adjacent column, the reduction of ambulation is tied to inability to carry out their normal job, work occupation of some hobbles or housework activities. The person is still able to walk and transfer on their own but at PPS 60% needs occasional assistance.

FIGURE 3.4 Palliative Performance Scale, version 2 (*continued*).

2. Activity & Extent of disease

'Some,' 'significant,' and **'extensive'** disease refer to physical and investigative evidence which shows degrees of progression. For example in breast cancer, a local recurrence would imply 'some' disease, one or two metastases in the lung or bone would imply 'significant' disease, whereas multiple metastases in lung, bone, liver, brain, hypercalcemia or other major complications would be 'extensive' disease. The extent may also refer to progression of disease despite active treatments. Using PPS in AIDS, 'some' may mean the shift from HIV to AIDS, 'significant' implies progression in physical decline, new or difficult symptoms and laboratory findings with low counts. 'Extensive' refers to one or more serious complications with or without continuation of active antiretrovirals, antibiotics, etc.

The above extent of disease is also judged in context with the ability to maintain one's work and hobbies or activities. Decline in activity may mean the person still plays golf but reduces from playing 18 holes to 9 holes, or just a par 3, or to backyard putting. People who enjoy walking will gradually reduce the distance covered, although they may continue trying, sometimes even close to death (eg. Trying to walk the halls).

3. Self-Care

'Occasional assistance' mean that most of the time patients are able to transfer out of bed, walk, wash, toilet and eat by their own means, but that on occasion (perhaps once daily or a few times weekly) they require minor assistance.

'Considerable assistance' means that regularly every day the patient needs help, usually be one person, to do some of the activities noted above. For example, the person needs help to get to the bathroom but is then able to brush his or her teeth or wash at least hands and face. Food will often need to be cut into edible sizes but the patient is then able to eat of his or her own accord.

'Mainly assistance' is a future extension of 'considerable.' Using the above example, the patient now needs help getting up but also needs assistance washing his face and shaving, but can usually eat with minimal or no help. This may fluctuate according to fatigue during the day.

'Total care' means that the patient is completely unable to eat without help, toilet or do any self-care. Depending on the clinical situation, the patient may or may not be able to chew and swallow food once prepared and fed to him or her.

4. Intake

Changes in intake are quite obvious with **'normal intake'** referring to the person's usual eating habits while healthy.

'Reduced' means any reduction from that and is highly variable according to the unique individual circumstances.

'Minimal' refers to very small amounts, usually pureed or liquid, which are well below nutritional sustenance.

FIGURE 3.4 Palliative Performance Scale, version 2 (*continued*).

5. Conscious Level

'Full consciousness' implies full alertness and orientation with good cognitive abilities in various domains of thinking, memory, etc. 'Confusion' is used to denote presence of either delirium or dementia and is a reduced level of consciousness. It may be mild, moderate or severe with multiple possible etiologies. **'Drowsiness'** implies either fatigue, drug side effects, delirium or closeness to death and is sometimes included in the term stupor. **'Coma'** in this context is the absence of response to verbal or physical stimuli; some reflexes may or may not remain. The depth of coma may fluctuate throughout a 24 hour period.

FIGURE 3.4 Palliative Performance Scale, version 2 (*continued*).

ECOG PERFORMANCE STATUS	
Grade	ECOG
0	Fully active, able to carry on all pre-disease performance without restriction
1	Restricted in physically strenuous activity but ambulatory and able to carry out work of a light or sedentary nature, e.g., light house work, office work
2	Ambulatory and capable of all selfcare but unable to carry out any work activities. Up and about more than 50% of waking hours
3	Capable of only limited selfcare, confined to bed or chair more than 50% of waking hours
4	Completely disabled. Cannot carry on any selfcare. Totally confined to bed or chair
5	Dead

Note: These scales and criteria are used by doctors and researchers to assess how a patient's disease is progressing, assess how the disease affects the daily living abilities of the patient, and determine appropriate treatment and prognosis. They are included here for health care professionals to access.

FIGURE 3.5 Eastern Cooperative Oncology Group assessment.

Source: Oken, M. M., Creech, R. H., Tormey, D. C., Horton, J., Davis, T. E., McFadden, E. T., & Carbone, P. P. (1982). Toxicity and response criteria of the Eastern Cooperative Oncology Group. *American Journal of Clinical Oncology, 5,* 649–655.

One such document is a physician (or provider) orders for life-sustaining treatment (POLST), which is called a medical orders for life-sustaining treatment (MOLST) in some states. This form is created during a conversation with a medical provider and lays out the patient's end-of-life wishes. It is considered a medical order, and is most useful in times of emergency. Typically, POLST or MOLST forms are intended for patients who have a life expectancy of 1 year or less (Bomba, Kemp, & Black, 2012). The forms are often printed on brightly colored paper and the order remains in place regardless of the care setting (e.g., hospital, long-term care facility; Figure 3.6).

HIPAA PERMITS DISCLOSURE OF POLST TO OTHER HEALTH CARE PROVIDERS AS NECESSARY

Physician Orders for Life-Sustaining Treatment (POLST)

First follow these orders, then contact Physician/NP/PA. A copy of the signed POLST form is a legally valid physician order. Any section not completed implies full treatment for that section. POLST complements an Advance Directive and is not intended to replace that document.

EMSA #111 B
(Effective 4/1/2017)*

Patient Last Name:	Date Form Prepared:
Patient First Name:	Patient Date of Birth:
Patient Middle Name:	Medical Record #: *(optional)*

A	**CARDIOPULMONARY RESUSCITATION (CPR):** *If patient has no pulse and is not breathing.*
Check One	*If patient is NOT in cardiopulmonary arrest, follow orders in Sections B and C.*
	☐ **Attempt Resuscitation/CPR** (Selecting CPR in Section A **requires** selecting Full Treatment in Section B)
	☐ **Do Not Attempt Resuscitation/DNR** (Allow Natural Death)

B	**MEDICAL INTERVENTIONS:** *If patient is found with a pulse and/or is breathing.*
Check One	☐ **Full Treatment** – primary goal of prolonging life by all medically effective means.
	In addition to treatment described in Selective Treatment and Comfort-Focused Treatment, use intubation, advanced airway interventions, mechanical ventilation, and cardioversion as indicated.
	☐ *Trial Period of Full Treatment.*
	☐ **Selective Treatment** – goal of treating medical conditions while avoiding burdensome measures.
	In addition to treatment described in Comfort-Focused Treatment, use medical treatment, IV antibiotics, and IV fluids as indicated. Do not intubate. May use non-invasive positive airway pressure. Generally avoid intensive care.
	☐ *Request transfer to hospital only if comfort needs cannot be met in current location.*
	☐ **Comfort-Focused Treatment** – primary goal of maximizing comfort.
	Relieve pain and suffering with medication by any route as needed; use oxygen, suctioning, and manual treatment of airway obstruction. Do not use treatments listed in Full and Selective Treatment unless consistent with comfort goal. *Request transfer to hospital only if comfort needs cannot be met in current location.*
	Additional Orders: _____

C	**ARTIFICIALLY ADMINISTERED NUTRITION:** *Offer food by mouth if feasible and desired.*
Check One	☐ Long-term artificial nutrition, including feeding tubes. Additional Orders: _____
	☐ Trial period of artificial nutrition, including feeding tubes. _____
	☐ No artificial means of nutrition, including feeding tubes. _____

D	**INFORMATION AND SIGNATURES:**

Discussed with: ☐ Patient (Patient Has Capacity)   ☐ Legally Recognized Decisionmaker

☐ Advance Directive dated _____, available and reviewed →   Health Care Agent if named in Advance Directive:
☐ Advance Directive not available   Name: _____
☐ No Advance Directive   Phone: _____

Signature of Physician / Nurse Practitioner / Physician Assistant (Physician/NP/PA)
My signature below indicates to the best of my knowledge that these orders are consistent with the patient's medical condition and preferences.

Print Physician/NP/PA Name:	Physician/NP/PA Phone #:	Physician/PA License #, NP Cert. #:
Physician/NP/PA Signature: *(required)*		Date:

Signature of Patient or Legally Recognized Decisionmaker
I am aware that this form is voluntary. By signing this form, the legally recognized decisionmaker acknowledges that this request regarding resuscitative measures is consistent with the known desires of, and with the best interest of, the individual who is the subject of the form.

Print Name:	Relationship: *(write self if patient)*	
Signature: *(required)*	Date:	Your POLST may be added to a secure electronic registry to be accessible by health providers, as permitted by HIPAA.
Mailing Address: (street/city/state/zip):	Phone Number:	

SEND FORM WITH PATIENT WHENEVER TRANSFERRED OR DISCHARGED

*Form versions with effective dates of 1/1/2009, 4/1/2011, 10/1/2014 or 01/01/2016 are also valid

FIGURE 3.6 POLST form.

Source: The Coalition for Compassionate Care of California. (2018). *POLST California*. Retrieved from http://capolst.org/wp-content/uploads/2017/09/POLST_2017_Final.pdf. Materials used with permission from the Coalition for Compassionate Care of California, CoalitionCCC.org.

HIPAA PERMITS DISCLOSURE OF POLST TO OTHER HEALTH CARE PROVIDERS AS NECESSARY

Patient Information			
Name (last, first, middle):		Date of Birth:	Gender: M F

NP/PA's Supervising Physician	Preparer Name (if other than signing Physician/NP/PA)	
Name:	Name/Title:	Phone #:

Additional Contact	☐ None		
Name:	Relationship to Patient:	Phone #:	

Directions for Health Care Provider

Completing POLST

- **Completing a POLST form is voluntary.** California law requires that a POLST form be followed by healthcare providers, and provides immunity to those who comply in good faith. In the hospital setting, a patient will be assessed by a physician, or a nurse practitioner (NP) or a physician assistant (PA) acting under the supervision of the physician, who will issue appropriate orders that are consistent with the patient's preferences.
- **POLST does not replace the Advance Directive.** When available, review the Advance Directive and POLST form to ensure consistency, and update forms appropriately to resolve any conflicts.
- POLST must be completed by a health care provider based on patient preferences and medical indications.
- A legally recognized decisionmaker may include a court-appointed conservator or guardian, agent designated in an Advance Directive, orally designated surrogate, spouse, registered domestic partner, parent of a minor, closest available relative, or person whom the patient's physician/NP/PA believes best knows what is in the patient's best interest and will make decisions in accordance with the patient's expressed wishes and values to the extent known.
- A legally recognized decisionmaker may execute the POLST form only if the patient lacks capacity or has designated that the decisionmaker's authority is effective immediately.
- To be valid a POLST form must be signed by (1) a physician, or by a nurse practitioner or a physician assistant acting under the supervision of a physician and within the scope of practice authorized by law and (2) the patient or decisionmaker. Verbal orders are acceptable with follow-up signature by physician/NP/PA in accordance with facility/community policy.
- If a translated form is used with patient or decisionmaker, attach it to the signed English POLST form.
- Use of original form is strongly encouraged. Photocopies and FAXes of signed POLST forms are legal and valid. A copy should be retained in patient's medical record, on Ultra Pink paper when possible.

Using POLST

- Any incomplete section of POLST implies full treatment for that section.

Section A:

- If found pulseless and not breathing, no defibrillator (including automated external defibrillators) or chest compressions should be used on a patient who has chosen "Do Not Attempt Resuscitation."

Section B:

- When comfort cannot be achieved in the current setting, the patient, including someone with "Comfort-Focused Treatment," should be transferred to a setting able to provide comfort (e.g., treatment of a hip fracture).
- Non-invasive positive airway pressure includes continuous positive airway pressure (CPAP), bi-level positive airway pressure (BiPAP), and bag valve mask (BVM) assisted respirations.
- IV antibiotics and hydration generally are not "Comfort-Focused Treatment."
- Treatment of dehydration prolongs life. If a patient desires IV fluids, indicate "Selective Treatment" or "Full Treatment."
- Depending on local EMS protocol, "Additional Orders" written in Section B may not be implemented by EMS personnel.

Reviewing POLST

It is recommended that POLST be reviewed periodically. Review is recommended when:

- The patient is transferred from one care setting or care level to another, or
- There is a substantial change in the patient's health status, or
- The patient's treatment preferences change.

Modifying and Voiding POLST

- A patient with capacity can, at any time, request alternative treatment or revoke a POLST by any means that indicates intent to revoke. It is recommended that revocation be documented by drawing a line through Sections A through D, writing "VOID" in large letters, and signing and dating this line.
- A legally recognized decisionmaker may request to modify the orders, in collaboration with the physician/NP/PA, based on the known desires of the patient or, if unknown, the patient's best interests.

This form is approved by the California Emergency Medical Services Authority in cooperation with the statewide POLST Task Force. For more information or a copy of the form, visit www.caPOLST.org.

SEND FORM WITH PATIENT WHENEVER TRANSFERRED OR DISCHARGED

FIGURE 3.6 POLST form (*continued*).

Besides a POLST form, advance directives (ADs) can be used to allow patients to communicate what their goals of care and preferred treatments would be if they were unable to speak for themselves. There are two main types of ADs: living wills and medical power of attorney. A living will is a document in which the patient specifies which treatments they would want if they could no longer express their own wishes. Medical power of attorney differs in that the patient does not necessarily specify which treatments they would want. Rather, the patient designates someone else to make decisions for them if they are unable to do so (see Figure 3.7).

Once the patient's wishes are known, or a surrogate decision-maker is designated, an interdisciplinary team should plan supportive care and symptom management that is consistent with the patient's wishes. Palliative care can, and should, be incorporated into the treatment plan regardless of whether curative measures are underway or not.

Palliative Care

Palliative care is a holistic approach to promoting patient comfort within the limits of the disease process. It is a specialty practice centered on the management of symptoms, and can be incorporated into the plan of care at any stage of the disease process. Within the palliative care model, an interdisciplinary team plans interventions to meet the

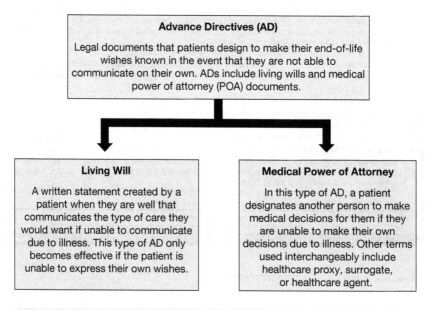

FIGURE 3.7 Advance directives.

Source: Wright, P. M. (2017). *Fast facts for the hospice nurse.* New York, NY: Springer Publishing Company. Copyright 2017 by Springer Publishing Company. Reprinted with permission.

patient's physical, emotional, spiritual, and psychological needs. The following eight domains of care were outlined in the National Consensus Project for Quality Palliative Care (2018):

1. Structure and processes of care
2. Physical aspects of care
3. Psychological and psychiatric aspects of care
4. Social aspects of care
5. Spiritual, religious, and existential aspects of care
6. Cultural aspects of care
7. Care of the patient at the end of life
8. Ethical and legal aspects of care

The palliative care nurse is responsible for assessing the patient's needs in each of these domains and for planning appropriate interventions. Some examples of the nurse's role include the following:

- Participating in quality improvement initiatives
- Utilizing evidence-based interventions to manage symptoms
- Properly documenting care
- Offering assistance to patients and families regarding decision-making, use of medical equipment, coping mechanisms, medication use and side effects, and so on
- Effectively collaborating with all members of the interdisciplinary team
- Facilitating appropriate referrals as needed
- Promoting comfort at the end of life through assessing and managing symptoms
- Providing respectful postmortem care
- Offering grief support to the patient's family at the time of death
- Applying ethical and legal principles to the care of all patients (Dahlin, 2015)

Palliative care should be introduced to the patient and family at the time of diagnosis of a serious or potentially terminal condition. Since palliative care often bears the connotation of end-of-life care, education is needed so that the patient and family understand that palliative care is a type of supportive care that can be utilized in every care setting. If a patient's condition deteriorates to the point that palliative and end-of-life care will be the sole focus, then hospice care should be considered if it is consistent with the patient's goals (see Table 3.1).

Table 3.1 Differences Between Hospice and Palliative Care

Hospice Care	Palliative Care
A type of care for terminally ill and dying patients	A type of care aimed at promoting comfort for seriously ill patients whether their condition is terminal or not
Bereavement services are provided for up to 1 year after the death of the patient	Bereavement services are not always provided
Care is primarily delivered in the home	Care may be delivered in acute care, long-term care, or other settings
Patient chooses to forgo curative treatments	Palliative care is provided in conjunction with either curative or end-of-life treatments
Covered by the Medicare hospice benefit	May or may not be covered by Medicare or other health insurance plans
Life expectancy of patient is 6 months or less	Life expectancy is not a factor

Hospice Care

Hospice care is a holistic approach to supporting patients at the end of life. It is specifically designed for those have chosen to forgo curative treatment. Although hospice care incorporates the principles of palliative care, its scope is limited to the care of patients who have a life expectancy of 6 months or less, if the disease runs its normal course without curative intervention. General hospice eligibility guidelines have been established by the Centers for Medicare & Medicaid Services (2015; see Figure 3.8).

Local coverage determinations are guidelines only; other supporting data should be used to determine hospice eligibility. For example, diagnosis-specific criteria are available to help determine when a disease is end stage (see Figure 3.9).

Many of the disease-specific criteria refer to scales such as the FAST scale, the Palliative Performance Scale, or others. The information from the scales, the local coverage determinations, the disease-specific criteria, and the expected disease trajectory all help to make a case for hospice admission. After the patient is admitted to hospice care, palliative care should continue throughout the disease trajectory and extend throughout the dying process.

Key points regarding recertification	• Document decline as needed but not less than every 15d • Recertification is based on ongoing documented evidence of decline and patient instability. If the patient's condition partially meets or does not meet LCD criteria, consider physician, assessment, diagnosis change, and/or discharge.
Types of disease trajectory	• Rapid decline: short period of steady decline (eg, cancer) • Saw-toothed decline: episodes of exacerbations, never back to previous baseline (eg, chronic obstructive pulmonary disease [COPD]) • Slow insidious decline: prolonged dwindling (eg, dementia, frailty)
Key questions to ponder	**Pain and symptom management** • What are the symptoms we are managing? What does it take to keep them under control? • How often are these symptoms escalating or the patient is having a crisis? **Disease progression/change in quality of life** • What evidence of decline are we seeing, reading, observing (eg, food intake, weight, physical assessment, arm circumference, mental status, change in medications/O_2)? • What is the patient/family telling us about decline (as evidenced by) (eg, stamina, ADLs, sleep/rest, social engagement, activities, symptoms, pain, psychospiritual issues)? **LCD criteria** • Does the patient still meet LCD guidelines? • Does the disease trajectory (pattern and momentum of decline) still reflect a terminal condition? **Instability** • Is the patient relatively stable? What would happen if hospice services were removed? • Will the improvement be sustained? What is the course of care and caregiver challenge?
Clinical status guidelines (use if there are no LCD-specific disease guidelines)	• Intractable serious infections: pneumonia, pyelonephritis, septicemia, recurrent fevers • Progessive inanition (exhaustion, lethargy) evidenced by: • >↓ 10% Weight in past 6 mo or body mass index <22 kg/m² (not due to depression/diuretics) • ↓ Mid-arm circumference (acromion [shoulder] to olecranon [elbow]) or abdominal girth • ↓ Skin turgor, ill-fitting clothes, increasing skin folds if weight not documented • Laboratory: albumin <2.5; ↓ cholesterol • Dysphagia with measured aspiration (eg, history of choking/gagging with feeding) or ↓ intake as evidenced by decreasing cups of food consumed • Symptoms (intractable/poorly responsive): dyspnea with ↑ respiratory rate; cough; nausea/vomiting; diarrhea; pain requiring ↑ doses of major analgesic • Signs: ↓ systolic blood pressure >90 mm Hg or ↑ postural hypotension; ascites; edema; venous, arterial, lymphatic obstruction; weakness; ↓ level of consciousness • Laboratory: ↑ Pco₂ or ↓ PO₂/Sao₂; ↑ calcium, creatinine or liver function; ↑↓ serum Na⁺ or ↑ K⁺ • ↓ PPS due to disease progression • ↓ FAST: 7a >6 words; 7b ~ 1 word; unable to: walk-7c, sit up: 7d, smile-7e, hold head up: 7f • ↓ ADLs: ambulation, bathing, continence, dressing, feeding, transfer • Progressive stage 3-4 pressure ulcers despite optimal care • ↑ ED visits, hospitalization, physician visits related to 1st diagnosis prior to election of hospice
Baseline to use with specific disease guidelines	• Documented clinical progression of disease: multiple ED visits, hospitalizations, home visits • PPS <70% (PPS for stroke or HIV <50%) • Partial/full dependence for 2+ ADLs: ambulation, bathing, continence, dressing, feeding, transfer • Significant comorbidities, eg, congestive heart failure, COPD, DM, ischemic heart, renal, liver, HIV dementia, neurological (cerebrovacular accident, amyotrophic lateral sclerosis, Parkinson disease), autoimmune (lupus, rheumatoid arthritis) • Receiving supportive, palliative, comfort care or treatment to comfort/improve functional level (eg, intravenous fluids, nasogastric tubes, transfusions, palliative chemotherapy, or radiation therapy)
Additional guidelines for neuromuscular diseases, multiple sclerosis, Parkinson disease	• Rapid disease progression or complications in the last 12 mo • Independent ADLs ↓ to assistance/dependency, eg, walker, wheelchair, bed-bound • Clear speech ↓ to unintelligible • Critical nutritional impairment: ↓ progression eating > pureed; ↓ intake fluids/food to sustain life; continuing weight loss; dehydration; without artificial feeding methods • ↓ Breathing capacity, dyspnea/O_2 at rest, declines ventilator • Signs and symptoms of infection: upper urinary tract infection (kidney infection); sepsis; recurrent aspiration pneumonia or fevers after antibiotics • Stage 3/4 decubitus

FIGURE 3.8 Local coverage determination.

ADLs, activities of daily living; DM, diabetes mellitus; FAST, Functional Assessment Staging scale; LCD, local coverage determination; PPS, Palliative Performance Scale.
Source: Jones, M., Harrington, T., & Mueller, G. (2013). Hospice admission eligibility: A staff education project. *Journal of Hospice & Palliative Nursing, 15*(2), 114–122. doi:10.1097/NJH.0b013e31826d743c. Used with permission.

Disease	All of These Criteria	At Least One of These Criteria	Supportive Factors
ALS	Disease progression in last 12 mo by one of following: • ↓ To wheelchair/bed • ↓ ~ Unintelligible speech • ↓ ~ Pureed diet • ↓ Most ADLs	• Vital capacity <30% or <60% with two symptoms (dyspnea at rest, unable to lie supine use of accessory muscles, weak cough, sleep-disordered breathing) + declines ventilator • ↓ Nutrition within last 12 mo: intake < sustain life, ↓ weight, dehydration, no TF	See also "One of These Criteria" for dementia
Cancer	Disease with distant metastases or CA with poor prognosis (eg, pancreatic)	• Continued decline on therapy • Declines further therapy	
Dementia	• FAST score 7 • ↓ Communicate 7A, 7B • ADLs with assistance • Walk with assistance • ↑ Incontinent urine/stool	• Aspiration pneumonia, UTI • Food/fluids < sustain life • Not a candidate for TF • Weight loss > 10% • Fever recurrent on antibiotics • Stage 3-4 decubitus • Laboratory: albumin <2.5	
Heart	New York Heart Association class IV: symptomatic at rest on diuretics and vasodilators	• Ejection fraction <20% • Refractory angina	• Symptomatic arrhythmias • Not a candidate for transplant • Past cardiopulmonary resuscitation, syncope, HIV
HIV	PPS <50% Laboratory: CD4 <25 cells/µL or > 100,000 copies/ml	• Central nervous system/ Systemic lymphoma • Loss of > 10% body mass • *Mycobacterium avium* complex bacterium • Refractory Cryptosporidium, Kaposi, toxoplasmosis • Encephalopathy, ↓ renal	• Persistent diarrhea ~ 1 y • Laboratory: albumin <2.5 • Age >50 y • Active substance abuse • No AIDS prescription • ↓ CHD, ↓ liver, ↓ AIDS dementia
Kidney	• No dialysis • No renal transplant	Laboratory: creatinine clearance • <10 mL/min • <15 mL/min DM or CHF • <20 mL/min DM + CHF Laboratory: serum creatinine • >8.0 mg/dL • >6.0 mg/dL, diabetes	Acute renal failure • Comorbidities: heart, lung, AIDS, disseminated intravascular coagulation, sepsis, ventilator • Laboratory: albumin <3.5 • Laboratory: platelets <25,000 Chronic renal failure: uremia, oliguria, K+ >7.0, pericarditis, fluid overload
Liver	Laboratory: international normalized ratio >1.5 Laboratory: albumin <2.5	• Ascites • History: peritonitis • History: variceal bleeding • Hepatic encephalopathy • Laboratory: ↑ blood urea nitrogen,↑ creatinine urine: Na <10 mEq/l, <400 mL/d	• Progressive malnutrition • ↓ Muscle, ↓ strength, ↓ endurance • Active alcoholism >80 g/d • Liver cancer • Hepatitis B, C (refractory to interferon)
Pulmonary	• Dyspnea at rest = bed to chair, cough fatigue • ↑ ED/hospital for upper respiratory tract infection • Room air saturation <88%		• Right heart failure (cor pulmonale) • Weight loss > 10% over 6 mo • Resting tachycardia > 100/min
Stroke	• PPS <40% • Acute >3 d: coma or obtunded and myoclonus • Chronic: FAST score 7, KPS and PPS <50%, no ADLs, weight loss > 10%, albumin <2.5	Coma: any three of the following on day 3 of coma: • Abnormal brain stem response • Abnormal/no verbal response • Absent withdrawal from pain • Laboratory: creatinine >1.5 mg/dL	

FIGURE 3.9 Disease-specific guidelines.

ADL, activities of daily living; ALS, amyotrophic lateral sclerosis; CA, cancer; CHF, congestive heart failure; COPD, chronic obstructive pulmonary disease; DM, diabetes mellitus; ED, emergency department; FAST, Functional Assessment Staging Scale; KPS, Karnofsky Performance Scale; PPS, Palliative Performance Scale; TF, tube feeding; UTI, urinary tract infection.
Source: Jones, M., Harrington, T., & Mueller, G. (2013). Hospice admission eligibility: A staff education project. *Journal of Hospice & Palliative Nursing, 15*(2), 114–122. doi:10.1097/NJH.0b013e31826d743c. Used with permission.

▪ NURSING CARE OF THE DYING PATIENT

Approaching Death

In the last days and hours of life, patients generally experience physical, psychosocial, and spiritual changes that are indicative of approaching death. The hospice nurse must be especially astute in differentiating signs of approaching death from other symptoms of the disease process. Usually signs of imminent death occur in clusters rather than as individual symptoms. However, individual symptoms may appear one by one over time in some patients. End-of-life symptoms depend on the terminal diagnosis, other concomitant illnesses, and the patient's overall condition. The manifestation and severity of symptoms is also influenced by the expected length of time to the patient's death.

Weeks to Months Prior to Death

In the final months, up to weeks before the patient's death, several changes take place that alert the nurse to the patient's changing condition. One of the earliest signs of decline is the loss of appetite that leads to marked weight loss and cachexia (Berry & Griffie, 2015). This decrease in the patient's desire to eat is often challenging for the patient's family to accept because it is a harbinger of further decline. Also, in most cultures, the preparation and sharing of food is a sign of wellness, happiness, love, and community. Thus the patient's anorexia can be very distressing to the caregivers. Family members and caregivers should be taught that the patient should not be force-fed, as this can lead to vomiting and aspiration.

Artificial nutrition can be considered when it is consistent with the patient's wishes. However, the hospice nurse should explain that artificial nutrition does little good at the end of life and may actually increase distressing symptoms (Heidrich, 2007). For patients who already have artificial nutrition orders in place, a decrease in the amount administered or discontinuation should be considered if the patient experiences untoward effects such as vomiting, aspiration, edema, congestive heart failure (CHF), pulmonary edema, or other signs of fluid overload.

Oral fluid intake should be encouraged for as long as possible (Heidrich, 2007). When the patient is no longer able to tolerate fluids, the hospice team should work closely with the family to determine if supplemental hydration is warranted. Most often, in the terminal phase, additional fluids are not necessary. However, there is some evidence that hypodermoclysis, the provision of subcutaneous fluids, may ease some end-of-life symptoms such as delirium, opioid toxicity, agitation, and dehydration when used judiciously. Family wishes for hydration related to cultural or religious beliefs can be met through hypodermoclysis or proctoclysis, the rectal administration of supplemental fluids (Kinzbrunner & Nguyen, 2011).

Days to Weeks Prior to Death

As the patient's condition continues to decline, psychological and spiritual distress may ensue. Patients often experience depression, anxiety, grief, and feelings of isolation during their final weeks. In a recent study, patients who had a diagnosis of COPD reported the highest levels of anxiety, likely due to acute episodes of dyspnea. Feelings of hopelessness, general dissatisfaction with life, and an overall sense of suffering were comparable among patients who had advanced disease (Chochinov et al., 2015).

> **Key Point**
>
> *Cachexia* involves not only weight loss but also muscle wasting, anorexia, fatigue, and weakness. The diagnostic criteria for cachexia are as follows:
>
> - Unintentional weight loss of ≥5% of body weight
> - Body mass index (BMI) <20 (patients <65) or BMI <22 (patients >65)
> - <10% total body fat
> - Increased cytokine levels (an increase in circulating cytokines leads to muscle tissue breakdown, or catabolism)
> - Albumin level of <35 g/L

In addition to psychological and spiritual distress, progressive physical weakness and increased dependence on caregivers are also expected in the terminal phase. As the patient's condition deteriorates, dysphagia or aphagia may occur. The hospice nurse may refrain from administering routine oral medications, but should then confer with the prescriber to discuss the discontinuation of unnecessary medications. Medications that are needed to promote comfort such as pain medications, anxiolytics, antiemetics, anticholinergics, and antipyretics should be administered through alternate routes such as the subcutaneous or rectal route when the patient is no longer able to swallow oral medications.

Care begins to focus narrowly on symptom management and comfort as the patient's condition continues to decline. Often asthenia leads to bedbound status, which compromises skin integrity due to pressure on bony prominences. Incontinence and malnutrition may

> **Key Point**
>
> A Kennedy ulcer, also called a Kennedy terminal ulcer, is a form of decubiti that develops suddenly in patients who are near death. The ulcer may begin as a discoloration or a blister and then quickly deteriorate to a full-thickness ulcer. The ulcer usually appears on the sacral area and is often pear or butterfly shaped.

also follow, which further contribute to skin breakdown. Proper skin care and frequent repositioning help to prevent decubiti. However, Kennedy ulcers often appear in the final days of a patient's life despite proper skin care. Caregivers and members of the hospice team must work in concert to address the multidimensional needs of the patient as death draws nearer.

Final Hours to Days

Hospice nurses are experts at assessing key signs of impending death and have an obligation to sensitively prepare families for what will ensue in the patient's finals days and hours. The hospice nurse should work with the hospice team to provide education on

- Saying goodbye and resolving conflicts
- Creating mementos by recording the patient's voice, taking photographs, making hand casts, and so on
- Finalizing funeral arrangements
- Gathering loved ones who wish to be present at the time of the patient's death (Bodtke & Ligon, 2016)

As the patient's death nears, assessment and aggressive symptom management remain key priorities for the hospice nurse (Berry & Griffie, 2015). Common signs of approaching death include the following (Berry & Griffie, 2015; Kehl & Kowalkowski, 2012; Kerr et al., 2014):

- Confusion and sometimes visions of loved ones who have passed away
- Terminal agitation followed by increased somnolence, often leading to unresponsiveness
- Changes in respirations including apnea, Cheyne–Stokes respirations, agonal breathing, and terminal secretions
- Temporal wasting
- Dehydration
- Pain
- Cyanosis of extremities or lips, cooling of extremities, hypertension leading to hypotension, peripheral edema, mottling
- Incontinence, oliguria, and eventually anuria

As death approaches, patients begin to withdraw from their loved ones and lose the ability to communicate verbally. Despite this, hearing is thought to remain intact. Thus, the caregivers should continue to talk with the patient and provide soothing sounds such as relaxing music throughout the dying process.

Caregivers should also be taught to assess nonverbal indications of pain and discomfort. Pain in the patient's final days is often related to tumor pressure, gastrointestinal distress, frailty, joint stiffness, immobility, or bladder distention. Kinzbrunner and Nguyen (2011) recommend use of the Face, Legs, Activity, Cry, Consolability (FLACC) scale (see Figure 3.10) for the assessment of pain in dying patients who are unable to verbalize their pain and discomfort.

CATEGORIES	SCORING		
	0	**1**	**2**
FLACC Behavioral Pain Assessment Scale			
Face	No particular expression or smile	Occasional grimace or frown; withdraw, disinterested	Frequent to constant frown, clenched jaw, quivering chin
Legs	Normal position or relaxed	Uneasy, restless, tense	Kicking or legs drawn up
Activity	Lying quietly, normal position, moves easily	Squirming, shifting back and forth, tense	Arched, rigid, or jerking
Cry	No cry (awake or sleep)	Moans or whimpers, occasional complaint	Crying steadily, screams or sob; frequent complaints
Consolability	Content, relaxed	Reassured by occasional touching, hugging, or being talked to; distractable	Difficult to console or comfort

How to Use the FLACC

In patients who are awake: observe for 1 to 5 minutes or longer. Observe legs and body uncovered. Reposition patient or observe activity. Assess body for tenseness and tone. Initiate consoling interventions if needed.

In patients who are asleep: observe for 5 minutes or longer. Observe body and legs uncovered. If possible, reposition the patient. Touch the body and assess for tenseness and tone.

Face
➤ Score 0 if the patient has a relaxed face, makes eye contact, shows interest in surroundings.
➤ Score 1 if the patient has a worried facial expression, with eyebrows lowered, eyes partially closed, cheeks raised, mouth pursed.
➤ Score 2 if the patient has deep furrows in the forehead, closed eyes, an open mouth, deep lines around nose and lips.

Legs
➤ Score 0 if the muscle tone and motion in the limbs are normal.
➤ Score 1 if patient has increased tone, rigidity, or tension; if there is intermittent flexion or extension of the limbs.
➤ Score 2 if patient has hypertonicity, the legs are pulled tight, there is exaggerated flexion or extension of the limbs, tremors.

Activity
➤ Score 0 if the patient moves easily and freely, normal activity or restrictions.
➤ Score 1 if the patient shifts positions, appears hesitant to move, demonstrates guarding, a tense torso, pressure on a body part.
➤ Score 2 if the patient is in a fixed position, rocking; demonstrates side-to-side head movement or rubbing of a body part.

Cry
➤ Score 0 if the patient has no cry or moan, awake or asleep.
➤ Score 1 if the patient has occasional moans, cries, whimpers, sighs.
➤ Score 2 if the patient has frequent or continuous moans, cries, grunts.

Consolability
➤ Score 0 if the patient is calm and does not require consoling.
➤ Score 1 if the patient responds to comfort by touching or talking in 30 seconds to 1 minute.
➤ Score 2 if the patient requires constant comforting or is inconsolable.

Whenever feasible, behavioral measurement of pain should be used in comjuction with self-report. When self-report is not possible, interpretation of pain behaviors and decisions regarding treatment of pain require careful consideration of the context in which the pain behaviors are observed.

Interpreting the Behavioral Score

Each category is scored on the 0–2 scale, which results in a total score of 0–10.

0 = Relaxed and comfortable	4–6 = Moderate pain
1–3 = Mild discomfort	7–10 = Severe discomfort or pain or both

FIGURE 3.10 FLACC scale.

Source: Merkel, S. I., Voepel-Lewis, T., Shayevitz, J. R., & Malviya, S. (1997). The FLACC: A behavioral scale for scoring postoperative pain in young children. *Pediatric Nursing, 23*(3), 293–297. The FLACC scale was developed by Sandra Merkel, MS, RN, Terri Voepel-Lewis, MS, RN, and Shobha Malviya, MD, at C. S. Mott Children's Hospital, University of Michigan Health System, Ann Arbor, MI. Used with permission.

Management of distressing symptoms should be based on the needs of the patient and family. When symptoms such as decreased appetite, increased somnolence, and cyanosis arise, a priority intervention is education of the family. It is important for families to understand that these changes are the normal aspects of the dying process and do not cause pain or distress for the patient.

Any symptoms that appear to cause the patient distress should be managed promptly. First, the nurse should determine whether medications or a change in routine could be the root cause of the symptoms. If identified, the cause of the symptoms should be promptly removed, or the effect mitigated as much as possible. Some symptoms, such as terminal agitation, may or may not be distressing for the patient but can have a potentially negative effect on the patient's safety and, therefore, must be addressed through

- Provision of a therapeutic environment
- Music therapy
- Activity as tolerated
- Medications such as haloperidol, chlorpromazine, risperidone, or lorazepam

Another common end-of-life symptom, terminal secretions (also called death rattle), is generally not thought to be painful or disturbing to the patient. But, since the sound of the secretions moving with each respiration can be distressing to family members, steps are often taken to diminish the sound or reduce the secretions. The hospice nurse should teach the family that terminal secretions are caused by the patient's inability to swallow saliva and clear secretions in the airway. Repositioning the patient as needed and suctioning the oropharynx may help to decrease the sound of secretions moving with respirations. If the secretions are causing dyspnea or distress to the patient, anticholinergic medications such as hyoscamine (subcutaneously [SQ]), atropine (sublingually [SL]), glycopyrrolate (SL), or scopolamine (topically or SQ) can be used to dry excess secretions.

As terminal symptoms progress, most patients will gradually experience asthenia and increasing somnolence, leading to coma. For others, multiple symptoms will arise, which lead to a period of agitation prior to the onset of a coma (Berry & Griffie, 2015). During the final hours, the focus of care should shift to

> **Key Point**
>
> Oropharyngeal suctioning may help to remove secretions that cause the sound of the "death rattle," but deep suctioning is not a recommended intervention for terminal secretions.

- Adhering to the patient's advance care plan
- Avoiding unnecessary interventions, such as vital sign monitoring and monitoring of pulse oximetry
- Treating fever
- Discontinuing unneeded routine medications (Berry & Griffie, 2015)

In the final hours, the patient will likely exhibit profound weakness and fatigue; gaunt and pale appearance; withdrawal from others; reduced awareness of surroundings; glassy or cloudy eyes; inability to swallow food, liquids, or medications; little to no urine output; agonal respirations and/or apnea; unresponsiveness; and tachycardia (Berry & Griffie, 2015; Bodtke & Ligon, 2016).

Caregivers should be aware that the patient may have a "predeath rally," which is a sudden reawakening involving coherent conversations, increased appetite, and an abrupt awareness of surroundings. The patient then returns to a semicomatose state within hours, which is often distressing to family members (Bodtke & Ligon, 2016). The hospice team must work closely with family members to avert false hope during a predeath rally and to prepare them for the patient's impending death.

The death trajectory and the symptoms involved are as individualized as the person who is transitioning toward death. The underlying disease(s), intractability of terminal symptoms, caregiver support, and goals of care all have bearing on the final trajectory. The hospice team must be prepared to manage symptoms associated with the terminal diagnosis as well as unexpected symptoms (see Table 3.2). Family and caregiver education should be individually tailored, with emotional and spiritual support provided by the hospice team before, during, and after the patient's death.

Table 3.2 Common Symptoms and Interventions at the End of Life	
Symptoms	**Interventions**
Agitation	Administer benzodiazepines, provide music, massage, dim lighting, and a cool environment
Dehydration	Provide frequent oral care and ice chips as tolerated, consider initiation of hypodermoclysis or proctoclysis, if consistent with goals of care
Dry mouth	Provide frequent oral care and frequent application of lip balm. Offer ice chips and oral swabs as tolerated. Artificial saliva may be used
Dyspnea	Treat cause, if possible. Administer opioids as prescribed. Reposition patient for comfort. Use a fan to provide moving air and provide cool environment
Edema	Elevate extremities as tolerated, use diuretics as indicated, consider decreasing or discontinuing artificial nutrition and/or hydration if symptoms of fluid overload arise
Fever	Administer acetaminophen suppository as prescribed, use fan to circulate air, dress patient in light clothing, and apply cool washcloths to forehead
Incontinence	Use disposable briefs and change promptly. Provide skin care after each incident of incontinence. Reposition patient frequently to prevent decubiti

(continued)

Table 3.2 Common Symptoms and Interventions at the End of Life *(continued)*	
Symptoms	**Interventions**
Pain	Administer oral medications until no longer tolerated. If patient is unable to swallow, provide pain medications subcutaneously or rectally. Use adjuvant medications as needed. Reposition patient for comfort, use distraction, massage, and/or heat/cold for comfort
Terminal secretions	Reposition patient for comfort. Administer anticholinergic medications to dry excess secretions if necessary. Oral suctioning may be implemented but deep suctioning should be avoided
Decubitus ulcers	Provide skin care with repositioning and when patient is incontinent. Provide appropriate wound care, and consider use of topical lidocaine to reduce pain

Afterdeath Care

At the time of a patient's death, the nurse will conduct a thorough assessment and will document the following:

- General appearance of the patient

- Absence of heart and lung sounds on auscultation (for 1 full minute)

- Lack of pupillary response to light

- Absence of response to verbal and tactile stimuli

- Time of death

- Who was notified of the death

- What time the family or caregiver notified the hospice agency (for home care patients)

- To whom the body was released (i.e., morgue, funeral director; Berry & Griffie, 2015)

> **Key Point**
>
> Family members of patients who have esophageal varices or tumors should be prepared for the possibility of terminal hemorrhage. Hemorrhaging is not usually painful for the patient, but the visual imagery is very distressing for families and caregivers. Hemostatic dressings may be used in cases of chronic bleeding. For acute bleeding, dark-colored towels and blankets should be available to minimize the visual impact. Sedation may be necessary if the patient is awake and alert. The family will also need focused attention and emotional support throughout the hemorrhagic event (Kinzbrunner and Nguyen, 2011).

Postmortem care should be provided in a respectful and culturally sensitive way, with attention to the patient's and family's religious preferences. The family members and caregivers should be invited to participate in postmortem care if they so desire.

> **Key Point**
>
> In accordance with federal law, if a patient's death occurs in a hospital setting, the primary decision-maker must be approached regarding organ donation.

The hospice nurse should prepare the death certificate as required by state law and should notify the primary care provider of the patient's death. Emotional support should be provided for the patient's family at the time of the patient's death. They should also receive assurance that the hospice team will provide bereavement support for up to one year after the patient's death.

▥ CONCLUSION

Conceptualizations of illness trajectories allow clinicians to predict the typical ups and downs of disease progression. The models can also be used as teaching tools when working with patients and families. However, each terminal disease bears specific characteristics that are critical for the hospice professional to understand when conducting assessments or planning care. The final stages of any disease process involve a series of declinatory events. Symptoms related to the terminal illness may intensify, and new symptoms may manifest. Care should be guided by the patient's end-of-life wishes and symptoms should be managed for the comfort of both the patient and the family. Education for the patient and family should include information on the symptoms that will likely arise and treatments. There must also be recognition that even though the family is aware that their loved one is terminally ill, the signs of impending death bring this reality closer and emotional support is needed throughout the dying process as well as after the patient's death.

Chapter Summary

- Cancer diagnoses typically follow a trajectory of relative wellness for a period of time followed by a short, but predictable, period of decline.

- Long-term chronic illnesses such as COPD and CHF are associated with acute exacerbations of the disease. After the acute episodes, the patient does not return to the previous level of health and an overall decline in condition is noted over time.

- A gradual declinatory disease trajectory over a period of 6 to 8 years, without acute exacerbations, is associated with diseases such as dementia, debility, and frailty.

- A POLST form is a medical order that ensures the patient's wishes will be followed, even in emergency situations.

- ADs allow patients to make their end-of-life wishes known either through documentation of a living will or through naming a medical power of attorney to make decisions when the patient is no longer able to do so.

- Palliative care is a holistic approach to promoting comfort through the efforts of an interdisciplinary team. It can be incorporated into any stage of the disease process and into any care setting.

- Palliative care is a component of hospice, but hospice focuses exclusively on end-of-life care.

- Patients who are admitted to hospice must choose to forgo curative treatments.

- Clinicians can use local coverage determinations, disease-specific criteria, prognostication tools, and knowledge of disease trajectories to estimate life expectancy.

(continued)

Chapter Summary (*continued*)
• Symptoms related to imminent death vary by the patient's expected mortality, underlying disease processes, and concomitant illnesses.
• In the final weeks and months before death, patients often experience loss of appetite and weight loss, which may lead to cachexia.
• Artificial nutrition and hydration can be considered when consistent with the goals of care.
• Spiritual distress, anxiety, and feelings of hopelessness should be addressed by the hospice team as they arise.
• As physical dependence increases, caregivers should be taught proper repositioning and skin care techniques.
• Kennedy ulcers may appear quickly in patients who are nearing death.
• Common signs of approaching death include terminal agitation, respiratory changes, temporal wasting, dehydration, pain, cyanosis, cooling of extremities, incontinence and/or anuria.
• When patients become nonverbal, the FLACC scale should be used to assess pain.
• Terminal agitation should be managed to ensure the safety of the patient.
• Although terminal secretions are not thought to be distressing or painful for the patient, interventions can be initiated to diminish the sound of noisy respirations or to reduce excess secretions.
• Some patients experience a predeath rally, but then return to a comatose state within several hours.
• The patient's death should be pronounced in accordance with state law.
• Bereavement care should be provided to the patient's family for up to one year following the patient's death.

▨ PRACTICE QUESTIONS

1. A 67-year-old patient who has end-stage pancreatic cancer reports a progressively decreased ability to perform activities of daily living and significant weight loss. The hospice nurse knows that

   a. The patient's symptoms are consistent with the beginning of a predictable period of decline commonly associated with cancer diagnoses

   b. The patient will recover from this exacerbation but will not return to the previous level of functioning

   c. The symptoms that the patient has reported are not related to the cancer diagnosis

   d. The interdisciplinary team should discuss appetite-enhancing medications and the use of a stimulant to combat fatigue

2. A patient who has recently been diagnosed with early-onset Alzheimer's-type dementia asks, "How long do I have before things get really bad?" The nurse's best response is

   a. Patients who have dementia often live for many years and experience a gradual decline in functioning over time

    b. You will most likely notice severe cognitive and physical changes within the next few months

    c. In early-onset dementia, there is a lengthy period of relative wellness followed by a rapid decline

    d. Over the next few years, you will experience periods of wellness with acute exacerbations from time to time

3. For the patient in the previous question, which tool would be the best choice for evaluating the patient's condition over time?

    a. The Palliative Performance Scale

    b. The Karnofsky Scale

    c. The FAST scale

    d. The Eastern Cooperative Oncology Group Performance Scale

4. A 76-year-old palliative care patient who has end-stage chronic obstructive pulmonary disease (COPD) lives alone and is concerned that emergency responders will perform cardiopulmonary resuscitation (CPR) if they are called to her home. At this time, the nurse should discuss

    a. Legal guardianship

    b. Medical power of attorney

    c. A living will

    d. A physician (or provider) orders for life-sustaining treatment (POLST)

5. A living will ensures that

    a. A designated person can make decisions for the patient when the patient is no longer able to speak for himself or herself

    b. A patient's wishes will be known when the patient can no longer speak for himself or herself

    c. A healthcare provider can order end-of-life care

    d. Emergency responders can forego life-saving treatments

6. A patient is very distraught and tells the nurse that she has just been diagnosed with breast cancer and her doctor recommended palliative care. She asks, "Does this mean it's terminal?" The nurse's best response is

    a. Palliative care is the same as end-of-life care; the goal is to keep you comfortable

    b. Palliative care is aimed at managing symptoms and can be incorporated into your other treatments

    c. A recommendation for palliative care means that your cancer is very advanced

    d. There is no way to determine how advanced the cancer is right now.

7. Patients who have end-stage dementia usually have a Functional Assessment Staging (FAST) scale score of

    a. 1

    b. 3

    c. 7

    d. 10

8. To be eligible for hospice, a patient who has cancer must

    a. Have another end-stage disease

    b. Choose to forego curative treatments

    c. Have an Eastern Cooperative Oncology Group (ECOG) score of 0

    d. Have a Palliative Performance Scale (PPS) score of ≥80

9. A 70-year-old patient who has end-stage renal disease stopped dialysis yesterday and has been referred to hospice. During the admission intake, he tells the nurse that he would like to pursue renal transplantation. The most appropriate intervention is to

    a. Request a referral for evaluation for transplantation

    b. Tell the patient he is not eligible for hospice

    c. Call the hospice medical director for advice

    d. Arrange a meeting for the patient and the interdisciplinary team

10. The wife of a critically ill patient in the intensive care unit asks the nurse about palliative care. The nurse's best response is

    a. "I'll request a referral and arrange a meeting for you with the palliative care team"

    b. "Do you think your spouse might die soon?"

    c. "Palliative care is not appropriate in the intensive care unit"

    d. "Tell me more about why you would request palliative care"

11. Which of the following is not a common sign of imminent death?

    a. Irregular breathing pattern

    b. Seizures

    c. Confusion

    d. Cyanosis

12. When evaluating a new hospice nurse during orientation, it is important to correct which of the following statements?

    a. "Terminal secretions don't indicate pain"

    b. "I will need to perform deep suctioning for a patient with terminal secretions"

    c. "When a patient has terminal secretions, I can reposition them to diminish the sound"

    d. "Families should know that terminal secretions are part of the normal dying process"

13. Martin is a 79-year-old patient who has end-stage lung cancer. Over the past few weeks, he has grown increasingly weak, has become incontinent, and has become bedbound. He has had no oral intake for the past 48 hours and is increasingly somnolent. On today's visit, the nurse notices that Martin responds only to tactile stimuli by muttering and turning his head. His respirations are also labored and respiratory secretions have increased. The most appropriate intervention is

    a. Suction the patient now and PRN

    b. Administer haloperidol

    c. Discuss intravenous fluid replacement with the family

    d. Teach the family about the dying process

14. For the patient in the preceding scenario, which of the following medications would the nurse recommend having on hand?

    a. Acetaminophen suppositories

    b. Morphine

    c. Scopolamine

    d. Lidocaine

15. A patient whose death is imminent exhibits deep respirations that are rapid and labored. The hospice nurse should

    a. Start supplemental oxygen

    b. Reposition the patient

    c. Administer an anticholinergic medication

    d. Suction the patient's oropharynx

16. An 86-year-old home care hospice patient with end-stage breast cancer is actively dying and is no longer able to take fluids orally due to dysphagia. The patient appears comfortable. Her family is concerned that she will suffer from dehydration. Which of the following should the nurse do now?

    a. Assure the patient's family that she appears to be comfortable at present

    b. Start intravenous (IV) access

    c. Encourage the family to provide ice chips for the patient

    d. Discuss transfer to an inpatient hospice setting

17. Which of the following medications should not be discontinued for an actively dying hospice patient who can no longer swallow?

    a. Oral extended-release morphine

    b. Oral calcium supplement

    c. Lactulose

    d. Scopalomine

18. An assessment of a home care hospice patient who is actively dying reveals a quarter-sized blister in the sacral area. The nurse should

    a. Cleanse the area vigorously with warm water

    b. Apply a barrier cream every 2 hours

    c. Teach the family that the blister can deteriorate into a full-thickness ulcer very quickly

    d. Contact the hospice social worker to discuss possible neglect

19. A patient in an inpatient hospice setting has terminal secretions. Which intervention should the nurse implement first?

    a. Assess the patient for distress

    b. Administer glycopyrrolate

    c. Auscultate the patient's lungs

    d. Provide supplemental oxygen

20. A patient who has esophageal varices is admitted to the hospice inpatient unit. Which of the following should the nurse have at the bedside?

    a. Ice chips

    b. An obturator

    c. Suction equipment

    d. Dark towels

■ REFERENCES

Berry, P., & Griffie, J. (2015). Planning for the actual death. In B. R. Ferrell, N. Coyle, & J. A. Paice (Eds.), *Oxford textbook of palliative nursing* (4th ed., pp. 515–530). New York, NY: Oxford University Press.

Bodtke, S., & Ligon, K. (2016). *Hospice and palliative medicine handbook: A clinical guide.* Retrieved from http://www.hpmhandbook.com/

Bomba, P., Kemp, M., & Black, J. S. (2012). POLST: An improvement over traditional advance directives. *Cleveland Clinic Journal, 79*(7), 457–464. doi:10.3949/ccjm.79a.11098

Centers for Medicare and Medicaid Services. (2015). *Local Coverage Determination (LCD): Hospice–Determining terminal status (L33393).* Retrieved from https://www.cms.gov/medicare-coverage-database/details/lcd-details.aspx?LCDId=33393&ver=2&kc=59c12399-6&bc=AAAAAAQAAAAAAA%3d%3d&#0

Chochinov, H. M., Johnston, W., McClement, S. E., Hack, T. F., Dufault, B., Enns, M., . . . Kredentser, M. S. (2015). Dignity and distress towards the end of life across four non-cancer populations. *PLOS ONE*, *12*(11), e0188141. doi:10.1371/journal.pone.0188141

Coalition for Compassionate Care of California. (2018). *POLST California*. Retrieved from http://capolst.org/wp-content/uploads/2017/09/POLST_2017_Final.pdf

Dahlin, C. M. (2015). National consensus project for quality palliative care: Promoting excellence in palliative nursing. In B. R. Ferrell, N. Coyle, & J. A. Paice (Eds.), *Oxford textbook of palliative nursing* (4th ed., pp. 11–19). New York, NY: Oxford University Press.

Heidrich, D. E. (2007). The dying process. In K. K.,Kuebler, D. E. Heidrich, & P. E. Esper (Eds.), *Palliative and end-of-life care: Clinical practice guidelines* (2nd ed., pp. 33–45). St. Louis, MO: Saunders Elsevier.

Jones, M., Harrington, T., & Mueller, G. (2013). Hospice admission eligibility: A staff education project. *Journal of Hospice & Palliative Nursing*, *15*(2), 114–122. doi:10.1097/NJH.0b013e31826d743c

Karnofsky, D. A., & Burchenal, J. H. (1949). *The clinical evaluation of chemotherapeutic agents*. New York, NY: Columbia University Press.

Kehl, K., & Kowalkowski, J. A. (2012). A systematic review of the prevalence of signs of impending death and symptoms in the last 2 weeks of life. *American Journal of Hospice & Palliative Medicine*, *30*(6), 601–616. doi:10.1177/1049909112468222

Kerr, C. W., Donnelly, J. P., Wright, S. T., Kusczak, S. M., Banas, A., Grant, P. C., . . . Luczkiewicz, D. L. (2014). End-of-life dreams and visions: A longitudinal study of hospice patients' experiences. *Journal of Hospice and Palliative Medicine*, *17*(3), 296–303. doi:10.1089/jpm.2013.0371

Kinzbrunner, B. M., & Nguyen, V. D. (2011). The last days: The actively dying patient. In B. M. Kinzbrunner & J. S. Policzer (Eds.), *End of life care: A practical guide* (2nd ed., pp. 309–330). New York, NY: McGraw Hill.

Merkel, S. I., Voepel-Lewis, T., Shayevitz, J. R., & Malviya, S. (1997). The FLACC: A behavioral scale for scoring postoperative pain in young children. *Pediatric Nursing*, *23*(3), 293–297.

Murray, S. A., Kendall, M., Boyd, K., & Sheikh, A. (2005). Illness trajectories and palliative care. *BMJ*, *330*, 1007–1011. doi:10.1136/bmj.330.7498.1007. Retrieved from www.bmj.com

National Consensus Project for Quality Palliative Care. (2018). *Clinical practice guidelines for quality palliative care* (4th ed.). Richmond, VA: National Coalition. Retrieved from https://www.nationalcoalitionhpc.org/wp-content/uploads/2018/10/NCHPC-NCPGuidelines_4thED_web_FINAL.pdf

Oken, M., Creech, R., Tormey, D., Horton, J., Davis, T. E., McFadden, E. T., . . . Carbone, P. P. (1982). Toxicity and response criteria of the Eastern Cooperative Oncology Group. *American Journal of Clinical Oncology*, *5*, 649–655. doi:10.1097/00000421-198212000-00014. Retrieved from https://journals.lww.com/amjclinicaloncology/Pages/default.aspx

Reisberg, B. (1987). Functional assessment staging (FAST). *Psychopharmacology Bulletin*, *24*(4), 653–659. Retrieved from https://www.researchgate.net/journal/0048-5764_Psychopharmacology_bulletin

Victoria Hospice Society. (2001). *Palliative Performance Scale (PPSv2)*. Retrieved from http://www.npcrc.org/files/news/palliative_performance_scale_PPSv2.pdf

Wright, P. M. (2017). *Fast facts for the hospice nurse*. New York, NY: Springer Publishing Company.

4 End-Stage Cancer

Cancer turns a patient's world upside down. In one moment, time goes from being counted forward from birth, to being counted backwards from death.
—Fong (2013, p. v)

LEARNING OBJECTIVES

After completing this section, the nurse will be able to

1. Discuss key features of terminal cancer
2. Identify risk factors for common forms of cancer
3. Determine interventions appropriate for oncologic emergencies

CANCER

Cancer refers to a group of diseases that are characterized by genetic mutations in normal cells that cause them to become malignant. These genetic mutations involve the following

- Oncogenes, which are mutant genes that regulate cell proliferation
- Tumor suppressor genes, which impede cell proliferation and suppress or prevent cell mutations

Cancer involves inactivation of tumor suppressor genes, allowing replication of mutated cells. Oncogenes allow accelerated proliferation of the mutated cells, resulting in the rapid growth of cancerous tumors (Rote & Virshup, 2014). The number of newly diagnosed cancers and the mortality rate for all cancers varies by type (see Table 4.1).

Regardless of cancer type, the greatest risk for cancer is advancing age. However, certain cancers are more common in certain age groups (see Figure 4.1). Gender also plays a role in cancer prevalence. However, the leading cause of cancer deaths in American men and women is lung cancer. For men, this is followed by colorectal and prostate cancers. And, for women, this is followed by breast and colorectal cancers (National Cancer Institute, 2017).

Table 4.1 Overview of Common Cancers

Cancer Type	New Cases Annually	Annual Mortality
Thyroid	56,870	2,010
Pancreatic	53,670	43,090
Breast	Female: 252,710 Male: 2,470	Female: 40,610 Male: 460
Lung	222,500	155,870
Liver	40,710	28,920
Kidney	63,990	14,400
Colorectal	135,430	50,260
Prostate	161,360	26,730
Endometrial	61,380	10,920
Melanoma	87,110	9,730
Leukemia	62,130	24,500
Non-Hodgkin lymphoma	72,240	20,140

Source: National Cancer Institute. (2017). Common cancer types. Retrieved from https://www.cancer.gov/types/common-cancers

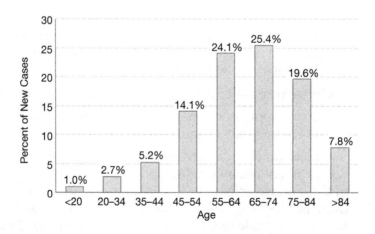

FIGURE 4.1 Percentages of new cancer cases by age.

Source: National Cancer Institute (2015a). Age and cancer risk. Retrieved from https://www.cancer.gov/about-cancer/causes-prevention/risk/age

Key Assessments

Nursing assessment of the patient who has incurable or untreated cancer involves determination of the stage of the cancer and performance measures. The staging of tumors commonly follows the tumor, node, and metastasis (TNM) system. The presence, absence, or extent of the primary tumor (T) is noted. Lymph node involvement, if present, is denoted by the letter N. If metastasis is present, its extent is denoted by the letter M (see Table 4.2).

Key Terms
Malignancy: Characterized by uncontrolled growth
Metastasis: Transference of cancer cells from the primary site to other areas of the body through the bloodstream or lymphatic system
Neoplasm: Literally meaning "new growth," as in uncontrolled tumor growth
Oncogenesis: The transformation of normal, healthy cells into cancer cells
Angiogenesis: The formation of vessels from the tumor

Table 4.2 Tumor Staging		
Primary Tumor (T)	**Regional Lymph Node (N)**	**Distant Metastasis (M)**
TX: Primary tumor cannot be measured	**NX:** Cancer in nearby lymph nodes cannot be measured	**MX:** Metastasis cannot be measured
T0: No evidence of tumor	**N0:** No evidence of cancer in nearby lymph nodes	**M0:** No evidence that cancer has spread to other parts of the body
T1, T2, T3, T4: Refers to the size and/or extent of the main tumor. The higher the number after the T, the larger the tumor or the more it has grown into nearby tissues. T's may be further divided to provide more detail, such as T3a and T3b.	**N1, N2, N3:** Refers to the number and location of lymph nodes that contain cancer. The higher the number after the N, the more lymph nodes that contain cancer.	**M1:** There is evidence that the cancer has spread to other parts of the body.

Source: National Cancer Institute. (2015b). Cancer staging. Retrieved from https://www.cancer.gov/about-cancer/diagnosis-staging/stagin

Treatment of Cancer

Treatment of cancer is multifaceted and involves the expertise of the interdisciplinary team to address the physical, psychosocial, emotional, and spiritual needs of the patient and family. Treatment often involves surgery, radiation, and/or chemotherapy.

> **Key Terms**
>
> Other terms used to describe or stage tumors include the following:
>
> **In situ (Tis):** Abnormal cells are present but have not spread to nearby tissue
>
> **Localized:** Cancer cells are present but have not spread to other parts of the body
>
> **Regional:** Cancer has spread to areas near the primary tumor site such as lymph nodes, tissues, or organs
>
> **Distant:** Cancer has spread to areas of the body that are not near the primary tumor site
>
> **Unknown:** Not enough information is available to stage the tumor
>
> *Source:* National Cancer Institute. (2015b). Cancer staging. Retrieved from https://www.cancer.gov/about-cancer/diagnosis-staging/staging

- Surgery can be curative, palliative, invasive, minimally invasive, or reconstructive. However, some patients are not surgical candidates due to the extent of metastasis, concomitant disease processes, or inability to tolerate anesthesia.

- Radiation can be curative or palliative. Radiation can be delivered externally (teletherapy) or internally (brachytherapy).

  - Teletherapy involves delivery of external beams of radiation from a source outside of the body to the tumor site. Low-energy radiation is used for cancers that are topical, such as melanomas. High-energy radiation is necessary for treating tumors deeper in the body tissue. Stereotactic radiation is used for the treatment of brain, head, and neck tumors because it allows a very high-dose radiation to be targeted at a specific body area. Another method of using concentrated radiation is through Gamma Knife surgery, which destroys tumor tissue, does not harm healthy tissue, and requires no incision.

  - Brachytherapy involves the insertion of radioactive material directly into the tumor site. The radioactive isotopes may be delivered via rods, seeds, molds, or wires. The radioactive sources may be removed or may remain in place permanently.

- Chemotherapy is the use of chemical agents to hinder the replication of malignant cells. Some chemotherapeutic agents interfere with DNA synthesis, others prevent cell division. Chemotherapeutic agents affect both cancerous and noncancerous cells, which leads to the destruction of rapidly reproducing healthy cells such as hair follicles, cells in the digestive and reproductive tracts, and bone marrow.

Destruction of these cells leads to alopecia, nausea, vomiting, diarrhea, neutropenia, thrombocytopenia, and anemia (National Institutes of Health, 2017).

Types of Cancers

Hospice nurses encounter patients with many different types of cancer. Therefore, it is important to understand the risk factors related to various forms of cancer, as well as the symptoms the patient will likely report. In this way, the hospice nurse can determine whether symptoms are likely related to cancer progression or to another disease process. Similarly, patients who have an end-stage cancer diagnosis often experience pain at sites of metastasis. Thus, the hospice nurse must be aware of the most common sites of metastasis for common cancers. Table 4.3 provides a summary of important considerations for common forms of cancer.

> **Key Point**
>
> Chemotherapy can decrease the functioning of bone marrow. Blood cells formed in the bone marrow are affected, leading to neutropenia (low number of white blood cells), anemia (low number of red blood cells), and/or thrombocytopenia (low number of platelets).
>
> Neutropenia increases the patient's risk for infection; anemia increases risk for fatigue, lethargy, tachycardia, dizziness, and/or chest pain; and thrombocytopenia increases the risk of bleeding.

End-of-Life Care

When curative measures fail, or when a patient chooses to forgo curative treatment, a discussion regarding the patient's goals of care should be initiated by the healthcare provider. If the patient declines curative interventions, then hospice transition should be discussed. Regardless of whether the patient chooses to transition to hospice, palliation of distressing symptoms should be integrated into the plan of care. The goal of palliative care is to promote comfort and quality of life and to maintain functional status to the greatest extent possible within the limitations of the disease process. Maintenance of quality of life and comfort includes not only addressing physical symptoms but also psychosocial and spiritual issues as well.

The most common distressing symptoms experienced by patients who have end-stage cancer are fatigue, pain, decreased appetite, and dyspnea (American Cancer Society, 2016). Each of these symptoms should be managed using pharmacological or nonpharmacological interventions. The hospice nurse is responsible for monitoring the patient's symptoms and the effects of interventions. Importantly, tumor growth and metabolic changes related to cancer can cause acute changes in the patient's condition that necessitate a reevaluation of the patient's overall condition and desired goals of care. Each of these acute problems are summarized in Table 4.4.

Table 4.3 Advanced Cancer Considerations

Type	Main Risk Factors	Symptoms	Prevalence (2014)	Common Sites of Metastasis	5-Year Survival Rate (2007–2013)
Brain	Cancer at another body site (brain is common site of metastasis) The cause of most adult brain tumors is unknown	Morning headache Headache that resolves with vomiting Seizures Changes in vision, hearing, or speech Decreased appetite Nausea/vomiting Changes in mood, personality, behavior, or ability to focus on tasks Balance changes Muscle weakness Changes in sleep patterns	162,341	Primary brain tumors originate in the brain tissue and rarely spread to other parts of the body. Secondary brain tumors arise when cancer spreads from a primary site, such as the colon or liver, to the brain.	33.6%
Esophageal	Tobacco abuse Alcohol abuse	No early signs or symptoms Painful swallowing/dysphagia Weight loss Hoarseness/cough Indigestion/heartburn Pain behind sternum	45,547	Retroperitoneal or celiac lymph nodes; liver and/or lungs	18.8%

(continued)

Table 4.3 Advanced Cancer Considerations (*continued*)

Type	Main Risk Factors	Symptoms	Prevalence (2014)	Common Sites of Metastasis	5-Year Survival Rate (2007–2013)
Thyroid	Exposure to radiation to the head or neck during childhood Genetic predisposition	Palpable nodes or tumor in the neck Difficulty breathing or swallowing Pain with swallowing Hoarseness	726,646	Lymph nodes, lungs, bone	98.2%
Breast	Personal history of breast cancer or first-degree relative with breast cancer (mother, daughter, sister) Genetic predisposition (*BRCA1* or *BRCA2*) Early or late menarche Radiation therapy to breast or chest Alcohol abuse Obesity Advanced maternal age at birth of first child or nulliparity Dense breast tissue (on mammography)	Lump or thickening in the breast or axilla Change in the size or the shape of the breast Inverted nipple (new onset) Dimpling or puckering of the skin over the breast Discharge from nipple Scaly, red, swollen skin around areola Dimpling of the skin over the breast that looks like an orange peel (this is called peau d'orange)	3,327,552	Lungs, pleura, liver, brain	89.7%

(continued)

Table 4.3 Advanced Cancer Considerations (continued)

Type	Main Risk Factors	Symptoms	Prevalence (2014)	Common Sites of Metastasis	5-Year Survival Rate (2007–2013)
Lung	Tobacco abuse Exposure to environmental carcinogens such as air pollution, asbestos, radiation, or radon Radiation therapy to chest Family history of lung cancer HIV	Cough/hemoptysis Chest pain Malaise Weight loss Dyspnea/hoarseness	527,228	Opposite lung, adrenal gland, bone, brain, liver	18.1%
Liver	Hepatitis B and/or C Alcohol abuse Metabolic syndrome Hemochromatosis Ingestion of aflatoxin (a carcinogen produced by certain fungi that be found on corn, nuts, and grain)	Palpable lump or pain in right upper quadrant of abdomen Pain in right shoulder or back Jaundice, dark urine, pale or chalky stools Increased bruising or bleeding Fatigue or weakness Nausea/vomiting, poor appetite or early satiety, weight loss Fever	66,771	Lung, portal vein, portal lymph nodes	17.6%
Pancreatic	Smoking Morbid obesity History of diabetes mellitus or chronic pancreatitis Genetic predisposition	Jaundice Pale stools Dark urine Mid-abdominal or mid-back pain Decreased appetite, weight loss Malaise	64,668	Adjacent organs such as the liver, lungs, or stomach. May also metastasize to bone and brain	8.2%

(continued)

Table 4.3 Advanced Cancer Considerations (*continued*)

Type	Main Risk Factors	Symptoms	Prevalence (2014)	Common Sites of Metastasis	5-Year Survival Rate (2007–2013)
Colorectal	Family history of colon or rectal cancer in first-degree relative Personal history of colon, rectal, or ovarian cancer or history of high-risk adenomas (colon polyps >1 cm or with abnormal microscopy) Genetic predisposition >3 alcoholic beverages daily Smoking Obesity African American heritage	Change in bowel habits, thin stools. Bowel fullness after defecation Hematochezia Diarrhea or constipation Fatigue/malaise Gas pains, bloating, cramping, or abdominal fullness, vomiting, weight loss	1,317,247	Lung, liver, peritoneum	64.9%
Stomach	*Helicobacter pylori* infection in stomach; chronic gastritis Pernicious anemia Intestinal metaplasia High dietary intake of highly salted or smoked foods and/or low fiber diet Smoking First-degree relative with history of stomach cancer; male gender	Indigestion, heartburn, and/or bloating. Stomach pain/mild nausea/vomiting Decreased appetite in advanced disease Hematochezia, jaundice, ascites, dysphagia	95,764	Liver, lung, peritoneum	30.6%

(continued)

Table 4.3 Advanced Cancer Considerations (*continued*)

Type	Main Risk Factors	Symptoms	Prevalence (2014)	Common Sites of Metastasis	5-Year Survival Rate (2007–2013)
Renal	Smoking Chronic misuse of pain medications Obesity Hypertension Family history of renal cancer Genetic conditions such as von Hippel–Lindau disease or hereditary papillary renal cell carcinoma	Hematuria Abdominal mass Flank pain Decreased appetite Unexplained weight loss Anemia	483,225	Adrenal gland, bone, brain, liver, lung	71.4%
Bladder	Tobacco use, especially smoking Family history of bladder cancer Exposure to occupational chemicals such as paints, dyes, metals, or petroleum products History of radiation to pelvis Treatment with cyclophosphamide or ifosfamide Use of *Aristolochia fangchi* Consumption of drinking water with high levels or arsenic or chlorine History of bladder infections; prolonged use of bladder catheter	Hematuria Dysuria Frequent urination Lower back pain	696,440	Bone, liver, lung	77.3%

(*continued*)

Table 4.3 Advanced Cancer Considerations *(continued)*

Type	Main Risk Factors	Symptoms	Prevalence (2014)	Common Sites of Metastasis	5-Year Survival Rate (2007–2013)
Cervical	HPV infection Exposure to DES in utero	Often asymptomatic but patient may experience: Vaginal bleeding or discharge (including postcoitus); dyspareunia Pelvic pain	256,078	Liver, lung, peritoneum	67.1%
Ovarian	Family history of ovarian cancer (first-degree relative and second-degree relative) Genetic predisposition	Pain or pressure in abdominal or pelvic area Heavy or irregular vaginal bleeding, especially after menopause Clear, white, or blood-tinged vaginal discharge Gas, bloating, or constipation	222,060	Liver, lung, peritoneum	46.5%
Uterine	Endometrial hyperplasia Obesity Metabolic syndrome Nulliparity Early menarche and/or late menopause PCOS	Vaginal bleeding unrelated to menstruation Postmenopausal bleeding Dysuria Dyspareunia Pelvic pain	710,228	Local pelvic recurrence, pelvic and paraaortic nodes, peritoneum, and lungs	81.3%

(continued)

Table 4.3 Advanced Cancer Considerations (*continued*)

Type	Main Risk Factors	Symptoms	Prevalence (2014)	Common Sites of Metastasis	5-Year Survival Rate (2007–2013)
Uterine (*continued*)	First-degree relative with uterine cancer; presence of genetic mutations linked to Lynch syndrome Hyperinsulinemia				
Prostate	Advanced age Family history of prostate cancer African American ethnicity Excessive intake of vitamin E, folic acid, and/or calcium Hormonal alterations	Weak or interrupted urine stream Urinary frequency/nocturia Incomplete emptying of bladder Hematuria Pelvic area pain Anemia and associated symptoms (dizziness, dyspnea, fatigue, pallor)	3,085,209	Adrenal gland, bone, liver, lung	98.6%
Melanoma	Fair complexion, light eye color (blue or green), light hair (blonde or red) Prolonged exposure to natural or artificial sunlight History of multiple blistering sunburns or personal history of melanoma Family history of atypical nevus syndrome Immunosuppression	Changes in the size, shape, or color of a mole Mole(s) with irregular borders and uneven pigment Asymmetric mole(s) Presence of satellite mole(s)(appearance of new mole[s] near an existing mole) Mole(s) that itch, bleed, ooze, or become ulcerated	1,169,351	Bone, brain, liver, lung, skin, muscle	91.7%

(continued)

Table 4.3 Advanced Cancer Considerations (*continued*)

Type	Main Risk Factors	Symptoms	Prevalence (2014)	Common Sites of Metastasis	5-Year Survival Rate (2007–2013)
Leukemia	Exposure to chemotherapy or radiation treatments Exposure to environmental radiation Male gender White race Genetic predisposition	Fever Fatigue, weakness Bleeding and bruising easily, petechiae Decreased appetite, weight loss Bone or stomach pain Recurrent infection Painless neck, axilla, abdomen, or groin mass	387,728	Spinal fluid, liver, spleen, lymph nodes, testicles	60.6%
Lymphoma	Advanced age Male gender Immune system disorders or autoimmune disease *H. pylori* infection Human T-lymphotropic virus type 1 or Epstein–Barr virus infection	Lymphadenopathy Fever, night sweats Fatigue Weight loss Urticaria Unexplained chest pain, bone pain, or abdominal pain	661,996	Lymph nodes, thymus, spleen	71.0%

(continued)

Table 4.3 Advanced Cancer Considerations *(continued)*

Type	Main Risk Factors	Symptoms	Prevalence (2014)	Common Sites of Metastasis	5-Year Survival Rate (2007–2013)
Multiple myeloma	Advanced age African American race Male gender Radiation exposure or exposure to toxic chemicals Personal history of MGUS or plasmacytoma	Can be asymptomatic Bone pain, especially in the back or ribs Dyspnea Bleeding and bruising easily Weakness in extremities Marked fatigue	118,539	Bone marrow, adjacent soft tissue or organs	49.6%

DES, diethylstilbestrol; HPV, human papilloma virus; MGUS, monoclonal gammopathy of undetermined significance; PCOS, polycystic ovarian syndrome.
Source: National Cancer Institute (2017). Common cancer types. Retrieved from https://www.cancer.gov/types/common-cancers

Table 4.4 Acute Complications of Advanced Cancer

Complication	Description	Symptoms	Diagnosis	Interventions
TLS (Sekeres, 2010)	Occurs when the by-products of tumor cell breakdown cannot be cleared quickly enough by the kidneys and remain in the bloodstream. This condition causes a buildup of metabolites, resulting in hyperkalemia, hyperphosphatemia, hyperuricemia, and hypocalcemia. TLS can result from cancer treatment and can be fatal.	Nausea, vomiting, diarrhea Weakness/fatigue Neuralgias Dysrhythmias Confusion/delirium/hallucinations Restlessness/irritability Seizures	CBC Chem 14 Uric acid levels Urinalysis	Allopurinol to reduce uric acid production IV hydration Diuresis Hemodialysis may be required
DIC (National Heart, Lung, and Blood Institute, 2017)	Results from the formation of blood clots in the body's small vessels. This condition can lead to organ damage. Because the platelets coagulate in the small vessels, fewer remain in circulation, which can lead to severe bleeding.	Chest pain, shortness of breath, dyspnea, myocardial infarction DVT, gangrene Headache, aphasia, paralysis Oliguria Hemorrhage	CBC Blood smear PT/PTT Serum fibrinogen	Supplemental oxygen Fluid replacement Whole blood or blood products, as indicated Heparin as indicated

(continued)

Table 4.4 Acute Complications of Advanced Cancer (*continued*)

Complication	Description	Symptoms	Diagnosis	Interventions
Hyperleukocytosis and leukocytosis (Riggiero, Rizzo, Amato, & Riccardi, 2016; Röllig & Ehninger, 2015)	Most commonly seen in patients who have acute leukemia or chronic myeloid leukemia. It is a blood abnormality characterized by a leukocyte count >50 × 10^9/L–100 × 10^9/L (normal range = 4 × 10^9/L– 11 × 10^9/L). This condition is caused by excessive proliferation of leukocytes and puts patients at risk for DIC and tumor lysis syndrome (TLS)	Respiratory distress Neurological deficits	Leukocyte count >50 × 10^9/L–100 × 10^9/L	Prevention of tumor Lysis Cytoreduction Blood or platelet transfusion, as indicated Anticoagulant therapy, as indicated Allopurinol to decrease uric acid IV hydration CBC BID
Neutropenia (Lustberg, 2012)	Neutropenia occurs when the ANC falls below 1,000/mm^3 (normal range 1,500–8,000/mm^3). Neutropenia increases the risk of infection. Chemotherapy is the most common cause.	Many be asymptomatic Fever Fatigue Lethargy	ANC below 1,000/mm^3 Anemia	Treatment with broad-spectrum antibiotics. Hospitalization may be required.
Metastatic spinal cord compression (Al-Qurainy, 2016)	The spread of bony metastasis into the spine causes displacement of the spinal nerves and/or vertebral collapse.	Acute-onset back pain Paraplegia or tetraplegia Cauda equine syndrome (neurological deficits in the lower extremities, bowel or bladder incontinence, lower back or leg pain, saddle anesthesia)	MRI	Corticosteroids Analgesia Palliative management is often the treatment of choice

(*continued*)

Table 4.4 Acute Complications of Advanced Cancer (*continued*)

Complication	Description	Symptoms	Diagnosis	Interventions
Superior vena cava syndrome (Borooah, 2018)	Occurs when the superior vena cava is compressed by an extrinsic tumor or metastatic lymph nodes.	Facial edema, venous dilation across chest and in upper extremities, dyspnea, hoarseness and dysphagia Patient may report feeling constriction in the neck or throat area Neurologic complications may include increased intracranial pressure, confusion, coma, brainstem herniation, and death	May be diagnosed empirically Chest x-ray or CT scan are useful for determining size and location of tumor or malignant lymph nodes	Reducing intracranial pressure, airway management, steroids to decrease edema Chemotherapy and radiation may be options to decrease size of tumors or malignant lymph nodes if consistent with goals of care
Septic shock (Canadian Cancer Society, 2018; Martin, Cheek, & Morris, 2014)	Cancer and cancer treatments deplete the immune system, which can lead to overwhelming systemic infection.	Severe hypotension, hypoxia, tachycardia, fluctuating temperature, restlessness, changes in mentation, tachypnea that can lead to ARDS	Often diagnosed empirically. The patient may have increased white cell count, lactic acidosis, and impaired coagulation Cultures should be obtained	Consistent with goals of care Artificial ventilation, cardiac support, and antibiotics are options

(*continued*)

Table 4.4 Acute Complications of Advanced Cancer (*continued*)

Complication	Description	Symptoms	Diagnosis	Interventions
Cardiac tamponade (Bodtke & Ligon, 2016; Borooah, 2018)	Accumulation of fluid in the pericardial sac that causes compression of the cardiac muscle.	Beck's triad: hypotension, increased jugular vein pressure and distention, muffled heart sounds Tachycardia, pulsus paradoxus (drop in systolic BP >10 mmHg with inspiration) New onset cardiomegaly on x-ray, low voltage on EKG Shortness of breath, chest pain, orthopnea, and general weakness	Chest x-ray EKG, two-dimensional Echocardiogram	Pericardiocentesis, percutaneous pericardiostomy If consistent with goals of care, indwelling pericardial catheter, VATS pericardial window, intrapericardial instillation of antineoplastic and sclerosing agents
SIADH (Borooah, 2018)	Characterized by hyponatremia that results from the production of arginine vasopressin by the tumor.	Many patients are asymptomatic. Early symptoms include anorexia, nausea, irritability or depression, muscle cramps, peripheral edema, lethargy, weakness, and behavioral changes. If sodium levels drop below 110 mEq/L, depressed deep tendon reflexes, seizures, and coma may occur.	Low serum sodium, normal CO_2, normal potassium, low urine osmolality	Fluid restriction to 0.5 to 1 L/day with increased sodium and protein intake. In severe cases, and when consistent with the patient's goals of care, serum sodium level can be corrected cautiously with 3% saline solution

(continued)

Table 4.4 Acute Complications of Advanced Cancer (*continued*)

Complication	Description	Symptoms	Diagnosis	Interventions
Hypercalcemia of malignancy (Bodtke & Ligon, 2016)	Increased serum calcium levels due to the breakdown of bone tissue from metastasis.	Use the mnemonic "moans, stones, groans, bones, thrones, psychiatric overtones" (p. 136) (muscle pains, renal calculi, bone pain, constipation, polyuria, confusion/depression/lethargy)	Serum calcium levels 12 mg/dL to ≥14 mg/dL Median survival is 30 days without intervention; only a few days if serum calcium level is >16 mg/dL	Treat symptoms in accordance with the patient's goals of care Interventions to reduce serum calcium may include isotonic saline hydration, calcitonin, bisphosphonates, loop diuretics, glucocorticoids, denosumab, and/or hemodialysis Avoid medications that increase serum calcium, such as theophylline, and calcium supplements (including antacids)

ADRS, adult respiratory distress syndrome; ANC, absolute neutrophil count; BP, blood pressure; CBC, complete blood count; DIC, disseminated intravascular coagulation; DVT, deep vein thrombosis; IV, intravenous; PT, prothrombin time; PTT, partial thromboplastin time; SIADH, syndrome of inappropriate secretion of antidiuretic hormone; TLS, tumor lysis syndrome; VATS, video-assisted thoracoscopic surgery.

CONCLUSION

A diagnosis of terminal cancer is devastating to patients and their families. The hospice nurse must have a command of the staging of cancers, cancer treatment options, how to approach conversations about goal setting, and how to address symptoms that arise as a result of cancer treatment or disease progression. Additionally, the hospice nurse must also incorporate cultural and religious family preferences when planning care. Since the patient and family are considered the unit of care in hospice, the plan of care must also include nursing interventions designed to prepare the family for the patient's approaching death and to support them emotionally and spiritually, in collaboration with the hospice team, throughout the entire course of the illness, and after the patient's death.

Chapter Summary

- Cancer is characterized by genetic mutations in normal cells.
- The greatest risk factor for cancer is aging.
- Tumor staging refers to the size of the tumor, lymph node involvement, and metastases.
- Common treatments for cancer include surgery, radiation, and chemotherapy. Not all patients are good candidates for these therapies, depending on age, extent of metastasis, and concomitant illnesses.
- End-of-life care for patients who have terminal cancer should be holistic and aligned with the patient's goals of care.
- Emotional support and teaching regarding the disease process should be provided for the patient and family throughout the course of the illness.

PRACTICE QUESTIONS

1. A 79-year-old patient has been diagnosed with breast cancer, stage T2, N0, M0. This means that
   a. The cancer has metastasized
   b. There is evidence of cancer in nearby lymph nodes
   c. The primary tumor cannot be measured
   d. There is no evidence that the cancer has metastasized

2. A 64-year-old palliative care patient who has end-stage chronic obstructive pulmonary disease (COPD) was recently diagnosed with lung cancer, T1, N0, M1. This means that
   a. There is no evidence of a tumor
   b. There is no evidence that the lymph nodes contain cancer cells
   c. There is no evidence of metastasis
   d. There is a very large tumor in the left lung

3. A 30-year-old patient who is genetically predisposed to lung cancer receives a report that what appeared to be a mass on her most recent x-ray was confirmed by CT scan to be T0, N0, M0. This should be explained in the following way

   a. There is a small tumor in the lung, but there is no lymph node involvement

   b. There is no metastasis, but there is lymph node involvement

   c. There is no tumor, but there may be cancer cells in the lymph nodes

   d. There is no tumor, no evidence of cancer in the lymph nodes, and no metastasis

4. A 45-year-old patient who has ovarian cancer tells the nurse that her oncologist described the cancer as "localized." The nurse explains that this means that

   a. Cancer cells are present but have not spread to other parts of the body

   b. The cancer has spread only to nearby lymph nodes

   c. The cancer has spread to distant sites

   d. There are abnormal cells present but not cancer cells

5. An 88-year-old palliative care patient with a history of end-stage chronic obstructive pulmonary disease, heart failure, type 2 diabetes mellitus, and hypertension was recently diagnosed with colon cancer. The patient asks the nurse if she might consider surgery "to take the cancer out." The nurse's best response is

   a. "I'm sure there are many curative options for you"

   b. "I'd like to talk with you about hospice care"

   c. "Is your goal to be completely cured of the cancer?"

   d. "Do you feel you are a good candidate for surgery?"

6. The patient in the previous question tells the nurse she would like to talk with her oncologist about palliative chemotherapy. The potential side effect of chemotherapy that poses the greatest risk to this patient is

   a. Lethargy

   b. Anemia

   c. Dizziness

   d. Alopecia

7. A patient who has throat cancer reports that she has woken with a headache several days this week but if she vomits the pain goes away. The hospice nurse suspects that the patient has

   a. Increased intracranial pressure

   b. Esophageal varices

    c. Metastasis to the brain

    d. Severe migraines

8. A 51-year-old patient is referred to palliative care after being diagnosed with thyroid cancer. A significant risk factor for this type of cancer is

    a. Smoking

    b. Numerous dental x-rays during childhood

    c. Obesity

    d. History of type I diabetes mellitus

9. A patient who has spinal cord compression is referred for palliative care. Which of the following findings, if noted on the initial assessment, would be unexpected?

    a. Saddle numbness

    b. Constipation

    c. Hyperreflexia

    d. Facial edema

10. A 72-year-old hospice patient who has lung cancer reports increased dyspnea and chest pain. The nurse knows that these symptoms are most likely related to

    a. Spread of the cancer to the opposite lung

    b. Tuberculosis

    c. Metastasis to the esophagus

    d. Formation of a saddle clot

◼ REFERENCES

Al-Qurainy, R. (2016). Metastatic spinal cord compression: Diagnosis and management. *BMJ, 353,* 1–7. doi:10.1136/bmj.i2539

American Cancer Society. (2016). *Managing symptoms of advanced cancer.* Retrieved from https://www.cancer.org/treatment/understanding-your-diagnosis/advanced-cancer/managing-symptoms.html

Bodtke, S., & Ligon, K. (2016). *Hospice and palliative medicine handbook: A clinical guide.* Retrieved from http://www.hpmhandbook.com/

Borooah, B. (2018). Oncologic emergencies: A review. *International Journal of Research in Medical Sciences, 6*(5), 1484–1490. doi:10.18203/2320-6012.ijrms20181492

Canadian Cancer Society. (2018). *Septic shock.* Retrieved from http://www.cancer.ca/en/cancer-information/diagnosis-and-treatment/managing-side-effects/septic-shock/?region=sk

Fong, Y. (2013). A review of: Bitter and sweet: A family's journey with cancer. In D. Thiel (Ed.), *Bitter and sweet: A family's journey with cancer* (pp. 5–6, v–vi). Seneca, NY: West.

Lustberg, M. (2012). Management of neutropenia in cancer patients. *Advances in Hematology and Oncology, 10*(2), 825–826. Retrieved from https://www.ncbi.nlm.nih.gov/pmc/articles/PMC4059501/

Martin, L., Cheek, D. J., & Morris, S. E. (2014). Shock, multiple organ dysfunction syndrome, and burns in adults. In L. K. McCance, S. E. Huether, V. L. Brashers, & N. S. Rote (Eds.), *Pathophysiology: The biologic basis for diseases in adults and children* (7th ed., pp. 1669–1698). St.Louis, MO: Elsevier Mosby.

National Cancer Institute (2015a). *Age and cancer risk.* Retrieved from https://www.cancer.gov/about -cancer/causes-prevention/risk/age.

National Cancer Institute. (2015b). *Cancer staging.* Retrieved from https://www.cancer.gov/about -cancer/diagnosis-staging/staging

National Cancer Institute. (2017). *Common cancer types.* Retrieved from https://www.cancer.gov/ types/common-cancers

National Heart, Lung, and Blood Institute. (2017). *Disseminated intravascular coagulation.* Retrieved from https://www.nhlbi.nih.gov/health-topics/disseminated-intravascular-coagulation

National Institutes of Health. (2017). *SEER training: Cancer treatment.* Retrieved from https://training.seer.cancer.gov/treatment/

Röllig, C., & Ehninger, G. (2015). How I treat hyperleukocytosis in acute myeloid leukemia. *Blood, 125,* 3246–3252. doi:10.1182/blood-2014-10-551507

Rote, N. S., & Virshup, D. M. (2014). Cellular proliferation: Cancer. In K. L. McCance, S. E. Huether, L. V. Brashers, & N. S. Rote (Eds.), *Pathophysiology: The biologic basis for diseases in adults and children* (7th ed., pp. 363–395). St. Louis, MO: Elsevier Mosby.

Riggiero, A., Rizzo, D., Amato, M., & Riccardi, R. (2016). Management of hyperleukocytosis. *Current Treatment Options in Oncology, 17*(7), 1–10. doi:10.1007/s11864-015-0387-8

Sekeres, M. (2010). *Oncologic emergencies.* Retrieved from http://www.clevelandclinicmeded.com/medical pubs/diseasemanagement/hematology-oncology/oncologic-emergencies/

5 Neurological Disorders

*Neurosurgery attracted me as much for its intertwining of brain
and consciousness as for its intertwining of life and death.*
—Kalanithi (2016, p. 81)

■ LEARNING OBJECTIVES

After completing this section, the nurse will be able to

1. Differentiate between neurological and neurovascular disorders
2. Identify the main causes of neurological disorders
3. Identify the disease trajectories for neurological and neurovascular disorders

■ THE NEUROLOGIC SYSTEM

The nervous system functions seamlessly as an integrated whole. But to facilitate understanding of how various processes occur, the nervous system is typically described according to specific structures or functions. For example, the central nervous system (CNS) includes the brain and spinal cord. The peripheral nervous system (PNS) includes the cranial nerves (see Table 5.1), which emanate from the brain and the spinal nerves (Figure 5.1). The spinal nerves emanate from the spinal cord (Sugerman, 2014).

The PNS can be further divided into the somatic nervous system and the autonomic nervous system. The somatic nervous system regulates voluntary movement of skeletal muscles and the autonomic nervous system regulates involuntary muscle functions, such as organ systems and viscera. The autonomic nervous system is further divided into the sympathetic and parasympathetic pathways (Sugerman, 2014).

Sympathetic and parasympathetic responses are usually opposite of each other. The sympathetic nervous system is responsible for the "fight or flight" reaction. When stimulated, the sympathetic nervous system causes mental alertness, increased heart rate and increased cardiac

Table 5.1 Cranial Nerves

Cranial Nerve	Function	Test
I. Olfactory	Sense of smell	Ask patient to distinguish a variety of smells
II. Optic	Vision	Check vision using Snellen chart
III. Occulomotor	Pupillary reflex Eyelid closure	Check pupillary reflex using a pen light. Pupils should constrict when exposed to light). Observe patient's ability to fully open and close eyelid
IV. Trochlear	Eye movement	Ask patient to follow finger with eyes through the cardinal movements
V. Trigeminal	Movement of facial muscles, including jaw. Sense of pain, touch, and temperature of face	Ask patient to clench teeth and then move jaw from side to side. Use blunt and sharp and objects and cold and warm objects to test facial sensations. Test corneal reflex with a sterile cotton wisp (patient should blink when eye is lightly touched with the cotton wisp)
VI. Abducens	Lateral movement of the eyes	Test ability to move eyes laterally
VII. Facial	Sense of taste Facial expressions	Assess patient's sense of taste using salty, sour, sweet and bitter substances. Ask patient to smile and close eyes
VIII. Vestibu-locloclear (acoustic)	Hearing and sense of equilibrium	*Rinne test:* Hold tuning fork near ear to determine conduction of sound by air *Weber test:* Place tuning fork on top of patient's head to determine conduction of sound through bone. Air conduction should be greater than bone conduction.
IX. Glossopha-ryngeal	Ability to swallow, speak, and cough Gag reflex	Check gag reflex and ask patient to swallow saliva and then a small amount of liquid. Ask patient to speak and to cough
X. Vagus	Sensory and motor function of the pharynx. Also innervates smooth muscles of the abdominal organs and viscera	Same as glossopharyngeal nerve testing
XI. Spinal Accessory	Function of trapezius and sternocleidomas-toid muscles as well as soft palate, larynx, and pharynx	Ask patient to shrug shoulders, and turn head from side to side against resistance
XII. Hypoglossal	Innervates tongue	Assess position of tongue and patient's ability to move tongue

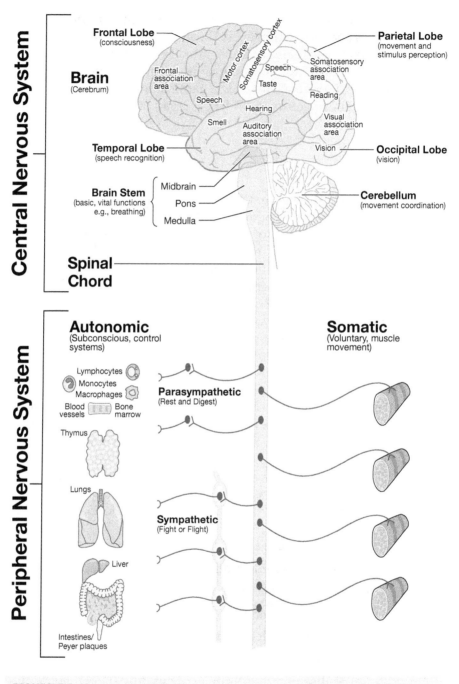

FIGURE 5.1 Neurons, the cells.

contractility, bronchodilation, decreased digestion, and peripheral vasodilation. On the other hand, the parasympathetic nervous system activates the "rest and digest" response. It regulates digestion, promotes relaxation, decreases heart rate, and decreases peripheral vasodilation.

Neurons, the cells of the nervous system, are not contiguous. The spaces between neurons, the synapses, are the spaces in which electrical or chemical signals are transmitted between neurons. The depletion or overproduction of neurotransmitters such as "norepinephrine, acetylcholine, dopamine, histamine, gamma-amino butyric acid (GABA), and serotonin" (Sugerman, 2014, p. 452) can cause neurological and or mood disorders.

Neurological Disorders

Neurological disorders that are included in the "neurological disease" category of hospice admission criteria are chronic degenerative conditions such as amyotrophic lateral sclerosis, Parkinson's disease (PD), muscular dystrophy, myasthenia gravis, and multiple sclero-

> **Key Point**
>
> Pseudobulbar affect is characterized by episodes of sudden uncontrollable and inappropriate laughing or crying. It is common in patients who have neurological disorders. The treatment for this affect is dextromethorphan 20 mg with quinidine 10 mg (Schwartz, 2015).

sis. Each of these disorders is caused by dysfunction within the neurological system and is progressive and degenerative. The trajectory of neurological disorders typically involves gradual functional decline over a period of 6 to 8 years. But in some cases, the disease trajectory can take a rapid turn when respiratory muscles are affected, leading to respiratory arrest. In other cases, an acute illnesses such as pneumonia or a sudden cardiac event may precede the patient's death.

The hospice admission criteria for all of the neurological diseases are essentially the same and presume evidence of the following:

The patient must meet at least one of the following criteria (1 or 2A or 2B):

1 OR 2A OR 2B, below:

1. Critically impaired breathing capacity evidenced by
   - Dyspnea at rest
   - Vital capacity <30%
   - Need for supplemental oxygen at rest
   - Patient refusing artificial ventilation

2. Rapid disease progression evidenced by the following changes
   - Independent ambulation to wheelchair or bedbound status
   - Normal to barely intelligible or unintelligible speech
   - Normal to pureed diet
   - Independence in most activities of daily living (ADLs) to needing major assistance in all ADLs

And either A OR B:

A. Critical nutritional impairment demonstrated by *all* of the following in the preceding 12 months:

- Oral intake of nutrients and fluids insufficient to sustain life
- Continuing weight loss
- Dehydration or hypovolemia
- Absence of artificial feeding methods

B. Life-threatening complications in the past 12 months as demonstrated by more than one of the following:

- Recurrent aspiration pneumonia
- Pyelonephritis
- Sepsis
- Recurrent fever
- Stage 3 or 4 pressure ulcer(s)

A brief review of each of the neurological disorders will be provided in the following sections with an overview of signs, symptoms, diagnostic criteria, treatments, palliative approaches to care, and finally, end-of-life considerations.

Amyotrophic Lateral Sclerosis or Lou Gehrig Disease

Amyotrophic lateral sclerosis (ALS) is a rare, debilitating, and incurable neurologic disease characterized by progressive muscle atrophy with hyperreflexia that results from denervation (amyotrophy; Boss & Huether, 2014a; Gorman, 2015). Although it is the most common neurologic disease, the exact etiology remains unknown. Risk factors include familial predisposition, female gender, and age over 40 years (Boss & Huether, 2014a; Gorman, 2015; Mazzini, DeMarchi, Corrado, & D'Alfonso, 2017).

Early symptoms of ALS include (Boss & Huether, 2014a; Gorman, 2015) the following:

- Impaired fine motor skills
- Muscle cramping
- Muscle weakness
- Paresis that typically begins with a single muscle group
- Slurred speech
- Incoordination
- Dysphagia

According to Brooks, Miller, Swash, and Munsat (2000), diagnosis of ALS presumes the following:

- Evidence of lower motor neuron (LMN) degeneration by clinical, electrophysiological, or neuropathologic examination
- Evidence of upper motor neuron (UMN) degeneration by clinical examination
- Progressive spread of symptoms or signs within a region or to other regions, as determined by history or examination
- **Together with the absence of**
    - ▩ Electrophysiological or pathological evidence of other disease processes that might explain the signs of LMN and/or UMN degeneration
    - ▩ Neuroimaging evidence of other disease processes that might explain the observed clinical and electrophysiological signs (p. 293)

Diagnosis of ALS is largely based on the patient's medical history and clinical examination. Symptoms can mimic several other neurologic disorders, so electrodiagnostic, neurophysiological, neuroimaging, and clinical laboratory studies can be used to rule out other diagnoses and confirm the diagnosis of ALS (Brooks et al., 2000).

Although there is no cure for ALS, multiple strategies have been used to both promote comfort and extend the patient's life. The only pharmacological intervention that has been found to extend survival and time to tracheostomy is riluzole (Boss & Huether, 2014a; Schwartz, 2015). Interventional medical options depend on the patient's goals of care. For example, decisions regarding the use of artificial nutrition, mechanical ventilation, and diaphragm pacing must be considered. In addition to these treatments, interventions to preserve function and comfort, such as physical, occupational, speech, and respiratory therapy should be initiated early in the disease process. Further, communication barriers can be overcome through the use of traditional phonetic boards or the more advanced eye-tracking or brain–computer interface systems (Hwang, Weng, Wang, Tsai, & Chang, 2014).

As ALS progresses, the patient's speech becomes increasingly impaired, dyspnea becomes more pronounced, and movement impossible. Cognitive impairment is present in some, but not all, patients (Beeldman et al., 2016). Senses such as touch, hearing, taste, smell, and vision remain largely intact, as does cardiac function (The ALS Association, 2018; Boss & Huether, 2014a). The prognosis for patients diagnosed with ALS is approximately 3 to 5 years (Connolly, Galvin, & Hardiman, 2015; Gorman, 2015). Throughout the disease process, the multidisciplinary palliative care team should be involved to manage symptoms, promote comfort, and provide emotional and spiritual support to the patient and family (Kovach & Reynolds, 2015; Schwartz, 2015). Most patients who have ALS eventually succumb to respiratory failure, which can ensue quickly and unexpectedly. In the terminal phase of ALS, the hospice team must work with the patient and family to make determinations regarding respiratory support and to provide guidance to the family when symptoms rapidly progress.

Parkinson's Disease

PD is the second most commonly diagnosed neurodegenerative disorder. Symptoms often begin on one side of the body and then progress to the other side. It is characterized by progressive degeneration of

Key Point
Parkinsonism is a term used to describe symptoms similar to those associated with PD but are not associated with the loss of dopaminergic neurons in the substantia nigra (Schwartz, 2015).

dopaminergic neurons in the substantia nigra and the presence of Lewy bodies, which results in both motor and nonmotor symptoms. Hallmark motor symptoms are bradykinesia, muscle rigidity, postural instability or unbalance, and resting tremor. Tremor, rigidity, and movement disorder are the three components of the "classic triad" of PD symptoms. Ultimately, the disease leads to paralysis and complete physical dependence (Kovach & Reynolds, 2015; Schwartz, 2015).

Nonmotor symptoms associated with PD include depression, decreased sense of smell, emotional lability, bladder incontinence, constipation, dermatologic problems, sleep disturbances, dementia, orthostatic hypotension, muscle cramping and pain, and lethargy. As PD progresses, dysphagia often results from an inability to completely chew food and to swallow it without choking. Aspiration may result, so protection of the patient's airway is a priority.

The exact causes of PD are not known, but onset is usually associated with aging. It is most commonly diagnosed in adults over the age of 40, with the majority of cases diagnosed in those over 60. Initial care should be focused on stabilizing functional capacity and enhancing safety with transfers or ambulation. The time from diagnosis to death in patients who have PD varies. Management of PD usually involves medications such as levodopa, dopamine receptor agonists, catechol-O-methyltransferase inhibitors, selective MAO-B inhibitors, muscarinic receptor agonists, and amantadine (Robertson, 2018), as well as diligent management of symptoms as they arise. Additionally, safety planning is a priority as the patient's ability to ambulate independently becomes compromised.

Patients can live with PD for many years before the onset of the terminal phase. In the terminal phase, rigidity and immobility are increased. Because of the lengthy course of the illness, nursing care should include emotional support of the patient and family. Education must be provided to prepare for each part of the terminal phase. The palliative care or hospice team should work closely with the patient and family to appropriately manage symptoms as they arise, with particular attention given to assessing for hypotensive episodes and gastric immotility (Kovach & Reynolds, 2015; Schwartz, 2015).

Muscular Dystrophy

Muscular dystrophy (MD) is an umbrella term for genetic conditions that lead to progressive muscle weakness and atrophy. The two types of MD that affect the skeletal and cardiac muscles are Duchenne and Becker; both types occur primarily in males. The sequelae of MD include cardiac enlargement, dyspnea, extreme fatigue, and lower extremity edema. Management of MD involves the use of medications such as eteplirsen (Exondys 51), steroids, angiotensin-converting enzyme (ACE) inhibitors, or beta-blockers.

Duchenne MD (DMD) is caused by a mutation of the dystrophin gene. It is characterized by muscle weakness that is first noted in early childhood and progressively worsens, leading to complete immobility and lack of muscle control by the teenage years. Patients who have DMD have a life expectancy of 20 to 30 years (Schwartz, 2015), with an average age of survival of 23 to 27.8 years (Van Ruiten et al., 2016). Management of DMD involves ongoing evaluation of the following four areas (Birkrant et al., 2018):

1. *Respiratory management* involves monitoring respiratory function, assisted coughing, routine assessment of pulse oximetry, determination of candidacy for tracheostomy, if needed, pulmonary function testing, and sleep studies.

2. *Ambulatory status* should be maintained through physical and occupational therapy for as long as possible because declination from ambulatory to nonambulatory status sets off a cascade of other potential health problems. For example, nonambulatory status leads to weak cough efforts, which then increases the risk for atelectasis, pneumonia, progression to respiratory failure, and increased risk for infection.

3. *Bone health* is serious concern for patients who have DMD because a staple in the management of the disease is long-term steroid use. Thus, it is not surprising that steroid use, in combination with limited ambulatory ability, contributes to osteoporosis. Osteoporosis contributes to a high prevalence of bone fragility and fractures. It is critical, then, for the nurse to assess for decreased bone density and fractures, particularly vertebral fractures. Caregivers should also be taught about the risk for fracture and how to safely reposition the patient in bed or transfer the patient out of bed.

4. *Cardiac health* is often compromised in patients who have DMD. The nurse must frequently assess for signs of heart failure such as marked dyspnea, dependent edema, hypoxia, orthopnea, jugular vein distention, activity intolerance, and marked fatigue. The presence and severity of dysrhythmias and the feasibility of implantation of an automated implantable cardioverter defibrillator (AICD) device should be discussed. For patients who have an AICD device implanted, deactivation of the defibrillator during the terminal

phase of the disease must be taken into account. Finally, some patients who have DMD may be candidates for a left ventricular assist device (LVAD) as a destination therapy (Iodice et al., 2015). If the patient and family are interested in taking this route, then proper referrals should be made for evaluation and treatment.

Ultimately, the cause of death for patients who have DMD is most often related to cardiac failure or respiratory failure. Because of the availability of noninvasive ventilation, the cause of death for those who have DMD is predominantly cardiomyopathy (Van Ruiten et al., 2016).

Becker MD is a milder form of MD than DMD. It is caused by a genetic mutation that severely reduces dystrophin levels. The lack of the dystrophin protein leads to muscle fiber damage and muscle weakness (van den Bergen et al., 2014). Muscle weakness may become so severe in the later stages of the disease that the patient loses ambulatory ability.

The course of BMD is somewhat unpredictable and the symptoms vary from patient to patient. The first signs of the disease usually appear in the teenage years or early adulthood and include cramps with exercise, difficulty with walking or running, marked fatigue, falls, and in some cases, mild learning problems. The testing involved in the diagnosis of BMD can include genetic testing, needle electromyography (to determine whether the problem is related to the muscles themselves or to nerve signal conduction), and nerve conduction studies (American Association of Neuromuscular & Electrodiagnostic Medicine, 2018). Patients who have Becker MD may live into their 40's or beyond (National Institutes of Health, 2018).

For both DMD and BMD, a team-based approach to care and expertly coordinated support services are necessary. Family caregivers should be provided with extensive education on the disease process, goals of care, and advance directives. Palliation of symptoms should begin very early in the disease process to lessen the disease burden. Because of the lengthy disease process, family caregivers may normalize the care of their loved one as well as the management of symptoms within the ongoing family dynamic. After years of managing numerous exacerbations, infections, and other challenges, caregivers have likely cultivated hope that most problems are surmountable. Thus, when faced with the prospect that the patient's condition is in the terminal stage, caregivers may feel shocked and devastated.

Extensive discussions regarding advance directives, airway management options (i.e., tracheostomy and ventilator support), goals of care, and preferred place of death must be discussed. As the patient's condition worsens, the family should be prepared for the likelihood that the patient's death will be related to pulmonary arrest or cardiac arrest secondary to pulmonary complications (Birkrant et al., 2018). Bereavement care for the family should involve the patient's family caregivers as well as siblings, particularly for patients with DMD, whose life expectancy is limited beyond their teenage years.

Myasthenia Gravis

Myasthenia gravis (MG) is an autoimmune disease that primarily affects the neurological system. It is characterized by intermittent muscle weakness that often follows activity and is

Key Point
The term myasthenia gravis is derived from Latin and Greek words meaning "grave muscular weakness" (Myasthenia Gravis Foundation of America, 2018).

alleviated by rest. Symptoms of MG result from degradation of the acetylcholine receptors at the neuromuscular junctions, which interferes with transmission of signals from the brainstem to the muscles. Thus, MG causes skeletal muscle weakness and fatigability. The first sign of MG is ptosis. Other symptoms may include diplopia, dysphagia, and dyspnea. Chewing and speaking are also affected (American Academy of Ophthalmology, 2018). Involuntary muscles are not affected.

Apart from genetic predisposition, risk factors have not been definitively identified. The "most common comorbidities are thyroid disease, systemic lupus erythematosus and rheumatoid arthritis" (Gilhus, Nacu, Andersen, & Owe, 2014, p. 17). Women are more likely to develop initial symptoms of MG between the ages of 20 and 40, while men are more likely to develop symptoms of MG over the age of 60 (American Academy of Ophthalmology, 2018).

Treatment of MG involves the use of several pharmacological interventions to suppress the immune response and decrease inflammation. For example, glucocorticosteroids are used to combat systemic inflammation even though their exact mechanism in suppressing the symptoms of MG is not well understood. Medications such as azathioprine (AZT), mycophenolate mofetil (MMF), methotrexate (MTX), cyclosporine A (CSA), and tacrolimus (TAC) are used to suppress the immune response and inflammation by directly affecting the immune system. Acetylcholinesterase inhibitors are used to slow the hydrolysis of acetylcholine. This slowing increases the availability of acetylcholine at the synaptic cleft, which improves transmission of neuromuscular signal transmission (Urban, Jacobi, & Jander, 2018). Since MG is incurable, the goal of treatment is remission.

Between periods of remission, patients who have MG are at risk for exacerbations, commonly referred to as myasthenic crises. These exacerbations are characterized by muscle weakness that is so severe the patient is incapacitated with either quadriparesis or quadriplegia. Severe dysphagia and respiratory distress also occur. The decreased tidal volume and decreased tidal capacity that accompany the respiratory distress put the patient at risk for respiratory arrest (Boss & Huether, 2014b).

Myasthenic crisis usually occurs within 3 to 4 hours of administration of medications, but can also be precipitated by physical or emotional stress, aspiration pneumonitis, pregnancy, sleep deprivation, pain, or infection (Boss & Huether, 2014b; Wendell & Levine, 2011).

Myasthenic crisis requires immediate intervention if the symptoms are to be suppressed. During exacerbations of MG, apheresis and intravenous immunoglobulin therapy are used (Urban et al., 2018). Roughly 90% of patients who experience myasthenic crisis require intubation and mechanical ventilation (Wendell & Levine, 2011). Therefore, an advance directive should be in place for every patient who has MG so that invasive interventions that are contrary to the patient's stated goals of care are not initiated.

The treatments used to suppress MG also put the patient at risk for other complications. Specifically, even though use of anticholinesterase inhibitor medications is essential (Schwartz, 2015), overdose places the patient at risk for cholinergic crisis. Clinically, patients in cholinergic crisis present similarly to those in myasthenic crisis, except that symptoms such as "diarrhea, cramping, fasciculation, bradycardia, pupillary constriction, and increased salivation and increased sweating" (p. 625) may also accompany cholinergic crisis. Cholinergic crisis typically occurs 30 to 60 minutes after taking anticholinergic medications (Boss & Huether, 2014b). As in myasthenic crisis, the patient is at risk for respiratory arrest.

Because MG is not curable, palliative care delivered by an interdisciplinary team is useful to decrease anxiety and dyspnea, and to promote comfort. Further, the palliative care team can work with the patient and family to develop goals of care and advance directives, particularly in regard to airway management and ventilator support. In cases of refractory MG, hospice care should be initiated if the hospice admission criteria are applicable and it is consistent with the patient's and family's goals of care.

Multiple Sclerosis

Multiple sclerosis (MS) is a chronic, progressive, autoimmune disease. MS is most commonly diagnosed in middle-aged White women who have a first-degree relative with MS. Other risk factors include vitamin D deficiency, cigarette smoking, and infection with the Epstein–Barr virus (Boss & Huether, 2014b). The disease is characterized by demyelination of the neural sheath that surrounds nerve fibers in the CNS. When the myelin sheath is degraded, signals between nerves and muscles cannot be transmitted properly, which leads to muscle weakness, spasticity, and ultimately to paralysis. Additionally, plaque formation occurs in the periventricular white matter, optic nerves, and spinal cord, which leads to degeneration of axons (Boss & Huether, 2014b).

The impairment to nerve signal transmission causes symptomatology related to the affected nerves. Initial symptoms vary depending on the location of the lesions (Brownlee et al., 2017, p. 1338), but often include visual and motor deficits because the optic nerve and motor centers in the brainstem are commonly affected. Other symptoms include overwhelming fatigue, functional impairment, bowel and bladder incontinence, visual disturbances, dizziness and vertigo, pain, cognitive changes, depression, spasticity, and sexual dysfunction (Kovach & Reynolds, 2015; Schwartz, 2015). Symptoms often occur in clusters.

Prior to the onset of initial symptoms, there is usually a precipitating event, such as infection, trauma, or pregnancy. If symptoms are precipitated by pregnancy, they usually occur around 12 weeks postpartum. This onset is most likely related to the stress and fatigue of childbirth rather to the pregnancy itself (Boss & Huether, 2014b).

Symptom onset can be categorized as relapsing or progressive. Relapsing MS is generally characterized by an acute episode of "unilateral optic neuritis, a partial myelitis, or a brainstem syndrome" (Brownlee et al., 2017, p. 1338) that occurs over hours or days with peak symptomatology within of 4 weeks of onset. Remission is usually spontaneous. Progressive onset of MS symptoms is insidious, occurring over the course of months or even years. Most often, initial presentation involves asymmetric paraparesis, progressive hemiparesis, and cerebellar ataxia. Rarely, blindness or dementia can occur (Brownlee et al., 2017, p. 1338).

A diagnosis of MS should be suspected if the patient's reported symptoms and physical examination are suggestive of the disease. Confirmation of the diagnosis requires "objective evidence of CNS lesions disseminated in time and space, and. . . that there is no better explanation for the clinical presentation and that alternative diagnoses are considered and excluded" (Brownlee et al., 2017, p. 1338). Upon initial diagnosis, treatment should be initiated to restore function as quickly as possible and to slow disease progression. Treatment modalities for MS may include the use of the following:

- Subcutaneous injection of interferon beta or pegylated interferon beta-1a to reduce inflammation

- Oral administration of teriflunomide, which inhibits the proliferation of autoreactive T and B cells

- Intravenous infusion of natalizumab every 4 weeks to prevent lymphocytes from crossing the blood–brain barrier

- Intravenous infusion of ocrelizumab every 6 months to suppress the immune response (Comi, Radaelli, & Sørenson, 2017)

Pharmacological treatment of MS should be augmented with physical and occupational therapy to preserve functional status. The rate of declination varies, but the patient's age, comorbidities, and response to therapy account for some of the variation in disease progression. Patients who have MS often experience "progressive dwindling" as the disease trajectory. However, one notable turning point is the loss of ambulatory ability, which precipitates rapid disease progression.

In the terminal stage of MS, care should focus on ensuring comfort and safety, as well as the emotional support of the patient–family unit. Holistic care must be provided using a team approach. Ultimately, the cause of death is often related to interminable MS or its complications (i.e., aspiration pneumonia or urinary tract infection) or the onset or exacerbation of another disease process such as cancer or a cardiac event (Martin, Raffel, & Nicholas, 2016).

Neurovascular Disease

Neurovascular disorders result from occlusion or damage to the cerebral vessels. Neurovascular disorders include intracranial aneurysms, arteriovenous malformations (AVMs), carotid artery disease, and intracranial atherosclerotic disease. Each of these disorders will be reviewed in the following sections.

Intracranial aneurysms occur when an intracranial vessel bulges outward from the vessel wall. Because of this weakness in the vessel, there is a risk for bleeding into the cerebral tissue, which in turn, leads to increased intracranial pressure, cranial nerve compression, and varied

> **Key Point**
>
> Aging causes structural and functional changes in the nervous system such as increased permeability of the blood–brain barrier, neurotransmitter imbalances, sleep disturbances, altered tendon reflexes, deficits in taste, smell, and memory impairment (Sugerman, 2014).

neurological symptoms that depend on the location of the aneurysm. Unfortunately, aneurysms are usually asymptomatic until an acute event such as a subarachnoid hemorrhage, intracerebral hemorrhage, or both occur. In such cases, unless invasive therapy is feasible and reasonable, a ruptured cerebral aneurysm can result in the patient's death (Boss & Huether, 2014b).

AVMs are relatively rare congenital vascular conditions in which arteries flow directly to veins through a network of malformed vessels that lack a true capillary bed. Because the blood flow through the malformed vessels is impeded, the patient is at risk for aneurysm or thrombus formation at the site of the AVM. The AVM is present at birth, but most patients will not experience symptoms until later in life. Rupture of the vessel, which can be fatal, is most likely to occur in patients between the ages of 20 and 30 (Boss & Huether, 2014b).

Vascular and atherosclerotic diseases cause narrowing of the vessels. Cardiac artery disease (CAD) is a vascular disease characterized by narrowing of the cardiac vessels. This narrowing of the vessels is most often related to hypercholesteremia, which can cause fatty plaques to lodge within the vessels. With the vessel diameter narrowed, cardiac workload is increased, and hypertension ensues. Hypertension is a key risk factor for stroke. Further, plaque particles may break away from the vessel wall and become lodged in the narrow cerebral vessels, leading to transient ischemic attack (TIA) or stroke.

Atherosclerosis can also occur within the vessels of the brain due to hypercholesterolemia. Cerebral vessels can become narrowed or obstructed by plaque, resulting in symptoms of TIA or stroke. Additionally, thrombi may become caught on plaque within a cerebral vessel and obstruct the vessel, leading to stroke or TIA. Treatment is dependent on the cause of the patient's symptoms, the patient's condition, and the presence and severity of other medical conditions.

Although hospice admission criteria do not specifically address AVMs, sclerosis, or cerebral aneurysms, any of these illnesses can result in stroke, coma, or death, which are considered potentially terminal conditions that may warrant hospice admission.

Cerebrovascular Accident/Stroke

Cerebrovascular accidents (CVAs) are the third leading cause of death in the United States. The incidence of stroke is twice as high in Blacks as in Whites and there is a genetic predisposition to CVA. Some of the common risk factors for CVA include hypertension, atherosclerosis, type 2 diabetes mellitus, congestive heart failure, peripheral vascular disease, carotid stenosis, sickle cell disease, smoking, obesity, postmenopausal hormone replacement therapy, and high sodium intake. Potential consequences of CVA include hemiplegia, aphasia, coma, and death (Boss & Huether, 2014b). Strokes are classified according to the cause:

1. *Thrombotic stroke* is caused by a blood clot that formed in the brain or intracranial vessels.

2. *TIA* is most often caused by a temporary infarction of a vessel within the brain. This can cause stroke-like symptoms that resolve within 24 hours. Although the symptoms resolve, steps must be taken to prevent CVA, as roughly 30% of patients who experience TIA will have a CVA within one year of the TIA.

3. *Embolic stroke* occurs when a fragment of an embolism breaks loose from a clot that formed in a cardiac vessel, a carotid artery, or another vessel outside of the brain. Embolic stroke increases the risk for a subsequent stroke when the original clot deteriorates even further and more fragments move to the brain.

4. *Cerebral infarction* is caused by a lack of blood supply to an area of the brain secondary to a vascular infarction.

5. *Lacunar stroke* is caused by a microinfarct (<1 cm in diameter) in the cerebral vessels that result in microaneurysms. Lacunar strokes are associated with a history of smoking, type 2 diabetes mellitus, hyperlipidemia, and hypertension. Lacunar strokes most often result in strictly motor or sensory deficits.

6. *Hemorrhagic stroke* occurs with spontaneous bleeding in the brain. It is the most common cause of CVA and accounts for up to 18% of CVAs in Whites and up to 30% of CVAs in Blacks and Asians. The most common cause of hemorrhagic stroke is hypertension, followed by ruptured aneurysms and AVMs (Boss & Heuther, 2014b).

In the acute phase of CVA, the patient is often unable to speak for themselves or to make decisions regarding their care. Family members and loved ones, then, are usually tasked with decisions regarding initiation, withholding, or withdrawing treatments such as thrombolysis, mechanical ventilation, artificial nutrition and hydration, management of infections, and initiation of rehabilitation therapies (de Boer et al., 2015).

The burden of decision-making on the family in end-stage disease cannot be underestimated. According to de Boer et al. (2015), relatives who are tasked with making life-and-death decisions in the acute phase after a severe stroke feel immense pressure because they need to make critical decisions under time constraints, question whether they have the right to decide what happens to the patient, are reluctant to end life-sustaining treatments, and have difficulty coping with unexpected changes in the patient's condition. Decision-making may be made more complex if the patient has no advance directive because acute CVA often results in coma.

Coma

Coma is an altered state of consciousness in which the patient is unable to respond to verbal or tactile stimuli. Altered levels of consciousness can be categorized as follows (Boss & Huether, 2014b):

> **Key Point**
>
> "Level of consciousness is the most critical clinical index of nervous system function or dysfunction" (Boss & Huether, 2014b, p. 529).

- *Confusion:* Patient is unable to think clearly. Judgement and decision-making capacity are impaired
- *Disorientation:* Patient first becomes disoriented to time, then to place, and then to person
- *Lethargy:* Decrease in spontaneous speech or movement. Patient responds to verbal or tactile stimuli but may be disoriented
- *Coma:* Patient has no verbal response to verbal or tactile stimuli. Patient has no motor response to noxious or painful stimuli. Coma can categorized as follows:
  - Light coma: Patient exhibits purposeful movement in response to verbal or tactile stimuli
  - Coma: Patient may respond to verbal or tactile stimuli but response is not purposeful
  - Deep coma: Patient is unresponsive to any stimuli

The prognosis for a comatose patient is dependent on the cause and the level of severity of the coma. Poor outcomes are specifically associated with the following (Kovach & Reynolds, 2015):

- Coma after cardiac arrest
- Lack of pupillary response or lack of purposeful movement within 72 hours of the onset of the coma
- Age 60 years or more
- Coma related to traumatic head injury
- Multiple comorbidities
- Medical complications

Coma as a result of stroke is almost always fatal. The majority of patients who die from coma die in the acute care setting (Kovach & Reynolds, 2015). Palliative care for comatose patients in the acute care setting should focus on pain management, management of secretions, and respiratory support as appropriate, management of restlessness, nutrition and hydration, elimination, and skin care. Family support from the entire palliative care team is necessary, especially as families become involved in end-of-life decision-making.

When discussing care options with families, education should include information about irreversible coma, which occurs with the death of the cerebral hemispheres. The patient may not be able to respond meaningfully to stimuli, but if the brainstem is not involved, the respiratory, cardiac, and gastrointestinal systems will continue to function and the body temperature will be maintained (Boss & Huether, 2014b). Without intervention, the most likely cause of death will be an infection, such as pneumonia (Kovach & Reynolds, 2015). Families may consider hospice care if the patient meets the following admission criteria:

Hospice Admission Criteria for CVA and Coma

The patient with stroke or coma patient has **both** 1 and 2:

1. Poor functional status Palliative Performance Scale (PPS) ≤40%
2. Poor nutritional status with inability to maintain sufficient fluid and calorie intake

The patient who suffered a stroke **also** has *one or more* of the following:

- ≥10% weight loss in past 6 months
- ≥7.5% weight loss in past 3 months
- Serum albumin <2.5 gm/dL
- Current history of pulmonary aspiration without effective response to speech therapy interventions to improve dysphagia and decrease aspiration events

Supporting documentation for a patient with coma as a terminal diagnosis includes **three** of the following on the **third day** of the coma:

- Abnormal brain stem response
- Absent verbal responses
- Absent withdrawal response to pain
- Serum creatinine >1.5 gm/dL

CONCLUSION

End-of-life care for patients who have neurological disorders varies widely and is dependent on the etiology. In all cases, though, goals of care should include preservation of mental and physical function, safety management, and caregiver support. An interdisciplinary team approach is necessary to meet the complex care needs of the patient and family. In cases of slowly progressing neurological disorders, advance care planning should take place as early as possible. In acute neurological disease, the interdisciplinary team must work closely with the family members and other decision-makers to determine appropriate care strategies within the context of the disease process.

Chapter Summary

- The nervous system consists of the central and peripheral systems and is further divided into the somatic and autonomic systems. The nervous system pathways are responsible for sympathetic (fight or flight) and parasympathetic (rest and digest) responses.
- Depletion or overproduction of neurotransmitters can cause neurological disorders.
- Degenerative neurological disorders include ALS, PD, MD, MG, and MS.
- Neurovascular disorders result from occlusion or damage to the cerebral vessels. Examples include intracranial aneurysms, AVMs, carotid artery disease, and intracranial atherosclerotic disease.
- End-of-life care for all neurological disorders is dependent on the patient's goals of care. Palliative care should be introduced as early as possible to minimize symptom burden. Hospice care should be considered when the patient meets hospice admission criteria and when it is consistent with the patient's goals of care.

PRACTICE QUESTIONS

1. A patient who has chronic obstructive pulmonary disease (COPD) is given a handheld nebulizer treatment with albuterol. The patient then reports rapid heart rate, increased mental alertness, and insomnia. The nurse knows that the medication has stimulated the

    a. Sympathetic nervous systems

    b. Autonomic nervous system

    c. Parasympathetic nervous system

    d. Central nervous system

2. Which of the following symptoms, if noted in a patient who has amyotrophic lateral sclerosis, is most predictive of the onset of the terminal phase of the disease process?

   a. Dysphagia

   b. Slurred speech

   c. Paresis

   d. Respiratory distress

3. The most effective long-term strategy to combat respiratory distress in a 65-year-old patient who has amyotrophic lateral sclerosis is

   a. Incentive spirometry

   b. Repositioning

   c. Continuous supplemental oxygen

   d. Diaphragmatic pacer

4. A 48-year-old patient with a history of cardiac disease, type 2 diabetes, and hypertension tells the palliative care nurse that she has recently noticed hand tremors at rest and has a hard time initiating ambulation. The patient should be evaluated for

   a. Diabetic neuropathy

   b. Parkinson's disease

   c. Intermittent claudication

   d. Medication side effects

5. Which of the following medication changes would the nurse expect for the patient in the previous question?

   a. Increase insulin at bedtime

   b. Discontinue antihypertensive medication

   c. Start levodopa

   d. Initiate anticoagulant therapy

6. Which of the following is the priority diagnosis for a patient who has end-stage muscular dystrophy?

   a. Knowledge deficit

   b. Incontinence

   c. Impaired gas exchange

   d. Impaired swallowing

7. During a palliative visit, the mother of a patient who has muscular dystrophy tells the nurse that the patient has cardiomegaly. The nurse knows that

   a. This is common among patients who have muscular dystrophy

   b. The patient's condition is now considered terminal

    c. Opioids should be kept in the home to treat potential dyspnea

    d. A stool softener should be added to the daily medication regimen to prevent straining

8. The family of a 17-year-old patient who has muscular dystrophy requests that the patient's advance directive indicate that mechanical ventilation should not be initiated. The nurse should

    a. Contact child protective services

    b. Recommend a hospice consult

    c. Relay the information to the palliative care team

    d. Document the information in the patient's chart

9. A nurse is caring for a hospice patient who has myasthenia gravis. The nurse should teach the caregiver that if the patient experiences myasthenic crisis

    a. Mechanical ventilation will be required

    b. The advance directive should be followed

    c. The patient should be transferred to a hospice inpatient unit

    d. 10 mg of morphine should be given

10. A palliative care patient who has multiple sclerosis (MS) reports the loss of vision in one eye. The nurse knows

    a. The patient is experiencing a focal seizure, which is common in patients who have MS

    b. This is an emergency and indicates an impending stroke

    c. This is a sign of MS exacerbation

    d. The patient's blindness is related to the MS and is irreversible

▪ REFERENCES

American Academy of Ophthalmology. (2018). *Myasthenia gravis: Causes, symptoms, and risk.* Retrieved from https://www.aao.org/eye-health/diseases/myasthenia-gravis-causes-symptoms-risk

American Association of Neuromuscular & Electrodiagnostic Medicine. (2018). *Becker muscular dystrophy.* Retrieved from http://www.aanem.org/Patients/Disorders/Becker-Muscular-Dystrophy

Beeldman, E., Raaphorst, J., Twennaar, M. K., deVisser, M., Schmand, B. A., & deHaan, R.J. (2016). The cognitive profile of ALS: A systematic review and meta-analysis update. *Journal of Neurological and Neurosurgical Psychiatry, 87*(6), 611–619. doi:10.1136/jnnp-2015-310734

Birkrant, D. J., Bushby, K., Bann, C. M., Alman, B. A., Apkon, S. D., Blackwell, A., & Ward, L. M. (2018, January 23). Diagnosis and management of Duchenne muscular dystrophy, part 2: Respiratory, cardiac, bone health, and orthopaedic management. *Lancet Neurology, 17*(4), 347–361. doi:10.1016/S1474-4422(18)30025-5

Boss, B. J., & Huether, S. E. (2014a). Alterations in cognitive systems, cerebral hemodynamics, and motor function. In K. L. McCance & S. E. Huether (Eds.), *Pathophysiology: The biologic basis for disease in adults and children* (7th ed., pp. 527–580). St. Louis, MO: Elsevier.

Boss, B. J., & Huether, S. E. (2014b). Disorders of the central and peripheral nervous systems and the neuromuscular junction. In K. L. McCance & S. E. Huether (Eds.), *Pathophysiology: The biologic basis for disease in adults and children* (7th ed., pp. 581–640). St. Louis, MO: Elsevier.

Brooks, B. R., Miller, R. G., Swash, M., & Munsat, T. L., for the World Federation on Neurology Research Group in Motor Neuron Diseases (2000). El Escorial revisited: Revised criteria for the diagnosis of amyotrophic lateral sclerosis. *Journal of the Neurological Sciences, 124S*, 96–107. doi:10.1016/0022-510X(94)90191-0

Brownlee, W. J., Hardy, T. A., Fazekas, F., & Miller, D. H. (2017). Diagnosis of multiple sclerosis: Progress and challenges. *The Lancet, 389*, 1336–1346. doi:10.1016/S0140-6736(16)30959-X

Comi, G., Radaelli, M., & Sørensen, P. S. (2017). Evolving concepts in the treatment of relapsing multiple sclerosis. *The Lancet, 398*, 1347–1356. doi:10.1016/S0140-6736(16)32388-1

Connolly, S., Galvin, M., & Hardiman, O. (2015). End-of-life management in patients with amyotrophic lateral sclerosis. *Lancet Neurology, 14*, 435–442. doi:10.1016/S1474-4422(14)70221-2

de Boer, EM., Depla, M., Wojtkowiak, J., Visser, M. C., Widdershoven, G. A. M., Francke, A. L., . . . Hertough, C. M. P. M. (2015). Life-and-death decision-making in the acute phase after a severe stroke: Interviews with relatives. *Palliative Medicine, 29*(5), 451–457. doi:10.1177/0269216314563427

Gilhus, N. E., Nacu, A., Andersen, J. B., & Owe, J. F. (2014). Myasthenia gravis and risks for comorbidity. *European Journal of Neurology, 22*(1), 17–23. doi:10.1111/ene.12599

Gorman, L. M. (2015). The palliative advanced practice registered nurse in the specialty outpatient setting. In C. Dahlin, P. J. Coyne, & B. R. Ferrell (Eds.), *Advanced practice palliative nursing* (pp. 151–158). New York, NY: Oxford University Press.

Hwang, C. S., Weng, H. H., Wang, L. F., Tsai, C. H., & Chang, H. T. (2014). An eye-tracking assistive device improves the quality of life for ALS patients and reduces caregivers' burden. *Journal of Motor Behavior, 46*(4), 233–238. doi:10.1080/00222895.2014.891970

Iodice, F., Testa, G., Averardi, M., Brancaccio, G., Amodeo, A., & Cogo, P. (2015). Implantation of a left ventricular assist device as a destination therapy in Duchenne muscular dystrophy patients with end stage cardiac failure: Management and lessons learned. *Neuromuscular Disorders, 25*, 19–23. doi:10.1016/j.nmd.2014.08.008

Kalanithi, P. (2016). *When breath becomes air*. New York, NY: Random House.

Kovach, C. R., & Reynolds, S. (2015). Neurological disorders. In M. Matzo & D. W. Sherman (Eds.), *Palliative care nursing: Quality care to the end of life* (4th ed., pp. 347–371). New York, NY: Springer Publishing Company.

Martin, J. E., Raffel, J., & Nicholas, R. (2016). Progressive dwindling in multiple sclerosis: An opportunity to improve care. *PLOS ONE, 11*(7), e0159210. doi:10.1371/journal.pone.0159210

Mazzini, L., DeMarchi, F., Corrado, L., & D'Alfonso, D. (2017). Genetics of amyotrophic lateral sclerosis: More than twenty years of studies. *The EuroBiotech Journal, 1*(s2), 131–132. doi:10.24190/ISSN2564-615X/2017/S2.05

Myasthenia Gravis Foundation of America. (2018). *What is myasthenia gravis (MG)?* Retrieved from http://myasthenia.org/WhatisMG.aspx

National Institutes of Health. (2018). *Duchenne and Becker muscular dystrophy*. Retrieved from https://ghr.nlm.nih.gov/condition/duchenne-and-becker-muscular-dystrophy

Robertson, E. D. (2018). Treatment of central nervous system degenerative disorders. In L. L. Brunton, R. Hilal-Dandan, & B. C. Knollman (Eds.), *The pharmacological basis of therapeutics* (13th ed., pp. 227–338). New York, NY: McGraw Hill.

Schwartz, M. A. (2015). Neurological disorders. In B. R. Ferrell, N. Coyle, & J. A. Paice (Eds.), *Oxford textbook of palliative nursing* (4th ed., pp. 349–365). New York, NY: Oxford University Press.

Sugerman, R. A. (2014). Structure and function of the neurologic system. In K. L. McCance & S. E. Huether (Eds.), *Pathophysiology: The biologic basis for disease in adults and children* (7th ed., pp. 447–483). St. Louis, MO: Elsevier.

The ALS Association. (2018). *Symptoms and diagnosis*. Retrieved from http://www.alsa.org/about-als/symptoms.html

Urban, P. P., Jacobi, C., & Jander, S. (2018). Treatment standards and individualized therapy of myasthenia gravis. *Neurology International Open, 2*, E84–E92. doi:10.1055/s-0043-124983

van den Bergen, J. C., Wokke, B. H., Janson, A. A., van Duinen, G., Hulsker, M. A., Ginjaar, H. B., . . . Verschuuren, J. J. (2014). Dystrophin levels and clinical severity in Becker muscular dystrophy patients. *Journal of Neurology, Neurosurgery, and Psychiatry, 85*, 747–753. doi:10.1136/jnnp-2013-306350

Van Ruiten, H. J. A., Bettolo, C. M., Cheetham, T., Eagle, M., Lochmuller, H., Bushby, K., . . . Guglieri, M. (2016). Why are some patients with Duchenne muscular dystrophy dying young?: An analysis of causes of death in North East England. *Journal of European Paediatric Neurology, 20*, 904–909. doi:10.1016/j.ejpn.2016.07.020

Wendell, L. C., & Levine, J. M. (2011). Myasthenic crisis. *The Neurohospitalist, 1*(1), 16–22. doi:10.1177/1941875210382918

6 Cardiac Disorders

Laughter and tears are the signs of an open heart.
—Beattie (1996, p. 155)

LEARNING OBJECTIVES

After completing this section, the nurse will be able to

1. Identify symptoms of heart failure
2. Distinguish between left-sided and right-sided heart failure
3. Identify pharmacological and nonpharmacological interventions for treating symptoms associated with heart failure

END-STAGE CARDIAC DISEASE

Heart disease causes roughly 610,000 deaths in the United States each year. It is the leading cause of death for American men and women (Centers for Disease Control and Prevention, 2017). Chronic cardiac disease leads to heart failure, which affects roughly 10% of American seniors (Brashers, 2014). Heart failure is a "condition in which the heart is unable to generate adequate cardiac output" (Brashers, 2014, p. 1175). This underperformance of the cardiac muscle leads to inadequate perfusion of all organs and tissues. Heart failure can be categorized as left heart failure or right heart failure.

Left Heart Failure

Left heart failure is often referred to as congestive heart failure (CHF). Defining characteristics of CHF include the following:

- Decreased ejection fraction (EF)
- Fatigue with minimal exertion
- Fluid retention
- Decreased appetite

- Dyspnea
- Arrhythmias
- Paroxysmal nocturnal dyspnea
- Cyanosis
- Tachycardia
- Orthopnea
- Pulmonary hypertension
- Restlessness
- Respiratory symptoms such as
  - Crackles
  - Wheezing
  - Tachypnea
  - Hemoptysis
  - Persistent cough

Right Heart Failure

Right heart failure is also called right ventricular failure. Defining characteristics of right heart failure include the following:

- Jugular vein distention
- Fatigue
- Ascites
- Hepatomegaly
- Splenomegaly
- Dependent edema
- Anorexia
- Gastrointestinal distress
- Fluid retention

> **Key Point**
>
> The primary causative factors of heart failure are ischemic heart disease and hypertension. Other predisposing factors include older age, diabetes, obesity, renal dysfunction, and a history of other cardiac disorders (Brashers, 2014).

Diagnosing Heart Failure

One frequently used criteria for determining whether a patient has heart failure was developed in the Framingham Heart Study (Kalon, Pinsky, Kannel, & Levy, 1993). The criteria indicate that a diagnosis of heart failure requires that two of the minor criteria be present, as well as two of the major criteria.

> **Key Point**
>
> The most common cause of right heart failure is left heart failure.

The minor criteria are as follows:

- Bilateral ankle edema
- Nocturnal cough
- Dyspnea on ordinary exertion
- Hepatomegaly
- Pleural effusion
- Decrease in vital capacity by 33% from the maximal value recorded
- Tachycardia (heart rate of ≥120 beats per minute)

The major criteria are as follows:

- Paroxysmal nocturnal dyspnea
- Neck vein distention
- Rales
- Cardiomegaly
- Acute pulmonary edema
- Third heart sound gallop
- Increased central venous pressure
- Circulation time ≥25 seconds (no longer used clinically)
- Hepatojugular reflux (see Figure 6.1)
- Pulmonary edema, visceral congestion, or cardiomegaly on autopsy

Regardless of the number of minor or major criteria, weight loss of ≥4.5 kg (about 10 pounds) in 5 days in response to treatment of CHF is usually indicative of heart failure.

Once a patient is diagnosed with heart failure, the extent of the disease can be further defined in terms of severity. The New York Heart Association's (NYHA) classification system for heart failure (The Criteria Committee of the New York Heart Association, 1994) is frequently used to document the extent of the patient's disease and terminality (see Table 6.1).

The NYHA's criteria addresses both the functional status of the patient and objective findings of the provider. Consistent with the hospice admission criteria, all hospice patients must meet NYHA criteria for class IV heart failure. That is, they exhibit significant cardiac symptoms even at rest and the inability to carry out minimal activities without dyspnea or angina. Other supporting assessment data for hospice admission with a terminal diagnosis of heart disease include the following points 1 and 2. Point 3 is used for supportive documentation.

1. Patient is or has been optimally treated for heart disease, has declined surgical procedures, or is not a candidate for such procedures.

2. Patient meets criteria for the NYHA class IV

Assessing for hepatojugular reflux

BY RICHARD L. PULLEN, JR., RN, EdD

ASSESSING FOR the presence of hepatojugular reflux is commonly done to detect heart failure. With right-sided heart failure, abdominal compression increases venous return to the heart and may markedly increase jugular vein distension (JVD) and pressure.

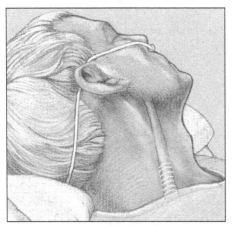

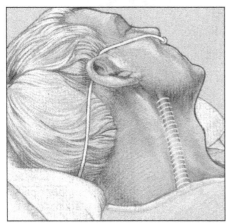

DO
• Explain the procedure to the patient and perform hand hygiene.
• Place him supine and elevate the head of his bed to 45 degrees. Stand at his right. Ask him to turn his head to the left and to breathe normally through his open mouth.

◀ Assess for distension of the internal and external jugular veins. Obvious bilateral distension when the head is elevated above 30 degrees indicates an abnormal increase in venous volume. Note the level of JVD for later comparison.

• With your right hand, apply firm pressure on your patient's midabdomen (at the periumbilical area) while assessing the highest point of oscillation in his right internal jugular vein.
• Continue applying firm pressure to his abdomen for 30 to 60 seconds. This moves venous blood from the liver sinusoids to the venous system. If the heart can pump this additional volume, the jugular veins will rise for a few seconds, then return to the previous level.

◀ If the patient has volume overload secondary to heart failure, jugular venous pressure rises and stays elevated for as long as you apply firm pressure. If the height of his neck veins increases by at least 3 cm throughout compression, he has positive hepatojugular reflux.

DON'T
• Don't let the patient hold his breath during the test.
• Don't perform the test if he exhibits abdominal guarding.
• Don't interpret a positive hepatojugular reflux as diagnostic of fluid overload unless it correlates with the patient's vital signs, breath and heart sounds, peripheral edema, and daily weights. ‹›

SELECTED REFERENCES
Dillon PM. *Nursing Health Assessment: A Critical Thinking, Case Studies Approach.* Philadelphia, Pa., F.A. Davis, 2003.
Jarvis C. *Physical Examination and Health Assessment,* 4th edition. St. Louis, Mo., W.B. Saunders Co., 2004.
Smeltzer SC, Bare BG. *Brunner & Suddarth's Textbook of Medical Surgical Nursing.* 10th edition. Philadelphia, Pa., Lippincott Williams & Wilkins, 2003.

Richard L. Pullen, Jr., is a professor of nursing at Amarillo (Tex.) College. Each month, *Clinical Do's & Don'ts* illustrates key clinical points for a common nursing procedure. Because of space constraints, it's not comprehensive.

FIGURE 6.1 Hepatojugular reflux.

Source: Pullen, R. I. (2006). Assessing for hepatojugular reflux. *Nursing2006, 36*(2), 28.

3. Significant CHF may be documented by an EF of ≤20%, but this documentation is not required if not already available

On assessment, objective signs of heart disease will be noted by the nurse.

Table 6.1 NYHA Classification of Functional Status

NYHA Class	Symptoms
I	Patients with heart disease but without limitation of physical activity
II	Patients with heart disease resulting in slight limitation of physical activity Comfortable at rest
III	Patients with heart disease resulting in marked limitation of physical activity. Comfortable at rest. Less than ordinary activity causes fatigue, dyspnea, palpitations, anginal pain.
IV	Patients with heart disease resulting in inability to carry out any physical activity without discomfort. Symptoms of cardiac insufficiency or of the anginal syndrome may be present even at rest. If any physical activity is undertaken, discomfort increases.

NYHA, New York Heart Association.
Source: Lammers, A. E., Adatia, I., del Cerro, M. J., Diaz, G., Freudenthal, A. H., Freudenthal, F., . . . Haworth, S. G. (2011). Functional classification of pulmonary hypertension in children: Report from the PVRI pediatric taskforce, Panama 2011. *Pulmonary Circulation, 1*(2), 280–285. doi:10.4103/2045-8932.83445

Cardiac Assessment

Inspection

- Assess overall skin color for pallor or rubor
- Inspect fingernails for clubbing and decreased capillary refill
- Assess neck veins for distension
- Assess for signs of cyanosis (lips, fingertips, lower extremities)
- Observe for dyspnea; note supplemental oxygen use

Auscultation

- Auscultate carotid artery for bruits
- Auscultate heart sounds (see Figure 6.2)
- Assess for abdominal bruit
- Measure blood pressure

Percussion

- Percussion of the heart is not usually necessary for hospice patients because most patients have had cardiac imaging
- Percussion of the liver may be indicated to assess for hepatomegaly
- Percussion of the abdomen indicates ascites if tympani is heard

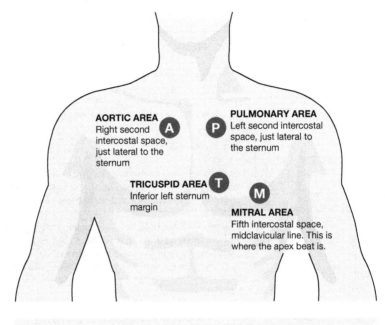

FIGURE 6.2 Heart auscultation.

Palpation

- Palpate peripheral pulses
- Determine point of maximal impulse (normally at the fifth intercostal space at the midclavicular line)
- Assess for hepatojugular reflux (if warranted)

End-Stage Heart Failure

Patients who have end-stage heart failure are debilitated and experience myriad symptoms such as dyspnea, rales, angina, murmurs, edema, ascites, constipation, orthopnea, nocturia, and paroxysmal nocturnal dyspnea and nocturnal cough. Often, the symptoms will be refractory despite traditional interventions. Therefore, the hospice nurse must be competent in taking a multimodal approach to the management of symptoms related to end-stage cardiac disease. Pharmacological interventions for patients who have heart failure can be found in Table 6.2. Nonpharmacological interventions to treat symptoms associated with heart failure may include the following:

- Using fans for overcoming feelings of breathlessness and dyspnea

> **Key Points**
>
> In adults, *systolic murmurs* are usually related to aortic stenosis or mitral valve regurgitation or mitral valve prolapse.
>
> *Diastolic murmurs* in adults are usually related to mitral valve stenosis or aortic regurgitation.

- Elevating lower extremities to combat edema
- Providing frequent skin care to reduce risk for skin breakdown related to poor circulation and edema
- Teaching energy conservation techniques to combat fatigue
- Arranging surroundings to provide easy access to food, drinks, medications, commode, and so on
- Elevating head when resting to provide relief from orthopnea
- Teaching meditation and relaxation exercises for anxiety
- Using supplemental oxygen as indicated
- Managing symptoms associated with comorbidities

Many patients who have a history of cardiac disease have had numerous medical interventions such as bypass surgeries, stent placement, and placement of internal pacemakers and/or automated implantable cardioverter defibrillators (AICDs). As the patient's final weeks and days approach, the AICD should be deactivated because "there is a significant risk that the patient will receive one or more shocks during the active dying process, which can be exceedingly disturbing to the patient, if she or he is aware, and to the family" (Kinzbrunner, 2011, p. 497). Therefore, even if the patient's terminal illness is not end-stage heart failure, the AICD should be deactivated prior to the patient's death.

To deactivate an AICD, a medical magnet can be placed over the AICD to prevent discharge. However, if the magnet is removed, the AICD will be reactivated. Therefore, the hospice agency should contact a professional who is trained in the deactivation of AICDs to arrange for the AICD to be permanently deactivated in the patient's home (National Hospice & Palliative Care Organization, 2008). The hospice nurse must ascertain the date the AICD was implanted, the manufacturer, and the model number in order to identify the correct method of deactivation (National Hospice & Palliative Care Organization, 2008). In many newer models of AICD/pacemaker devices, the pacemaker is magnetically shielded so that it can continue to work if the defibrillator is deactivated with a medical magnet. However, this might not be the case for older models (Kinzbrunner, 2011).

It is critical for the hospice nurse to determine whether the pacemaker is protected from magnetic deactivation because a pacemaker, unlike an AICD, should not be deactivated prior to the patient's death. Deactivation of a pacemaker can result in

> **Key Point**
>
> Deactivation of an AICD is not equivalent to physician-assisted suicide or euthanasia, and is unlikely to hasten a patient's death. It is the ethical equivalent of voluntarily withholding or withdrawing medical treatment (National Hospice & Palliative Care Organization, 2008).

Table 6.2 Pharmacological Interventions for Heart Failure

Category	Action	Examples
Aldosterone-blocking agents (also called aldosterone receptor antagonists or anti-mineralocorticoids)	Inhibit the sodium-retaining effects of aldosterone and increase the excretion of hydrogen and potassium, which leads to decreased blood pressure and a decrease in pericardial fluid	Eplerenone (Inspra) Spironolactone (Aldactone)
Anxiolytics	Prevent and treat anxiety, which is common in patients who have heart failure	Alprazolam (Xanax) Diazepam (Valium) Lorazepam (Ativan) Escitalopram (Lexapro)
ACE inhibitors	Reduce blood pressure by preventing the production of angiotensin, which constricts blood vessels. The overall effect is vasodilation (*Note:* these drugs all end with "pril")	Benazepril (Lotensin) Captopril Enalapril (Vasotec) Fosinopril Lisinopril (Prinivil, Zestril) Moexipril (Univasc) Perindopril (Aceon) Quinapril (Accupril) Ramipril (Altace) Trandolapril (Mavik)
ARBs	Block the vasoconstrictive effects of angiotensin II. They are used to treat hypertension and heart failure. They are also used in the prevention of renal disease in patients who have type 2 diabetes, and to prevent stroke (*Note:* These drugs end with "sartan")	Azilsartan (Edarbi) Candesartan (Atacand) Eprosartan (Teveten) Irbesartan (Avapro) Telmisartan (Micardis) Valsartan (Diovan) Losartan (Cozaar) Olmesartan (Benicar)
Antiarrhythmics	Prevent and treat abnormal cardiac impulses or abnormal conduction of impulses. There are four classes of antiarrhythmics, each with its own mechanism of action	*Class I:* Sodium channel blockers/blockage drugs (e.g., quinidine, lidocaine, propafenone) *Class II:* Beta-blockers (e.g., atenolol, metoprolol, propranolol, carvedilol) *Class III:* Potassium channel blockers (e.g., sotalol, amiodarone) *Class IV:* Calcium channel blockers (e.g., amlodipine, dilitiazem, verapamil)

(*continued*)

Table 6.2 Pharmacological Interventions for Heart Failure *(continued)*

Category	Action	Examples
Cardiac glycosides	Increase cardiac output and decrease heart rate, and ultimately improve ejection fraction by inhibiting sodium/potassium ATPase	Digoxin (Lanoxin) Digitoxin
Diuretics	Decrease cardiac workload by increasing water excretion. Loop diuretics act on the loop of Henle to decrease sodium and water reabsorption	Bumetanide (Bumex, Burinex) Furosemide (Lasix) Torsemide (Demadex)
Nitrates	Treat or prevent angina. Nitrates reduce vascular resistance, decrease left ventricular filling pressure, and increase cardiac output	Nitroglycerin (Nitrostat, Nitromist, Nitro-Bid) Isosorbide mononitrate or dinitrate (Isordil, Dilatrate-SR)
PDE-5 inhibitors	Inhibit the action of PDE-5, thus promoting pulmonary vessel dilation. They are used to treat pulmonary hypertension	Sildenafil (Viagra, Revatio) Tadalafil (Adcirca)
Statins	Prevent and treat atherosclerotic disease. They inhibit HMG-CoA reductase, which ultimately leads to a decreased cholesterol synthesis in the liver	Atorvastatin (Lipitor) Fluvastatin (Lescol) Lovastatin (Mevacor, Altocor) Pravastatin (Pravachol) Simvastatin (Zocor) Rosuvastatin (Crestor)

ACE, angiotensin-converting enzyme; ARBs, angiotensin II receptor blockers; HMG-CoA, ß-Hydroxy ß-methylglutaryl-CoA; PDE-5, phosphodiesterase 5.

immediate symptoms related to cardiac disease such as fatigue, dizziness, syncope, dyspnea, and bradycardia (Kinzbrunner, 2011).

▪ CONCLUSION

In hospice settings, the nurse works with patients who suffer acute cardiac events as well as the sequelae of chronic cardiac disease. Patients who are terminally ill due to end-stage heart failure often follow a trajectory of decline that includes exacerbations of heart failure manifested by dyspnea, angina, and edema. Management of the acute symptoms brings relief, but over time symptoms may become refractory, requiring a multifaceted approach to care. A hospice plan of care necessitates a team approach to address physical, spiritual, and psychological needs of the patient and family.

Chapter Summary

- Heart disease is the leading cause of death in the United States.
- Heart failure leads to low perfusion, which can have a negative effect on all body systems and organs.
- The primary causes of heart failure are ischemic heart disease and hypertension.
- Key characteristics of left-sided heart failure are decreased EF, fatigue with minimal exertion, tachycardia, orthopnea, and respiratory symptoms. Key characteristics of right-sided heart failure include jugular vein distention, ascites, and dependent edema. The most common cause of right-sided heart failure is left-sided heart failure.
- Key signs of heart failure include third heart sound gallop, hepatojugular reflux, pulmonary edema, cardiomegaly, lower extremity edema, nocturnal cough, and dyspnea on ordinary exertion.
- The NYHA's criteria for classification of heart failure is frequently used to document the extent of heart failure and the prognosis.
- Both pharmacological and nonpharmacological interventions should be used to relieve symptoms associated with heart failure.
- In the final stages of heart failure, the patient and family should consider deactivation of an internal defibrillator, if present. Pacemakers should not be deactivated.

■ PRACTICE QUESTIONS

1. A 70-year-old patient is admitted to hospice with a diagnosis of end-stage heart failure. Which of the following is not an expected finding?

    a. Jugular vein distension

    b. Oliguria

    c. Dependent edema

    d. Tachycardia

2. A patient who has heart failure is at risk for multisystem organ failure because heart failure causes

    a. Hypertension

    b. Edema

    c. Poor perfusion

    d. Pulmonary edema

3. An 80-year-old patient is seen for a hospice consult. She has a long history of ischemic heart disease, hypertension, cardiac bypass surgery, and an ejection fraction of 19%. She also has a history of breast cancer with left mastectomy (12 years ago) and was recently diagnosed with dementia. The patient's appetite is poor and she is dyspneic with minimal exertion. This patient meets hospice admission criteria for which of the following diagnoses?

a. Dementia

b. Debility

c. Cancer

d. Heart failure

4. On assessment, a patient is noted to have +3 lower extremity edema, ascites, and jugular vein distention. The most likely cause of these symptoms is

a. Recent myocardial infarction

b. Left-sided heart failure

c. Pulmonary hypertension

d. Right-sided heart failure

5. Patients admitted to hospice with a terminal diagnosis of heart failure are in which of the New York Heart Association's classes of heart failure?

a. I

b. II

c. III

d. IV

6. Patients who have marked limitation of activity due to cardiac disease, along with fatigue and dyspnea with less than ordinary exertion, meet the criteria for which of the New York Heart Association's classes of heart failure?

a. I

b. II

c. III

d. IV

7. The family member of a patient who is actively dying asks the hospice nurse if the patient's pacemaker should be deactivated. The nurse's best response is

a. "No. Deactivating the pacemaker will cause distressing symptoms."

b. "No. The pacemaker must be deactivated only if the device is a combination pacemaker/defibrillator."

c. "Only if the device was implanted prior to 1989."

d. "Yes, it should be deactivated with a medical magnet."

8. A patient with end-stage heart failure is taking sildenafil (Viagra) daily. The purpose of the drug for patients with heart failure is to

a. Decrease pulmonary hypertension

b. Correct arrhythmias

    c. Treat erectile dysfunction

    d. Treat angina

9. A 65-year-old patient who has heart failure tells the nurse in an inpatient hospice setting that he has difficulty breathing when lying flat in bed. What should the nurse do first?

    a. Explain that orthopnea is a very common symptom in heart failure patients

    b. Administer morphine for dyspnea

    c. Raise the head of the bed

    d. Check the patient's pulse oximetry

10. A patient who has heart failure is seen at home by the hospice nurse. The patient is experiencing new-onset, persistent cough and fatigue. These symptoms are most likely related to

    a. Pneumonia

    b. Heart failure

    c. Pulmonary hypertension

    d. Mitral valve regurgitation

■ REFERENCES

Beattie, M. (1996). *Journey to the heart*. New York, NY: Harper Collins.

Brashers, V. L. (2014). Alterations in cardiac function. In K. McCance, S. E. Huether, V. L. Brashers, & N. S. Rote (Eds.), *Pathophysiology: The biologic basis for diseases in adults and children* (7th ed., pp. 1129–1182). St. Louis, MO: Elsevier Mosby.

Centers for Disease Control and Prevention. (2017). *Heart disease in the United States*. Retrieved from https://www.cdc.gov/heartdisease/facts.htm

The Criteria Committee of the New York Heart Association. (1994). Functional capacity and objective assessment. In M. Dolgin (Ed.), *Nomenclature and criteria for diagnosis of the heart and great vessels*. Boston, MA: Little, Brown and Company.

Kalon, K. L., Pinsky, J. L., Kannel, W., & Levy, D. (1993). The epidemiology of heart failure: The Framingham Study. *Journal of the American College of Cardiology, 22*(Suppl. AJ), 6A–13A. Retrieved from http://www.onlinejacc.org/content/accj/22/4_Supplement_1/A6.full.pdf

Kinzbrunner, B. M. (2011). Invasive cardiac interventions. In B. M. Kinzbrunner & J. S. Policzer (Eds.), *End-of-life care: A practical guide* (pp. 495–505). New York, NY: McGraw Hill Medical.

Lammers, A. E., Adatia, I., del Cerro, M. J., Diaz, G., Freudenthal, A. H., Freudenthal, F., . . . Haworth, S. G. (2011). Functional classification of pulmonary hypertension in children: Report from the PVRI pediatric taskforce, Panama 2011. *Pulmonary Circulation, 1*(2), 280–285. doi:10.4103/2045-8932.83445

National Hospice & Palliative Care Organization. (2008). *Position statement on the care of hospice patients with automatic implantable cardioverter-defibrillators*. Retrieved from https://www.nhpco.org/sites/default/files/public/NHPCO_ICD_position_statement_May08.pdf

7 Pulmonary Disorders

Remember to breathe . . . It is after all, the secret of life.
—Maguire (2008, p. 12)

LEARNING OBJECTIVES

After completing this section, the nurse will be able to

1. Identify key symptoms associated with chronic obstructive pulmonary disease (COPD)
2. Determine the factors that increase risk of COPD exacerbation
3. Explain the hospice admission criteria for pulmonary disease

CHRONIC PULMONARY DISEASE

The most common end-stage pulmonary disease seen in hospice settings, after lung cancer, is chronic obstructive pulmonary disease (COPD; National Hospice and Palliative Care Organization, 2016). COPD is a preventable disease that involves chronic inhibition of airflow due to airway or alveolar abnormalities. COPD involves narrowing of the airways in the lungs due to chronic inflammation as well as diminishment of the alveoli to properly participate in air exchange (GOLD Science Committee, 2017).

COPD involves both emphysema and chronic bronchitis. Emphysema results from destruction of the gas-exchanging surfaces of the lung (alveoli). Chronic bronchitis is defined as "chronic cough and sputum production for at least 3 months in each of 2 consecutive years" (GOLD Science Committee, 2017, p. 6). Thus, COPD causes dyspnea due to a combination of restricted airways, decreased compliance of alveoli, and air trapping (see Figures 7.1 and 7.2).

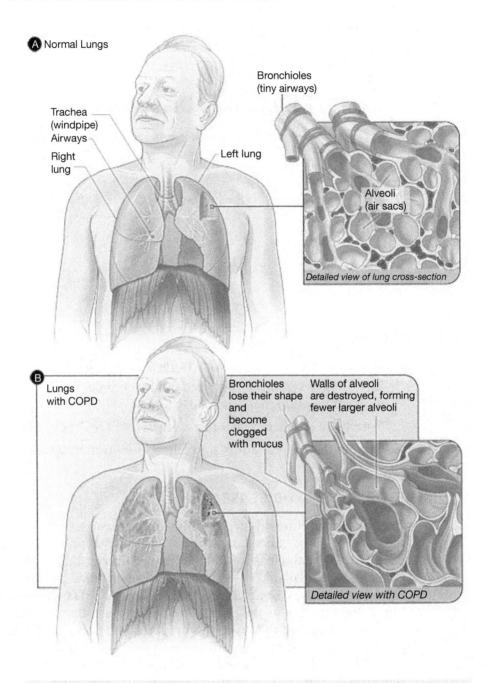

FIGURE 7.1 Effects of COPD.

COPD, chronic obstructive pulmonary disease.
Source: Kozak, K. (2017). The Body Show: COPD. Retrieved from http://hawaiipublicradio.org/post/body-show-copd-0

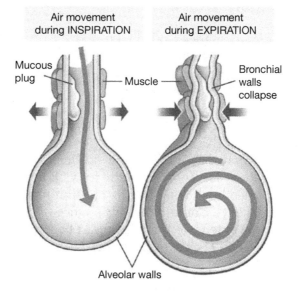

Air movement during INSPIRATION

Air movement during EXPIRATION

Mucous plug

Muscle

Bronchial walls collapse

Alveolar walls

FIGURE 7.2 Air trapping.

Source: Air trapping. (2013). *Mosby's medical dictionary* (9th ed.). St. Louis, MO: Mosby Elsevier. Used with permission from Mosby.

COPD is primarily caused by long-term exposure to air pollutants such as tobacco smoke or other pollutants that damage lung tissue. In the United States, nearly 15.7 million people have COPD. Risk factors for COPD include the following:

- Current or former smoker
- History of asthma
- Age ≥65 years
- American Indian/Alaska Native and multiracial non-Hispanic heritage
- Female gender
- Less than a high school education
- Unemployment
- Being divorced, widowed, or separated from spouse

  (Centers for Disease Control and Prevention, 2017)

Diagnosing of COPD

A definitive diagnosis of COPD can be made only with spirometry. Spirometry reveals the average forced expiratory volume over 1 second (FEV_1) as well as the forced vital capacity (FVC). The normal FEV_1/FVC ratio is

> **Key Point**
>
> In the United States, smoking is a key factor in the development and progression of COPD (Centers for Disease Control and Prevention, 2017).

approximately 70% to 85% and declines with age due to decreasing lung elasticity. Diagnostic criteria for COPD indicate the diagnosis can be confirmed by the presence of a postbronchodilator FEV_1/FVC <0.70 (GOLD Science Committee, 2017). Once COPD is diagnosed and confirmed, the extent of the disease can be determined using the criteria from the GOLD Science Committee (2017).

GOLD Stage 1 (Mild): FEV_1 is 80% normal predicted range
GOLD Stage 2 (Moderate): FEV_1 is 50% to 80% of normal predicted range
GOLD Stage 3 (Severe): FEV_1 is 30% to 50% of normal predicted range
GOLD Stage 4 (Very Severe): FEV_1 is less than 30% of the normal predicted range

Because stage level and symptomatology do not always align, it is important to assess and document the patient's symptoms regularly. Patients who have COPD, particularly end-stage COPD exhibit a host of symptoms such as

- Increased sputum production
- Dyspnea
- Debility due to dyspnea
- Weight loss, due to increased metabolic demands
- Fatigue, due to decreased oxygenation
- Anxiety and depression
- Syncope during coughing
- Rib fractures related to coughing (primarily in frail patients)
- Cor pulmonale (denoted by ankle edema)

Assessment of key symptoms should be monitored using valid and reliable tools. Over time, decreasing scores on the assessment measures helps to guide clinical interventions aimed at alleviating symptoms and also provides objective support for ongoing hospice care. Some commonly used tools to measure dyspnea include the following:

- Modified British Medical Council (mMRC) dyspnea scale (Fletcher, 1960)

- Baseline Dyspnea Index (BDI) (Mahler, Weinberg, Wells, & Feinstein, 1984).
- Transitional Dyspnea Index (TDI) (Mahler et al., 1984)
- Modified Borg Scale (Mahler & Horowitz, 1994)

Clinical assessment tools can also be used to assess a patient's risk for exacerbation of COPD symptoms. For patients with end-stage COPD, exacerbations can have serious consequences, particularly for patients with multiple comorbidities. Thus, risk for exacerbation should be carefully monitored and the patient's symptoms should be promptly addressed to ensure comfort within the limits of the disease process. Signs of elevated risk for exacerbation include the following (GOLD Science Committee, 2017):

- Higher than normal blood eosinophil count
- Presence of comorbidities
- Advancing spirometric grade (GOLD stage)
- Low arterial blood gas

Treating and Managing COPD

Smoking Cessation

All patients who have COPD should receive education about smoking cessation. Although COPD is incurable, smoking cessation reduces the risk of exacerbation of COPD symptoms. It also reduces the risk of fire due to dropped cigarettes or combustion with supplemental oxygen. Family members should also receive education on reducing the risk of exacerbations of COPD for the patient. The Agency for Healthcare Research and Quality (2012) advises all healthcare professionals to follow the five As to identify appropriate interventions for smokers. These are

Ask: Identify and document patient's tobacco use at every visit

Advise: Strongly encourage every tobacco user to quit

Assess: Determine whether the patient is willing to attempt to quit

Assist: If the patient is willing to attempt to quit, coordinate smoking cessation counseling and pharmacotherapeutic interventions, as necessary

Arrange: Schedule a follow-up visit or phone call within a week of the quit date to assess progress and provide support

Smoking cessation interventions should be carefully coordinated with the patient's primary care provider. Some smokers substitute e-cigarettes for cigarettes as a smoking cessation method, but the safety and efficacy of this substitution has not been established and should not be recommended. Several pharmacological interventions such as varenicline, bupropion, and nortriptyline have been shown to be effective components of a smoking cessation program. These pharmacological interventions can be initiated for patients who are addicted to nicotine but no longer have access to tobacco, such as during hospital stays, upon transfer to a hospice inpatient unit or upon admission to a long-term care facility.

Vaccines

Patients who have COPD should receive the annual influenza vaccine and the pneumococcal vaccine (PPSV23), as these reduce the risk of exacerbation of COPD as well as mortality (GOLD Science Committee, 2017).

Pharmacological Interventions

Patients who have stable COPD can be treated with a variety of medications to improve gas exchange, ease the work of breathing, and reduce the risk of COPD exacerbation. Several medications are also available to treat exacerbations of COPD. These medications are summarized in Table 7.1. For patients experiencing acute dyspnea, short-acting bronchodilators should be used to rapidly ease symptoms. When symptoms are refractory or severe, opioids should be initiated for dyspnea.

Nonpharmacological Interventions

In addition to pharmacological interventions, hospice nurses may implement nondrug interventions that alleviate symptoms of COPD. Some of these interventions include:

> **Key Point**
>
> Types of noninvasive positive-pressure ventilation devices include intermittent positive-pressure ventilator (IPPV), continuous positive-pressure airway device (CPAP), and bi-level positive airway pressure machines (Bi-PAP). These devices may be used in the home and are usually managed by the patient or a family member.

- Careful assessment of dyspnea (using a valid and reliable tool)
- Determination of factors that worsen or improve dyspnea
- Assessment of signs of poor perfusion such as cyanosis
- Repositioning
- Use of fans (or moving air)
- Meditation or relaxation techniques
- Aromatherapy
- Use of energy conservation techniques
- Chest physiotherapy

Table 7.1 Pharmacological Interventions for COPD

Types of Medications

Bronchodilators: Used to improve expiratory flow by widening airways. There are three types of bronchodilators:

1. *Beta-2 agonists:* Relax smooth muscle within the lungs to decrease bronchoconstriction. There are two types of beta-2 agonists, long acting and short acting. These drugs usually end in "terol."
   - LABAs are used as maintenance therapy to manage chronic disease. They are usually administered every 12 hours. *Examples:* formoterol, salmeterol, olodaterol.
   - SABAs are used to treat acute exacerbations of respiratory disease. They are usually administered every 4 to 6 hours as needed. *Examples:* fenoterol, levalbuterol, albuterol.
   - *Note:* Caution is warranted when using beta-2 agonists for patients who have concomitant cardiac disease. These medications can cause sinus tachycardia and other dysrhythmias. Other adverse effects include tremor, hypokalemia, and increased oxygen consumption.

2. *Anticholinergics, also called antimuscarinics:* Block M3 receptors. M3 receptors are found in various areas of the body and are responsible for, among other things, contraction of smooth muscle. When administered for bronchoconstriction, anticholinergics block the action of the M3 receptors, thereby causing the relaxation of smooth muscle around the airways, leading to bronchodilation. These medications are not specific to the M3 receptors around the airways; therefore, patients may experience other anticholinergic effects such as
   - Dry mouth
   - Constipation
   - Increased body temperature and sweating
   - Confusion or delirium
   - Tachycardia and flushing

   Anticholinergics (antimuscarinics) may be long acting (12–24 hours, depending on the drug) or short acting (6–9 hours, depending on the drug).

   > *Examples* of LAMA: glycopyrronium bromide, tiotropium, aclidinium bromide.
   > *Examples* of SAMA: ipratropium bromide, oxitropium bromide.

3. *Methylxanthines:* Enhance respiratory muscle function. These medications have a narrow therapeutic ratio, so blood levels must be monitored. Dosages must be lowered for older adults because drug clearance decreases with age. Drug interactions are numerous; the patient's drug profile must be carefully evaluated prior to initiation of methylxanthines. Potential adverse effects include the following:
   - Arrhythmias
   - Headaches
   - Nausea
   - Seizures
   Example: theophylline

Inhaled Corticosteroids: Used to decrease inflammation in the airways. ICSs are most effective for the management of COPD when combined with a LABA. Adverse effects include the following:
- Thrush
- Vocal changes
- Higher risk of pneumonia and TB (in patients with COPD)

(continued)

Table 7.1 Pharmacological Interventions for COPD *(continued)*

- Increased blood glucose
- Decreased bone density
- Development and/or thickening of subcapsular cataracts

Examples: beclomethasone dipropionate, budesonide, fluticasone, mometasone

Combination inhaled therapy: Include two or three medications given simultaneously. Combination medications promote medication compliance because they reduce the number of different medications a patient takes during the day. They also deliver a combination of medications that help to reduce the risk of COPD exacerbation.
- *Double inhaled therapy:* These medications are commonly a combination of a LABA and an ICS.

  Examples: budesonide/formoterol (Symbicort) and fluticasone/salmeterol (Advair)

- *Triple inhaled therapy:* These medications include a LABA, a LAMA, and an ICS. This combination of medications helps to improve overall lung function; however, demonstrable advantages of the three-drug combination over the two-drug combination will require further research.

  Example: fluticasone furoate/ umeclidinium/vilanterol

Oral glucocorticoids: Used to rapidly decrease inflammation during an acute exacerbation. They are not used in the long-term management of stable COPD. However, patients who have multiple exacerbations may take oral glucocorticoids repeatedly to manage their symptoms.

Examples: methylprednisolone, prednisolone, prednisone

Antibiotics: Used to decrease the risk of COPD exacerbation due to respiratory infection. Antibiotics may also be useful in managing acute exacerbations. Most commonly, aminoglycoside antibiotics are used. Adverse effects of aminoglycosides include the following:
- Nausea
- Vomiting
- Dizziness
- Seizures
- Dizziness
- Lethargy
- Muscle twitching or weakness
- Hearing loss due to ototoxicity (may be permanent)
- Hepatotoxicity

Examples: azithromycin, erythromycin

Phosphodiesterase-4 inhibitors: Reduce inflammation by inhibiting the effects of PDE4 on intracellular cAMP levels. PDE4 is responsible for breaking down cAMP. cAMP is responsible for activating PKA. PKA has a role in decreasing inflammation. Therefore, inhibiting PDE4 leads to an increase in cAMP, which then leads to an increase in PKA, which then decreases inflammation. Adverse effects of PDE4 inhibitors include the following:
- Nausea
- Vomiting
- Diarrhea

(continued)

Table 7.1 Pharmacological Interventions for COPD (*continued*)
• Headaches
• Neck pain
• Dizziness
• Anorexia
• Suicidality
• Atrial fibrillation
• Renal failure
Example: roflumilast

cAMP, cyclic adenosine monophosphate; COPD, chronic obstructive pulmonary disease; LABAs, long-acting beta-2 agonists; LAMAs, long-acting antimuscarinics; ICS, inhaled corticosteroids; M3 receptors, muscarinic acetylcholine receptors; PDE4, phosphodiesterase-4; PKA, protein kinase A; SABAs, short-acting beta-2 agonists; SAMAs, short-acting antimuscarinics, TB, tuberculosis.

End-of-Life Considerations

When patients who have respiratory disease are facing the end of life, symptoms must be identified and managed promptly to decrease feelings of breathlessness, which can lead to anxiety and panic. An advance directive should be discussed early in the disease process to determine the types of interventions the patient would want when the disease becomes very advanced. Depending on a patient's condition and wishes, mechanical ventilation may be an option as it can improve the patient's quality of life and maximize longevity.

Mechanical ventilation is an invasive form of respiratory support. It is not usually initiated for hospice patients, but some patients may already be using mechanical ventilation at the time of hospice admission. In such instances, a discussion regarding continuation or discontinuation of mechanical ventilation will become necessary as the pulmonary disease progresses.

When a patient or family chooses to discontinue mechanical ventilation, the primary goal is ensuring that the patient is not in distress during or after the procedure. Discontinuation of mechanical ventilation requires careful planning and family preparation. For patients in acute care settings, a decision will need to be made regarding whether the patient can or should be transferred home prior to the discontinuation of the mechanical ventilation.

If and when mechanical ventilation is discontinued, the hospice or palliative team should arrange the patient's environment so that the setting is as peaceful as possible. Unnecessary medical devices, particularly those with alarms, should be turned off. Necessary monitoring can take place outside of the room or monitors can be silenced and placed outside of the family's view so that they can be fully present with the patient.

Family and friends who wish to be present should be given time to arrive and should be fully educated on what to expect when the mechanical ventilation is discontinued (Negron & McInnis, 2011). Importantly, family members should be made aware that discontinuation of the mechanical ventilation may not immediately lead to the patient's death. In some cases, patients may continue to breathe on their own for hours or days. To support the family through the process, members of the hospice interdisciplinary team should be present if the family agrees.

The dying process for patients who have an end-stage pulmonary diagnosis usually involves tachypnea or bradypnea, changes in the depth of respirations, audible respirations, and the use of accessory muscles (Birkholz & Haney, 2018). End-of-life care through hospice may be arranged when it is consistent with the patient's goals of care and the patient meets admission criteria. The criteria used for determining hospice eligibility for patients with pulmonary disease include the following:

- Disabling dyspnea at rest
- Symptoms that are refractory to bronchodilators
- Decreased ability to perform activities of daily living (ADLs) due to disease
  and
  - Documented disease progression evidenced by increased need for medical office, urgent care, or emergency care visits and/or hospitalization
    and
    - Documentation of the following within the past 3 months:
      - pO_2 of <55 mmHg by ABG or O_2 sat $<88\%$ or pCO_2 >50 mmHg

Other supporting documentation may include diagnosis of cor pulmonale and right-sided heart failure, unintentional and progressive weight loss, and decreasing functional status (e.g., decreasing PPS or Karnofsky scores).

■ CONCLUSION

Patients who have end-stage pulmonary disease have a lengthy disease trajectory punctuated by periods of exacerbation and a return to a lower level of functioning following the exacerbation. Careful advance

> **Key Point**
>
> Guidelines for the discontinuation of mechanical ventilation in the acute care setting are available from the American College of Chest Physicians (CHEST) and the American Thoracic Society (ATS).

care planning should take place early in the disease process. Furthermore, excellent symptom management is required to treat symptoms as they arise to ensure the patient's comfort. In the later stages of the disease process, decisions about invasive interventions and the appropriateness of hospice care should be discussed by the patient, the family, and the hospice and/or palliative care team.

Chapter Summary

- The most common end-stage pulmonary disease seen in hospice settings, after lung cancer, is COPD.
- The main risk factor for COPD is smoking or other air pollutants.
- COPD is most common among those age 65 or older.
- COPD is diagnosed using spirometry.
- The GOLD Science Committee Criteria is used to stage COPD.
- Symptoms of COPD include productive cough, dyspnea, debility, weight loss, anxiety, and/or depression.
- Smoking cessation should be addressed with every patient who has COPD.
- Patients who have COPD should receive annual vaccinations to help prevent exacerbations of COPD.
- Both pharmacological and nonpharmacological interventions should be used to manage symptoms of COPD.
- An advanced care plan should be discussed early in the disease process.
- Hospice care should be discussed with the patient and family when it is consistent with the patient's goals.
- Patients who have end-stage pulmonary disease have a lengthy disease trajectory punctuated by periods of exacerbation and a return to a lower level of functioning following the exacerbation.

▨ PRACTICE QUESTIONS

1. The most common end-stage pulmonary disease seen in hospice settings is
   a. Lung cancer
   b. Chronic obstructive pulmonary disease (COPD)
   c. Cystic fibrosis
   d. Tuberculosis

2. Dyspnea caused by chronic obstructive pulmonary disease (COPD) is partially resultant from
   a. Severe mucous production
   b. Thrombosis
   c. Decreased alveolar compliance
   d. Left-sided heart failure

3. A risk factor for chronic obstructive pulmonary disease (COPD) is
   a. Age ≤65 years
   b. Asthma

    c. Advanced education

    d. Male gender

4. A palliative care patient has a forced expiratory volume over 1 second (FEV_1)/forced vital capacity (FVC) ratio of .65. This ratio is confirmatory for

    a. Asthma

    b. Bronchitis

    c. Chronic obstructive pulmonary disease (COPD)

    d. Emphysema

5. Weight loss in patients who have chronic obstructive pulmonary disease (COPD) is primarily related to

    a. Early satiety

    b. Nausea

    c. Dysphagia

    d. Increased metabolic demands

6. A frail, elderly hospice patient who has chronic obstructive pulmonary disease (COPD) is cared for at home by multiple caregivers. The patient reports new onset rib pain. The hospice nurse is aware that forcible coughing may cause rib pain and fractures in frail patients but should also assess for

    a. Hypocalcemia

    b. Delirium

    c. Hypoxia

    d. Abuse

7. A hospice nurse makes a home visit to a patient who has end-stage pulmonary disease. After determining that the patient is a smoker, the nurse should

    a. Assess for hypoxia

    b. Ask if anyone else in the home uses tobacco

    c. Strongly encourage the patient to quit smoking

    d. Teach the patient oxygen safety techniques

8. A patient who has end-stage chronic obstructive pulmonary disease (COPD) calls the hospice nurse to report increased dyspnea and increasing anxiety. After reviewing the patient's medications, the nurse recommends that the patient take which of the following now?

    a. Salmeterol

    b. Prednisone

    c. Alprazolam

    d. Albuterol

9. A palliative care nurse organizes a family meeting to discuss mechanical ventilation for a patient who has end-stage pulmonary disease. The primary consideration is the patient's

   a. Goals of care

   b. Eosinophil levels

   c. Carbon dioxide levels

   d. Religious beliefs

10. A patient is experiencing dyspnea that is refractory to bronchodilators. Which of the following should be initiated?

    a. Oxygen

    b. Opioids

    c. Anxiolytics

    d. Steroids

▪ REFERENCES

Agency for Healthcare Research and Quality. (2012). *Five major steps to intervention (The "5A's")*. Retrieved from https://www.ahrq.gov/professionals/clinicians-providers/guidelines-recommendations/tobacco/5steps.html

Birkholz, L., & Haney, T. (2018). Using a dyspnea assessment tool to improve care at the end of life. *Journal of Hospice & Palliative Care, 20*(3), 219–227. doi:10.1097/NJH.0000000000000432

Centers for Disease Control and Prevention. (2017). *Chronic obstructive pulmonary disease (COPD)*. Retrieved from https://www.cdc.gov/copd/index.html

Fletcher, C. M. (1960). Standardised questionnaire on respiratory symptoms: A statement prepared and approved by the MRC Committee on the Aetiology of Chronic Bronchitis (MRC breathlessness score). *BMJ, 2*, 1662.

GOLD Science Committee. (2017). *Global strategy for the diagnosis, management and prevention of COPD, global initiative for chronic obstructive lung disease (GOLD)*. Retrieved from http://goldcopd.org

Maguire, G. (2008). *A lion among men*. New York, NY: Harper Collins Press.

Mahler, D. A., & Horowitz, M. B. (1994). Perception of breathlessness during exercise in patients with respiratory disease. *Medicine & Science in Sports & Exercise, 26*, 1078–1081. doi:10.1249/00005768-199409000-00002

Mahler, D. A., Weinberg, D. H., Wells, C. K., & Feinstein, A. R. (1984). The measurement of dyspnea: Contents, inter-observer agreement, and physiologic correlates of two new clinical indexes. *Chest, 85*, 751–758. doi:10.1378/chest.85.6.751

Mosby. (2013). *Mosby's medical dictionary* (9th ed.). St. Louis, MO: Mosby Elsevier.

National Hospice and Palliative Care Organization. (2016). *Proposed FY 2017 hospice wage index and payment rate update and hospice quality reporting requirements*. Retrieved from https://www.nhpco.org/sites/default/files/public/regulatory/FY2017_Proposed_Wage-Index_Alert_042516.pdf

Negron, F. J., & McInnis, E. A. (2011). Dyspnea and other respiratory symptoms. In B. M. Kinzbrunner & J. S. Policzer (Eds.), *End-of-life care: A practical guide* (pp. 191–210). New York, NY: McGraw-Hill.

8

Renal Disorders

*Superficially, it might be said that the function of the kidneys is to
make urine; but in a more considered view one can say that the
kidneys make the stuff of philosophy itself.*
—Smith (1953, p. 3).

■ LEARNING OBJECTIVES

After completing this section, the nurse will be able to

1. Differentiate between acute and chronic renal disease
2. Explain the sequelae of chronic renal disease
3. Identify hospice admission criteria for chronic renal disease

■ KIDNEY DISEASE

The renal system maintains internal homeostasis, which is necessary for
metabolism. The kidneys maintain fluid balance, excrete waste products, conserve nutrients, ensure acid–base balance, help regulate glucose levels, and play a role in hormone secretion, which is key to blood
pressure regulation (Doig & Huether, 2014). Acute kidney injury (AKI)
can manifest in multiple ways, depending on the type and extent of the
damage to the renal system, but often includes oliguria, edema, nausea,
fatigue, and shortness of breath. AKI can be a consequence of medication toxicity, infection, obstruction of the urinary system, or metabolic
diseases. AKI is often reversible once the cause is identified, although
hemodialysis (HD) may be necessary for a short period of time. AKI is
characterized by the sudden (hours to days) onset of complete lack of
kidney function.

Conversely, chronic kidney disease (CKD) has a protracted onset and
results from chronic disease such as hypertension, diabetes, lupus, or
vascular disorders. It can also result from intrinsic kidney disease or

from the progression of renal injury, nephrolithiasis, chronic nephritis, or glomerulonephritis. Common signs of CKD include the following:

- Lethargy
- Seizures
- Mental status changes
- Epistaxis
- Anemia
- Pruritus
- Dyspnea
- Amenorrhea
- Impotence
- Infertility
- Myopathies
- Neuropathies
- Edema
- Hypertension
- Heart failure
- Bone pain
- Conjunctivitis

Symptoms associated with CKD may be also be associated with other health issues; therefore, it is important to carefully rule out other root causes.

Diagnosing CKD

Within the kidneys, the glomerular capillaries filter waste products from the blood. The glomeruli filter approximately 180 L/d, or roughly 120 mL/min. The rate at which the glomeruli are able to fil-

> **Key Point**
>
> Glomerular filtration rate (GFR) calculators are available online from the National Kidney Foundation (see www.kidney.org/professionals/kdoqi/gfr_calculator).

ter out waste is determined largely by the perfusion pressure in the glomerular capillaries. The filtration rate over a period of time is called the GFR (Doig & Huether, 2014). The GFR is calculated based on other measures, including the patient's serum creatinine, serum cysteine-C, age, gender, and race. The lower the patient's GFR, the lower the functionality of the kidneys (Figure 8.1).

The stage of a patient's CKD is determined using the GFR and the level of albuminuria. Albuminuria occurs when albumin, a type of protein normally found in the blood, passes through the kidneys and is identifiable in the urine. Albumin is a large protein molecule that should not be able to pass through the kidneys and into the urine. Therefore, if protein is detected in the urine using a simple urine dipstick test, further investigation using the albumin creatinine ratio (ACR) test may be necessary. The normal result of the ACR is ≤30 mg/g. Results above 30 mg/g may indicate CKD, even if the GFR is within normal range (National Kidney Foundation, 2017). Thus, if the patient's ACR results are above normal, consistent follow-up care is recommended. The severity of renal disease can be established using both the GFR and the level of albuminuria (Kidney Disease: Improving Global Outcomes CKD Workgroup, 2013; see Figure 8.2).

STAGES OF CHRONIC KIDNEY DISEASE		GFR*	% OF KIDNEY FUNCTION
Stage 1	Kidney damage with **normal** kidney function	90 or higher	90–100%
Stage 2	Kidney damage with **mild loss** of kidney function	89 to 60	89–60%
Stage 3a	**Mild to moderate** loss of kidney function	59 to 45	59–45%
Stage 3b	**Moderate to severe** loss of kidney function	44 to 30	44–30%
Stage 4	**Severe** loss of kidney function	29 to 15	29–15%
Stage 5	Kidney **failure**	Less than 15	Less than 15%

* Your GFR number tells you how much kidney function you have. As kidney disease gets worse, GFR number goes down.

FIGURE 8.1 GFR and renal disease.

GFR, glomerular filtration rate.
Source: Used with permission from the National Kidney Foundation. Retrieved from https://www.kidney.org/atoz/content/gfr

				Persistent Albuminuria Categories, Description and Range		
				Normal to mildly increased	Moderately increased	Severely increased
				<30 mg/g (<3 mg/mmol)	30–300 mg/g (3–30 mg/mmol)	>300 mg/g (>30 mg/mmol)
GFR Categories (mL/min/1.73 m²) Stage, Description, and Range	1	Normal or high	≥90	1 if CKD	1	2
	2	Mildly decreased	60–89	1 if CKD	1	2
	3a	Mildly to moderately decreased	45–59	1	2	3
	3b	Moderately to severely decreased	30–44	2	3	3
	4	Severely decreased	15–29	3	3	4+
	5	Kidney failure	<15	4+	4+	4+

FIGURE 8.2 Prognosis of CKD by GFR and albuminuria category.

CKD, chronic kidney disease; GFR, glomerular filtration rate.
Source: Used with permission from the National Kidney Foundation. Retrieved from: http://www.kdigo.org/clinical_practice_guidelines/pdf/CKD/KDIGO_2012_CKD_GL.pdf

Notably, patients may not exhibit signs of CKD until kidney function "declines to less than 25% of normal when normal adaptive renal reserves have been exhausted" (Doig & Huether, 2014, p. 1364). The symptoms will generally be related to alterations in creatinine, urea, potassium, and sodium levels (Doig & Huether, 2014). Alterations in kidney function affect every body system; therefore, the hospice nurse may see varied manifestations of renal failure (Table 8.1).

Treatment of CKD

After the diagnosis of CKD, patients and families will need accurate and honest information regarding treatment options in order to "decide on the care based on weighing of burdens and benefits and in accordance with their own values and preferences" (Kwok, Yuen, Yong, & Tse, 2016, p. 952). Treatments can be either aggressive or conservative; options are dependent on the patient's values, condition, and concomitant illnesses.

Treatment options for patients who have CKD include dietary management, medication, monitoring of fluids and electrolytes, laboratory testing, and cardiac evaluation. Dialysis or kidney transplantation may also be options (Couchoud, Beuscart, Aldigier, Brunet, & Moranne, 2015). The National Kidney Foundation (2015) has issued clinical practice guidelines for the initiation of HD. These guidelines indicate that

Table 8.1 Systemic Effects of Chronic Kidney Disease and Uremia

System	Manifestations	Mechanisms	Treatment
Skeletal	Spontaneous fractures and bone pain deformities of long bones	Chronic kidney disease–mineral bone disorder, bone inflammation with fibrous degeneration related to hyperparathyroidism, bone resorption associated with vitamin D and calcium deficiency	Control of hyperphosphatemia to reduce hyperparathyroidism; administration of calcium and aluminium hydroxide antacids, which bind phosphate in the gut, together with a phosphate-restricted diet; vitamin D replacement; avoidance of magnesium antacids because of impaired magnesium excretion
Cardiopulmonary	Pulmonary edema, Kussmaul respirations	Fluid overload associated with pulmonary edema and metabolic acidosis leading to Kussmaul respirations	ACE inhibitors; combination of propranolol, hydralazine, and minoxidil for those with high levels of renin; bilateral nephrectomy with dialysis or transplantation
Cardiovascular	Left ventricular hypertrophy, cardiomyopathy, and ischemic heart disease; hypertension, dysrhythmias, accelerated atherosclerosis; pericarditis with fever, chest pain, and pericardial friction rub	Extracellular volume expansion and hypersecretion of renin associated with hypertension; anemia increases cardiac workload; hyperlipidemia promotes atherosclerosis; toxins precipitate into pericardium	Volume reduction with diuretics that are not potassium sparing (to avoid hyperkalemia); lipid-lowering drugs; blood pressure–lowering strategies; dialysis

(continued)

Table 8.1 Systemic Effects of Chronic Kidney Disease and Uremia (*continued*)

System	Manifestations	Mechanisms	Treatment
Neurologic	Encephalopathy (fatigue, loss of attention, difficulty with problem-solving), peripheral neuropathy (pain and burning in the legs and feet, loss of vibration sense and deep tendon reflexes), loss of motor coordination, twitching, fasciculations, stupor, and coma with advanced uremia	Progressive accumulation of uremic toxins associated with end-stage renal disease Stroke or intracerebral hemorrhage associated with chronic dialysis	Dialysis or successful kidney transplantation
Endocrine	Restricted growth in children Higher incidence of goiter Osteomalacia	Elevated parathyroid hormone levels Decreased thyroid hormone	Endogenous recombinant human growth hormone; thyroid hormone replacement Same as skeletal described earlier
Hematologic	Anemia, usually normochromic normocytic; platelet disorders with prolonged bleeding times	Reduced erythropoietin secretion and reduced red cell production; uremic toxins shorten red blood cell survival and alter platelet function	Dialysis; recombinant human erythropoietin (controversial and iron supplementation; conjugated estrogens; DDAVP; transfusion)
Gastrointestinal	Anorexia, nausea, vomiting; mouth ulcers, stomatitis, urinous breath (uremic factor), hiccups, peptic ulcers, gastrointestinal bleeding, and pancreatitis associated with end-stage renal failure	Retention of metabolic acids and other metabolic waste products	Protein-restricted diet for relief of nausea and vomiting: Na^+ based alkali or alkali-inducing food

(continued)

Table 8.1 Systemic Effects of Chronic Kidney Disease and Uremia *(continued)*			
System	**Manifestations**	**Mechanisms**	**Treatment**
Integumentary	Abnormal pigmentation and pruritus	Retention of urochromes, contributing to sallow, yellow color; high plasma calcium levels and neuropathy associated with pruritus	Dialysis with control of serum calcium and phosphate levels
Immunologic	Increased risk of infection that can cause death; increased risk of carcinoma	Suppression of cell-mediated immunity; reduction in number and function of lymphocytes, diminished phagocytosis	Routine dialysis
Reproductive	Sexual dysfunction: menorrhagia, amenorrhea, infertility, and decreased libido in women; decreased testosterone levels, infertility, and decreased libido in men	Dysfunction of ovaries and testes; presence of neuropathies	No specific treatment

ACE, angiotensin-converting enzyme; DDAVP, 1-deamino-[8-c-arginine] vasopressin.
Source: Doig, A. K., & Huether, S. E. (2014). Structure and function of the renal and urologic systems. In K. L. McCance & S. E. Huether (Eds.), *Pathophysiology: The biologic basis for disease in adults and children* (7th ed., pp. 1319–1339). St. Louis, MO: Elsevier.

- Patients who reach CKD stage 4 (GFR <30 mL/min/1.73 m^2), including those who have intermittent need for maintenance dialysis at the time of initial assessment, should receive education about kidney failure and options for its treatment, including kidney transplantation, peritoneal dialysis (PD), HD in the home or in-center, and conservative treatment. Patients' family members and caregivers also should be educated about treatment choices for kidney failure.

- The decision to initiate maintenance dialysis in patients who choose to do so should be based primarily upon an assessment of signs and/or symptoms associated with uremia, evidence of protein energy wasting, and the ability to safely manage metabolic abnormalities and/or volume overload with medical therapy rather than on a specific level of kidney function in the absence of such signs and symptoms (p. 894).

Progression of CKD and Onset of End-Stage Renal Disease

Because the function of the kidneys impacts all body systems, kidney disease progression is often associated with imbalances of electrolytes or metabolic compounds, or by-products.

Key Point
The term *uremia* literally means urine in the blood (Matzo & Sherman, 2015).

Key factors that are associated with the progression of kidney disease are proteinuria, creatinine and urea clearance, sodium and water balance, phosphate and calcium balance, hematocrit and potassium balance, acid–base balance, and dyslipidemia (Doig & Huether, 2014). Patients who have CKD or end-stage renal disease (ESRD) often have long periods of stability with a rapid decline in functional capacity during the last 1 to 2 months of life. Cardiac failure–related volume expansion and the buildup of uremic toxins is the leading cause of death in patients with CKD (National Kidney Foundation, 2015).

The final trajectory of ESRD that includes long periods of stability followed by a rapid decline is different from the other trajectories related to end-stage organ failure. Thus, patients with ESRD should be conservatively managed until late in the disease process, with intense symptom management in the last weeks of life (Murtagh, Addington-Hall, & Higginson, 2014). During the last 72 hours of life, the symptoms most frequently experienced by patients with ESRD are dyspnea, fatigue, edema, pain (including angina), and anorexia. Most patients have more than one of these symptoms concomitantly (Kwok, Yuen, Yong, & Tse, 2016). Because of the unusual disease trajectory, patients may report feeling fairly well and may decline hospice admission until very late in the disease process.

End-of-Life Considerations

At the time that dialysis is offered, patients may consider PD or HD as viable options. Complications of dialysis may include infection, severe fatigue, and hypotension. For some patients, the risks of dialysis may substantially outweigh the potential benefits. For example, patients of advanced age or those who have multiple comorbidities may not be good candidates for dialysis. Likewise, patients who begin dialysis may experience significant burdens, particularly if HD is carried out frequently on an outpatient basis. Patients may choose to discontinue dialysis due to the burden of the treatments or due to unexpected complications.

Patients who decide to forego dialysis may consider hospice care. The criteria for hospice admission specify the following criteria:

- The patient is not seeking dialysis or transplantation
  and
  - Creatinine clearance is <10 mL/min (15 mL/min for patients with diabetes)
    and
    - Serum creatinine of >8 mg/dL (>6 for patients with diabetes)

Nurses documenting CKD should include evidence of uremia, oliguria (urine output <400 mL in 24 hours), intractable hyperkalemia (>7.0), uremic pericarditis, hepatorenal syndrome, and/or intractable fluid overload. In patients who have acute renal failure, supporting documentation should include the use of mechanical ventilation, malignancy (other than kidney), chronic respiratory disease, advanced cardiac disease, and/or advanced liver disease.

Family Support and Education

Hospice nurses provide much-needed support and education for families who are facing the loss of a loved one due to renal disease. Primarily, the hospice nurse must educate the patient's family regarding the trajectory of the illness. Because the typical trajectory includes lengthy periods of relative wellness, the family may question whether hospice care is necessary. Yet, preparing the family for an abrupt decline is essential. Additionally, both the patient and family should receive education regarding symptoms typically experienced by patients with ESRD, such as nausea and vomiting, pain, dyspnea, and pruritus (Matzo & Sherman, 2015) and the management of these symptoms.

■ CONCLUSION

End-of-life care for patients who have ESRD is dependent on a complex series of decisions by the patient and his or her family regarding treatment choices. The incorporation of dialysis may lead to a prolonged end-of-life trajectory. In some cases, patients may choose to forgo dialysis or may choose to discontinue dialysis if the burden of dialysis outweighs the benefits. In such cases, hospice care should be considered.

When a patient's terminality is related to ESRD, the patient and family should be aware that the typical trajectory of the disease may include periods of relative wellness followed by a rapid decline. Thus, planning should be undertaken to intervene as needed for terminal symptoms, which often include pain, cardiac symptoms, nausea and vomiting, pruritus, and dyspnea.

Chapter Summary

- The kidneys maintain internal homeostasis.
- AKI is usually caused by medication toxicity, infection, urinary obstruction, or metabolic diseases.
- AKI is characterized by sudden onset of kidney failure and is often reversible.
- CKD has a protracted disease trajectory. It is usually secondary to other disease processes such as hypertension, diabetes, lupus, or vascular disorders.
- Decreased GFR is a key sign of kidney disease.
- The severity of kidney disease is determined by GFR and albumin levels.
- Dialysis should be considered as part of the plan of care if it is consistent with the patient's goals of care.
- The trajectory of ESRD is often protracted with long periods of stability followed by a rapid decline.
- Palliative care should be initiated early in the disease process to minimize symptomatology.
- End-of-life care should be discussed when the burden of treatment outweighs the benefit or when it is consistent with the patient's goals.

■ PRACTICE QUESTIONS

1. A 76-year-old palliative care patient who has end-stage chronic obstructive pulmonary disease (COPD), hypertension, and a history of benign prostatic hypertrophy informs the nurse that he has been unable to void for the past 48 hours. Today, he noted edema of the lower extremities and nausea. The nurse suspects that the patient's symptoms are related to

   a. Exacerbation of COPD

   b. Acute renal failure secondary to urinary obstruction

   c. Cor pulmonale

   d. Hypertensive crisis

2. For the patient in the previous question, which of the following interventions is most appropriate?

   a. Recommend hemodialysis

   b. Insert a urinary catheter

   c. Administer a steroid medication

   d. Transfer the patient to the ED

3. A patient who has a terminal diagnosis of renal disease and a history of hypertension, hypercholestremia, type 2 diabetes, and cardiac disease has an acute episode of congestive heart failure. The priority nursing diagnosis is

   a. Ineffective coping

   b. Fluid volume excess

    c. Risk for unstable blood pressure

    d. Ineffective peripheral tissue perfusion

4. When caring for patients who have decreased kidney function, the dosages of most medications should be

    a. Increased due to poor absorption

    b. Increased due to greater metabolic demands

    c. Decreased due to enhanced renal filtration

    d. Decreased due to impaired elimination

5. Albuminuria indicates renal impairment because

    a. Nephrons should filter proteins out of urine

    b. Renal failure causes increased protein production

    c. Protein retention is a hallmark sign of renal disease

    d. Renal disease increases urinary elimination

6. Because of adaptive processes within the body, a patient who has chronic kidney disease may not manifest signs until they are at which stage of kidney disease?

    a. Stage 2

    b. Stage 3a

    c. Stage 3b

    d. Stage 4

7. Patients who are receiving hemodialysis may be admitted to hospice when

    a. The patient's glomerular filtration rate (GFR) is less than 170 L/d

    b. Palliative care has been initiated

    c. Dialysis is discontinued

    d. Creatinine clearance is less than 15mL/min

8. A patient who has end-stage renal disease and is receiving palliative care requests information about a renal transplant. The nurse's best response is

    a. "Transplantation is not advisable for patients receiving palliative care"

    b. "Tell me more about why you are interested in transplantation"

    c. "I'll arrange for a team meeting to discuss your goals of care"

    d. "There is a very long waiting list for transplant surgery. Have you considered peritoneal dialysis?"

9. A patient who has end-stage renal disease has been on hospice for 2 months. He is feeling well and asks the nurse whether hospice is really necessary. The nurse's best response is

   a. "End-stage renal disease often involves lengthy periods of relative wellness followed by an abrupt change in condition"

   b. "We should discuss the hospice criteria"

   c. "Are you unhappy with hospice services?"

   d. "I'll arrange for a team meeting to discuss this with you"

10. The family of a patient who is actively dying at home from renal disease calls the hospice nurse to report that the patient is experiencing dyspnea. The nurse should

    a. Immediately make a home visit for this hospice emergency

    b. Explain to the family that dyspnea is not related to end-stage renal disease

    c. Advise the family on steps to take to treat dyspnea at home

    d. Recommend transfer to an inpatient setting due to the change in condition

▪ REFERENCES

Couchoud, G. C., Beuscart, J. B. R., Aldigier, J. C., Brunet, P. J., & Moranne, O. P. (2015). Development of a risk stratification algorithm to improve patient-centered care and decision making for incident elderly patients with end-stage renal disease. *Kidney International, 88,* 1178–1186. doi:10.1038.ki.2015.245

Doig, A. K., & Huether, S. E. (2014). Structure and function of the renal and urologic systems. In K. L. McCance & S. E. Huether (Eds.), *Pathophysiology: The biologic basis for disease in adults and children* (7th ed., pp. 1319–1339). St. Louis, MO: Elsevier.

Kidney Disease: Improving Global Outcomes CKD Workgroup. (2013). KDIGO 2012 clinical practice guidelines for the evaluation and management of chronic kidney disease. *Kidney International Supplements, 3*(1), 1–150. Retrieved from http://www.kdigo.org/clinical_practice_guidelines/pdf/CKD/KDIGO_2012_CKD_GL.pdf

Kwok, A. O., Yuen, S. K., Yong, D. S., & Tse, D. M. (2016). The symptom prevalence, medical intervention, and health care service needs for patients with end-stage renal disease in a renal palliative care program. *American Journal of Hospice & Palliative Medicine, 33*(10), 952–958. doi:10.1177/1049909115598930

Matzo, M., & Sherman, D. W. (2015). *Palliative care nursing: Quality care to the end of life.* New York, NY: Springer Publishing Company.

Murtagh, F. E. M., Addinton-Hall, J. M., & Higginson, I. J. (2011). End-stage renal disease: A trajectory of functional decline in the last year of life. *Journal of the American Geriatrics Society, 58,* 304–308. doi:10.1111/j.1532-5415.2010.03248.x

National Kidney Foundation. (2015). KDOQI clinical practice guideline for hemodialysis adequacy: 2015 update. *American Journal of Kidney Disease, 66*(5), 884–030. Retrieved from http://www.ajkd.org/article/S0272-6386(15)01019-7/fulltext

National Kidney Foundation. (2017). *Albuminuria.* Retrieved from https://www.kidney.org/atoz/content/albuminuria

Smith, H. W. (1953). *From fish to philosopher.* Boston, MA: Little, Brown and Company.

9 Hepatic Disorders

The liver is an organ with a broad set of critical biologic functions, a unique dual vascular supply, and several distinct cell types that contribute to its physiologic functions as well as potential pathology.
—Schaffer and Friedman (2018, p. 3)

▨ LEARNING OBJECTIVES

After completing this section, the nurse will be able to

1. Identify key assessment findings indicative of liver disease
2. Explain end-of-life considerations for patients who have liver failure
3. Discuss end-of-care options for patients who have liver failure

▨ HEPATIC DISORDERS

The liver is the largest solid organ in the body. Located under the diaphragm on the right side of the body, the liver consists of two lobes: the right and the left. The liver is primarily involved in metabolism and digestion and secretes 700 to 1,200 mL of bile daily. Bile is an alkaline fluid that contains bile salts, electrolytes, and water. Bile is critical for digestive processes, especially absorption and metabolism of fats and fat-soluble vitamins. The liver also facilitates excretion of toxic substances from the blood such as alcohol, drugs, and hormones through the process of metabolic detoxification, also called biotransformation (Doig & Huether, 2014).

Damage to the liver can result from infection, especially viral hepatitis, autoimmune liver disease, genetic predisposition to liver disease, cancer, chronic alcohol abuse, or nonalcoholic fatty liver. Risk factors for liver disease include the following:

- Alcohol abuse

- Exposure to others' blood or body fluids through parenteral drug abuse, tattoos, or blood transfusion prior to 1982

- Exposure to hepatotoxic chemicals
- Diabetes
- Obesity (Mayo Clinic, 2019)

The primary cause of liver disease is hepatitis C, followed by alcohol abuse-related cirrhosis (American Liver Foundation, 2017). In the United States, nearly five million adults have been diagnosed with liver disease (Centers for Disease Control and Prevention, 2016). Death rates among those with chronic liver disease and cirrhosis are highest among men and those over the age of 65 (Centers for Disease Control and Prevention, 2017).

Liver Failure

Chronic liver failure (CLF) is a sequela of irreversible disease processes such as chronic viral hepatitis (A, B, or C), cancer, nonalcoholic fatty liver disease, or cirrhosis. Without liver transplantation, CLF progresses to end-stage liver disease (ESLD). Patients who have ESLD may

> **Key Point**
>
> Pruritus in liver disease often results from "the accumulation of pruritogenic bile acids and bile salts, modulation of itch pathways . . . imbalance between different types of receptors for endogenous opioids, and modulation of the perception of pruritus by serotonin and substance P" (Carrion, Rosen, & Levy, 2018, p. 517).

present with ascites, hepatic encephalopathy, poor immunity, anorexia and cachexia, portal hypertension, nausea, vomiting, electrolyte imbalances, pruritus, pain, malaise, and/or bleeding esophageal varices (see Chapter 16, Symptom Management; Mayo Clinic, 2019; Medici & Meyers, 2016). Patients may also be observed to have a protuberant abdomen related to ascites along with wasting of the extremities secondary to malnutrition and muscle wasting.

Patient Assessment

Assessment of the patient with liver disease should begin with a thorough history of symptoms such as pain, nausea, vomiting, altered bowel habits, rectal bleeding, abdominal distention, pruritus, or dysphagia. Inspection should include assessment of general appearance, and observation for jaundice, which involves inspection of the sclera and skin. The skin should further be inspected for rash, petechiae, open areas secondary to scratching, and nonhealing wounds. The facies should be examined for sunken eyes or facial features and temporal wasting, which indicate poor nutrition. If ascites is present, the nurse should observe for symmetry, presence of masses, bulges, or peristaltic waves (Swartz, 2014).

The nurse should auscultate the abdomen for bowel sounds and bruits. The nurse may then percuss the abdomen in all four quadrants, expecting to hear tympani over most of the abdomen due to the presence of gas in the stomach and intestines. Dullness is heard

> **Key Point**
>
> The disease trajectory for ESLD is often erratic with increasingly frequent, severe, and refractory exacerbation of symptoms. Death often occurs suddenly and is usually related to complications of the underlying disease process (Cox-North, Doorenbos, Shannon, Scott, & Curtis, 2013).

over solid organs such as the liver, allowing the nurse to approximate the liver borders, which should normally span no more than 10 cm (4 inches) or less. Palpation allows the nurse to identify areas of tenderness or rigidity. In patients who have generalized peritonitis, the abdomen is often described as "board-like." Rebound tenderness with palpation is indicative if there is local inflammation (Swartz, 2014).

Determining Prognosis in ESLD

Prognosis for patients who have ESLD can be estimated using validated prognostication tools such as the Model for End-Stage Liver Disease (MELD). The MELD accounts for the patient's international normalized ratio (INR), bilirubin, and creatinine levels. Patients with a MELD score of 10 to 19 have a 92% 6-month mortality (Potosek, Curry, Buss, & Chittenden, 2014).

Another widely used, valid tool to estimate prognosis in ESLD is the Child–Turcotte–Pugh (CTP), which takes into account the patient's total bilirubin, albumin, and INR, as well as the degree of encephalopathy and ascites. Patients whose liver disease is classified as Class A according to the CTP have a 95% 12-month mortality (Potosek et al., 2014).

In addition to the use of prognostic tools, ascites indicates a 50% 2-year mortality, with a 6-month median survival rate when it becomes refractory. Declining liver failure leads to renal failure, which is known as hepatorenal syndrome (HRS).

> **Key Point**
>
> The MELD calculator can be accessed at optn.transplant.hrsa.gov/resources/allocation-calculators/meld-calculator/
>
> The CTP calculator can be accessed at www.hepatitis.va.gov/provider/tools/child-pugh-calculator.asp

HRS type 1 heralds a 4-week survival rate, and type 2 HRS has a 6-month survival rate (Potosek et al., 2014).

Patients can be considered eligible for hospice services when symptoms such as ascites, hepatic encephalopathy, HRS, or bleeding esophageal varices become refractory to medical intervention. Further, the following criteria should be demonstrable:

- Prothrombin time (PT) more than 5 seconds over control, or INR >1.5
- Serum albumin <2.5 gm/dL
  and

- One or more of the following conditions:
  - Ascites, refractory to treatment or patient noncompliant
  - Spontaneous bacterial peritonitis
  - HRS, elevated creatinine and blood urea nitrogen (BUN), oliguria (<400 mL/d), urine sodium concentration (<10 mEq/L), cirrhosis, and ascites
  - Hepatic encephalopathy, refractory to treatment, or patient noncompliant
  - Recurrent variceal bleeding despite intensive therapy
- Supporting documentation may include the following:
  - Progressive malnutrition
  - Muscle wasting with reduced strength and endurance
  - Continued active alcoholism (>80 g ethanol per day)
  - Hepatocellular carcinoma
  - HBsAg (Hepatitis B) positivity (Stanford School of Medicine, 2019)

▪ CONCLUSION

Chronic liver disease is a debilitating condition that can lead to ESLD. The most common causes of liver disease include infection and alcohol abuse. When patients present with liver disease, a thorough assessment should be undertaken, including identification of risk factors. For patients who have signs of ESLD, valid prognostic tools such as the MELD or the CTP should be used to estimate terminality. Discussion regarding palliation of symptoms should be undertaken early in the disease process. Referral to hospice care should occur when it is consistent with the patient's goals of care.

Chapter Summary

- The liver is the largest solid organ in the body. Located under the right diaphragm, it secretes 700 to 1,200 mL of bile daily.

- Liver damage results from alcohol or drug abuse, medication toxicity, viral hepatitis, diabetes, and obesity.

- ESLD is a terminal condition. A liver transplant is needed to reverse the disease process.

- Palliation of symptoms is critical for patients who have ESLD. Hospice care should be initiated when the patient's condition is consistent with admission criteria and hospice admission is consistent with the patient's goals of care.

- At the end of life, patients who have ESLD experience increasingly refractory symptoms. Death often occurs suddenly and is usually related to complications of the underlying disease process.

▪ PRACTICE QUESTIONS

1. A 57-year-old patient who has end-stage liver disease is being treated for hepatic encephalopathy with 30 mL of lactulose BID. The patient is alert and oriented and reports several bouts of liquid diarrhea, one of which resulted in incontinence this morning. The nurse should

   a. Advise the patient to take 2 mg of loperamide orally after each loose stool

   b. Inform the patient that the diarrhea is a side effect of the lactulose

   c. Advise the patient to hold the next dose of lactulose

   d. Encourage the patient to replace fluids and electrolytes with sports drinks

2. A patient who has chronic renal failure reports severe generalized pruritus. The nurse knows that this symptom is most likely related to

   a. Alcohol abuse

   b. Allergic reaction

   c. Accumulation of bile salts

   d. Severe dehydration

3. End-stage liver disease is ideally treated with

   a. Lactulose

   b. Diphenhydramine

   c. Dialysis

   d. Transplantation

4. When percussing the abdomen of a patient who has end-stage liver disease, an expected finding would be a liver span of

   a. 15 cm

   b. 10 cm

   c. 8 cm

   d. 6 cm

5. A patient who has ascites secondary to end-stage liver disease had paracentesis yesterday but fluid has accumulated to an uncomfortable degree overnight. This indicates that the patient

   a. Should take a diuretic now

   b. Remains in supine position too frequently

   c. Must raise the lower extremities above the level of the heart

   d. Has a life expectancy of 6 months or less

⬛ REFERENCES

American Liver Foundation. (2017). *Liver disease statistics*. Retrieved from https://liverfoundation .org/liver-disease-statistics/#alcohol-related-liver-disease-and-cirrhosis

Carrion, A. F., Rosen, J. D., & Levy, C. (2018). Understanding and treating pruritus in primary biliary cholangitis. *Clinics in Liver Disease, 22*(3), 517–532. doi:10.1016/j.cld.2018.03.005

Centers for Disease Control and Prevention. (2016). *Chronic liver disease and cirrhosis*. Retrieved from https://www.cdc.gov/nchs/fastats/liver-disease.htm

Centers for Disease Control and Prevention. (2017). *QuickStats: Death rates for chronic liver disease and cirrhosis by sex and age group—National Vital Statistics System, United States, 2000 and 2015*. Retrieved from https://www.cdc.gov/mmwr/volumes/66/wr/mm6638a9.htm

Cox-North, P., Doorenbos, A., Shannon, S. E., Scott, J., & Curtis, J. R. (2013). The transition to end-of-life care in end-stage liver disease. *Journal of Hospice & Palliative Nursing, 15*(4), 209–215. doi:10.1097/NJH.0b013e318289f4b0

Doig, A. K., & Huether, S. E. (2014). Structure and function of the digestive system. In K. L. McCance & S. E. Huether (Eds.), *Pathophysiology: The biologic basis for disease in adults and children* (7th ed., pp. 1393–1422). St. Louis, MO: Elsevier.

Mayo Clinic. (2019). *Liver disease*. Retrieved from https://www.mayoclinic.org/diseases-ssconditions/ liver-problems/symptoms-causes/syc-20374502

Medici, V., & Meyers, F. J. (2016). Palliative care in end-stage liver disease. In S. Yennuralingam & E. Bruera (Eds.), *Oxford handbook of hospice and palliative medicine and supportive care* (2nd ed., pp. 385–396). New York, NY: Oxford University Press.

Potosek, J., Curry, M., Buss, M., & Chittenden, E. (2014). Integration of palliative care in end-stage liver disease and liver transplantation. *Journal of Palliative Medicine, 17*(11), 1271–1277. doi:10.1089/jpm.2013.0167

Schaffer, E. A., & Friedman, L. S. (2018). History taking and physical assessment for the patient with liver disease. In E. R. Schiff, W. C. Maddrey, & K. R. Reddy (Eds.), *Schiff's diseases of the liver* (12th ed., pp. 3–16). Oxford, UK: Wiley-Blackwell.

Stanford School of Medicine. (2019). *Liver disease*. Retrieved from https://palliative.stanford .edu/home-hospice-home-care-of-the-dying-patient/common-terminal-diagnoses/liver-disease/

Swartz, M. H. (2014). *Textbook of physical diagnosis* (7th ed.). Philadelphia, PA: Elsevier Saunders.

10 Dementia

Our brains do thousands of tasks, and we are usually not aware of most of them. We assume that other people's brains, like ours, are working as they should—but with a person who has dementia, we cannot make this assumption.
—Mace and Rabins (2011, p. 22)

LEARNING OBJECTIVES

After completing this section, the nurse will be able to

1. Differentiate types of dementia
2. Identify symptoms of dementia
3. Identify the disease trajectories for neurocognitive diseases

THE NEUROCOGNITIVE DISORDERS

Neurocognitive disorders (NCDs) "are those in which impaired cognition has not been present since birth or very early in life, and thus represents a decline from a previously attained level of functioning" (American Psychiatric Association, 2013, p. 591). Dementia is a form of major NCD, as defined in the *Diagnostic and Statistical Manual of Mental Disorders*, Fifth Edition (*DSM-5*; American Psychiatric Association, 2013). It is most common among those aged 60 years or older, with a sharp increase in incidence in those over 85 years (American Psychiatric Association, 2013; Boss & Huether, 2014). However, dementia is not strictly related to age; other risk factors include the following:

- Genetic predisposition
- Female gender
- Poor diet
- Obesity

- Diabetes
- Low education level
- Multiple comorbidities
- Living alone
- Depression

(American Psychiatric Association, 2013; Brody, 2015; Crowther & Costello, 2017)

Dementia is characterized by sometimes insidious changes in cognition and behavior. Key signs of dementia include the following:

- Memory changes
- Poor recognition
- Word searching
- Decreased executive function
- Poor attention span
- Alterations in behavior and mood
- Altered perceptions
- Decreased ability to perform activities of daily living

These symptoms are largely related to the structural and chemical changes that occur with neurodegeneration, atherosclerosis, inflammatory processes, trauma, cerebral lesions, or increased intracranial pressure (Boss & Huether, 2014; Crowther & Costello, 2017). The clinical manifestations of dementia can vary greatly. In cases of degenerative dementia, the diagnosis is largely based on thorough patient history, gathered over the course of several evaluations. Laboratory and diagnostic testing may also be used along with cognitive screenings (Brody, 2015; Crowther & Costello, 2017). According to the American Psychological Association (2013, p. 602), diagnostic criteria for dementia are as follows:

A. Evidence of significant cognitive decline from a previous level of performance in one or more domains (complex attention, executive function, learning and memory, language, perceptual-motor, or social cognition) based on

1. Concern for the individual, a knowledgeable informant, or the clinician that there has been a significant decline in cognitive function.

2. A substantial impairment in cognitive performance, preferably documented by standardized neuropsychological testing or, in its absence, another quantified clinical assessment.

B. The cognitive deficits interfere with independence in everyday activities (i.e., at a minimum, requiring assistance with complex instrumental activities of daily living, such as paying bills or managing medications)

C. The cognitive deficits do not occur exclusively in the context of a delirium

D. The cognitive deficits are not better explained by another mental disorder (e.g., major depressive disorder and schizophrenia)

Diagnosis of dementia presumes the exclusion of delirium and other mental disorders as well as the use or abuse of cognition-reducing drugs such as antipsychotics, anticholinergics, opioids, antiepileptics, sedatives, or hypnotics (American Psychiatric Association, 2013; Brody, 2015).

Since dementia is an umbrella term used to describe many forms of neurocognitive changes, the clinician should "specify whether the disorder is related to Alzheimer's disease, frontotemporal lobar degeneration, Lewy body disease, vascular disease, traumatic brain injury, substance/medication use, HIV infection, Prion disease, Parkinson's disease, Huntington's disease, another medical condition, multiple etiologies, or an unspecified reason" (American Psychiatric Association, 2013, p. 603).

The most common form of dementia is Alzheimer's-type dementia: It accounts for roughly 60% of cases. The next most common, in order, are Lewy body dementia, frontotemporal dementia, and vascular dementia (Brody, 2015). Some patients may have more than one type (Brody, 2015; Crowther & Costello, 2017). Each manifestation of dementia has different presenting symptoms and different disease trajectories (see Table 10.1).

Early diagnosis of dementia is crucial because, although it is incurable, several interventions are available to slow disease progression and maintain quality of life for as long as possible. Physical, occupational, and speech therapies should be initiated early in the disease process to maintain physical integrity and preserve speech and swallowing ability. Additionally, serious conversations about advance care plans, goals of care, and plans for long-term disease management, including the possibility of placement in a long-term care facility, should take place before the patient is mentally incapacitated.

Pharmacological therapy can also be initiated early in the disease process. For example, cholinesterase inhibitors, such as donepezil, are used to improve cholinergic transmission. Donepezil delays worsening of symptoms in the early stages of dementia by preventing the breakdown of acetylcholine, a chemical messenger important for learning and memory. In the later stages of dementia, N-methyl-D-aspartate (NMDA) receptor agonists, such as memantine, are used to improve memory, enhance reasoning skills, and maintain physical functioning for as long as possible. Cholinesterase inhibitors and NMDA receptor agonists can be used in combination (Alzheimer's Association, 2018; Boss & Huether, 2014).

Table 10.1 Symptoms Associated With Types of Dementia			
Alzheimer's	**Vascular**	**Lewy Body**	**Frontotemporal**
Short-term memory loss, forgetfulness, difficulty with new skills, decreased attention span, word searching, decreased recognition of persons, places, and things (Brody, 2015, p. 508). This type of dementia is characterized by its insidious onset and slow progression. Deterioration occurs over 6–8 years and is punctuated with periods of acute exacerbation of underlying diseases (Brody, 2015, p. 508).	Impaired executive function, motor deficits, decreased recall, aphasia, decreased problem-solving abilities (Brody, 2015, p. 508). This type of dementia involves irregular variability of symptoms accompanied by a stepwise decline. Onset of symptoms generally corresponds to transient ischemic attack or a cerebrovascular accident, or cerebral infarct (Crowther & Costello, 2017).	Variations in cognitive ability, visual hallucinations, parkinsonian movements, sleep disturbances, sensitivity to neuroleptics, numerous falls, autonomic disorders, systematic delusions (Brody, 2015, p. 508). Lewy body dementia results from abnormal deposits of the alpha-synuclein protein in the brain. Symptoms are progressive and include changes in memory and cognition, movement disorders, and/or neurocognitive changes (Lewy Body Dementia Association, 2018).	Disinhibition, aphasia, emotional distancing, obstinacy, apathy, egocentric behaviors, motor disturbances, decreased facial recognition (Brody, 2015, p. 508). Frontotemporal dementia is an umbrella term for cognitive and physical deterioration caused by nerve cell damage. The progression of symptoms is dependent on the underlying cause of the damage (Alzheimer's Association, 2018).

Note: Mixed-type dementia includes features of both Alzheimer's-type and vascular.

In the later stages of dementia, an interdisciplinary palliative care team should be involved to manage symptoms such as

- Serious motor impairment and safety issues
- Dysphagia, incontinence, and immobility that put the patient at risk for decubiti
- Communication barriers
- Infection and agitation
- Delirium

- Depression
- Lethargy
- Drowsiness
- Breathlessness
- Pain

(Crowther & Costello, 2017; Maxwell, 2015).

As dementia progresses, the patient becomes entirely dependent on others for physical care due to limb contractures and joint stiffness. Care must be taken to reduce pain with therapy, transfers, personal care, and procedures. Assessment of nonverbal manifestations of pain is a key nursing skill since pain is often underdetected and undertreated in patients who have dementia (Brorson, Plymouth, Örmon, & Bolmsjö, 2014; Crowther & Costello, 2017).

In the terminal phase of dementia, decisions regarding withholding or withdrawing interventions should be made in accordance with the patient's advance directive. If no advance directive is in place, the patient's family members or other decision-makers should work closely with the palliative care team to establish goals of care and appropriate interventions, carefully weighing the benefits of each intervention against the burdens. Discontinuation of interventions, including pharmacological treatments, should be considered when the disease progresses to the terminal phase, or when the intervention is inconsistent with the goals of care and/or the benefit is questionable (Crowther & Costello, 2017; Tija et al., 2014). The lengthy and sometimes unpredictable course of dementia can make prognostication challenging. Nonetheless, the hospice admission criteria for dementia provide guidance on the key factors in determining terminality.

The criteria for admission to hospice for dementia specify that the patient must be stage 7 or beyond according to the Functional Assessment Staging (FAST) scale (Figure 10.1) **and** have one or more of the following conditions:

- Aspiration pneumonia
- Septicemia
- Pyelonephritis
- Multiple pressure ulcers that are stage 3 or 4
- Recurrent fever
- Other significant condition that suggests limited prognosis

The patient's history should also reflect the inability to maintain sufficient fluid and calorie intake in the past 6 months (10% weight loss or albumin <2.5 gm/dL).

STAGE	SKILL LEVEL
1.	No difficulties, either subjectively or objectively.
2.	Complains of forgetting location of objects. Subjective word finding difficulties.
3.	Decreased job function evident to coworkers; difficulty in traveling to new locations. Decreased organizational capacity.*
4.	Decreased ability to perform complex tasks (e.g., planning dinner for guests), handling personal finances (forgetting to pay bills), difficulty marketing, etc.
5.	Requires assistance in choosing proper clothing to wear for day, season, occasion.
6a.	Difficulty putting clothing on properly without assistance.
6b.	Unable to bathe properly (e.g., difficulty adjusting bath water temperature), occasionally or more frequently over the past weeks.*
6c.	Inability to handle mechanics of toileting (e.g., forgets to flush the toilet, does not wipe properly or properly dispose of toilet tissue), occasionally or more frequently over the past weeks.*
6d.	Urinary incontinence, occasionally or more frequently over the past weeks.*
6e.	Fecal incontinence, occasionally or more frequently over the past week.*
7a.	Ability to speak limited to approximately a half dozen different words or fewer, in the course of an average day or in the course of an intensive interview.
7b.	Speech ability limited to the use of a single intelligible word in an average day or in the course of an interview (the person may repeat the word over and over).
7c.	Ambulatory ability lost (cannot walk without personal assistance).
7d.	Ability to sit up without assistance lost (e.g., the individual will fall over if there are no lateral rests [arms] on the chair).
7e.	Loss of the ability to smile.

FIGURE 10.1 Functional Assessment Staging of Alzheimer's Disease (FAST).

STAGE•• _____
*Scored primarily on the basis of information obtained from a knowledgeable informant and/or caregiver. ©1984 by Barry Reisberg, M.D. All rights reserved. Reisberg, B. (1988). Functional Assessment Staging (FAST). *Psychopharmacology Bulletin, 24,* 653–659.

▪ FAST SCALE ADMINISTRATION

The FAST scale is a functional scale designed to evaluate patients at the more moderate-severe stages of dementia when the Mini-Mental State Exam no longer can reflect changes in a meaningful clinical way. In the early stages the patient may be able to participate in the FAST administration, but usually the information should be collected from a caregiver or, in the case of nursing home care, the nursing home staff.

The FAST scale has seven stages:

1. which is normal adult
2. which is normal older adult
3. which is early dementia
4. which is mild dementia
5. which is moderate dementia
6. which is moderately severe dementia
7. which is severe dementia

FAST Functional Milestones

FAST stage 1 is the normal adult with no cognitive decline. FAST stage 2 is the normal older adult with very mild memory loss. Stage 3 is early dementia. Here memory loss becomes apparent to coworkers and family. The patient may be unable to remember names of persons just introduced to them. Stage 4 is mild dementia. Persons in this stage may have difficulty with finances, counting money, and travel to new locations. Memory loss increases. The person's knowledge of current and recent events decreases. Stage 5 is moderate dementia. In this stage, the person needs more help to survive. They do not need assistance with toileting or eating, but do need help choosing clothing. The person displays increased difficulty with serial subtraction. The patient may not know the date and year or where they live. However, they do know who they are and the names of their family and friends. Stage 6 is moderately severe dementia. The person may begin to forget the names of family members or friends. The person requires more assistance with activities of daily living, such as bathing, toileting, and eating. Patients in this stage may develop delusions, hallucinations, or obsessions. Patients show increased anxiety and may become violent. The person in this stage begins to sleep during the day and stay awake at night. Stage 6 is severe dementia. In this stage, all speech is lost. Patients lose urinary and bowel control. They lose the ability to walk. Most become bedridden and die of sepsis or pneumonia.

For most patients, the trajectory of dementia is a long period of deteriorating cognitive and physical function, generally over 6 to 8 years. This gradual decline is often punctuated with periods of acute exacerbation of underlying diseases. Some patients may succumb to acute events, such as myocardial or cerebral infarction, to complications of fractures or infections, such as pneumonia or urinary tract infections or malnutrition (Maxwell, 2015; Murray, Kendall, Boyd, & Sheikh, 2005).

Chapter Summary

- Dementia is a form of neurocognitive disorder.
- Incidence of dementia rises sharply with age.
- The most common forms of dementia are Alzheimer's, vascular, Lewy body, and frontotemporal.
- The FAST Scale is used to assess functional status in patients with dementia.
- Hospice eligibility requires a FAST scale score of 7+ for patients with dementia along with other criteria.
- The trajectory of decline for dementia involves slow deterioration over 6-8 years with exacerbations of any underlying diseases.

■ CONCLUSION

Dementia is a chronic, debilitating disease that can lead to terminality. Recognition of early signs of dementia and early palliation of symptoms can improve the patient's quality of life. As the disease progresses, palliative services, especially pain management, become a greater focus of care. In the final stage of the disease process, hospice care ensures focused patient care as well as family support and education from the hospice interdisciplinary team.

■ PRACTICE QUESTIONS

1. Neurocognitive disorders are
   a. Most common in those over 60 years
   b. Reversible
   c. Related to vascular problems
   d. Characterized by immobility

2. Which of the following, if observed in a patient who has dementia, is likely reversible?
   a. Memory loss
   b. Delirium
   c. Poor attention span
   d. Bladder incontinence

3. A patient with dementia may be eligible for hospice admission if their score on the Functional Assessment Staging (FAST) scale is

   a. 6e

   b. 5

   c. 3

   d. 7

4. A patient who has dementia is actively dying. His family asks the hospice nurse if he is in a coma because he is unresponsive to verbal or tactile stimuli but moans when turned in bed. The nurse's best response is

   a. "He is just lethargic from the medications."

   b. "The term 'coma' doesn't apply to patients who are actively dying."

   c. "Yes, most patients are comatose at this stage."

   d. "The dementia has progressed to the terminal phase."

5. A nurse is evaluating a patient for hospice admission. Which of the following provides the best support for a primary terminal diagnosis of dementia in an 88-year-old patient with a history of hypertension, diabetes, and obesity?

   a. Weight loss of 2 pounds over the past 3 months

   b. Evening blood glucose levels of less than 80

   c. Two recent hospitalizations for aspiration pneumonia

   d. Stage 1 pressure ulcer on the left heel

▪ REFERENCES

Alzheimer's Association. (2018). *Frontotemporal dementia.* Retrieved from https://www.alz.org/dementia/fronto-temporal-dementia-ftd-symptoms.asp#about

American Psychiatric Association. (2013). *Diagnostic and statistical manual of mental disorders* (5th ed.). Washington, DC: Author.

Boss, B. J., & Huether, S. E. (2014). Alterations in cognitive systems, cerebral hemodynamics, and motor function. In K. L. McCance & S. E. Huether (Eds.), *Pathophysiology: The biologic basis for disease in adults and children* (7th ed., pp. 527–580). St. Louis, MO: Elsevier.

Brody, A. A. (2015). Cognitive impairment. In C. Dahlin, P. J. Coyne, & B. R. Ferrell (Eds.), *Advanced practice palliative nursing.* (pp. 506–515). New York, NY: Oxford University Press.

Brorson, H., Plymouth, H., Örmon, K., & Bolmsjö, I. (2014). Pain relief at the end of life: Nurses' experiences regarding end-of-life pain relief in patients with dementia. *Pain Management Nursing, 15*(1), 315–323. doi:10.1016/j.pmn.2012.10.005

Crowther, J., & Costello, J. (2017). Palliative care for people with advanced major neuro-cognitive disorders. *International Journal of Palliative Nursing, 23*(10), 502–509. doi:10.12968/ijpn.2017.23.10.502

Mace, N. L., & Rabins, P. V. (2011). *The 36-hour day: A family guide to caring for people who have Alzheimer's disease, related dementias, and memory loss* (5th ed.). Baltimore, MD: The Johns Hopkins Press.

Maxwell, T. L. (2015). Caring for those with chronic illness. In B. R. Ferrell, N. Coyle, & J. A. Paice (Eds.), *Oxford textbook of palliative nursing* (4th ed., pp. 567–570). New York, NY: Oxford University Press.

Murray, S. A., Kendall, M., Boyd, K., & Sheikh, A. (2005). Illness trajectories and palliative care. *BMJ, 330,* 1007–1011. Retrieved from www.bmj.com

Reisberg, B. (1988). Functional Assessment Staging (FAST). *Psychopharmacology Bulletin, 24,* 653–659.

Tija, J., Briesacher, B. A., Peterson, D., Liu, Q., Andrade, S. E., & Mitchell, S. L. (2014). Use of medications of questionable benefit in advanced dementia. *JAMA Internal Medicine, 174*(11), 1763–1771. doi:10.1001/jamainternmed.2014.4103

11

Endocrine Disorders

There are a host of diseases and conditions that arise from endocrine gland dysfunction and these are generally discreet, with differing clinical presentation and management approaches depending on the endocrine gland of concern.
—Levesque (2012, p. 444)

■ LEARNING OBJECTIVES

After completing this section, the nurse will be able to

1. Identify risk factors and interventions for diabetes
2. Articulate the symptoms that are associated with thyroid disorders
3. Explain end-of-life considerations for endocrine disorders

■ ENDOCRINE DISORDERS

Endocrine disorders stem from dysfunction of one or more of the organs in the endocrine system. These organs are the pituitary, thyroid, parathyroid, pancreas, and adrenal glands (Levesque, 2012). The endocrine system is responsible for producing hormones and maintaining homeostasis. Hormones produced by the endocrine system include insulin, leptin, parathyroid hormone, prolactin, follicle-stimulating hormone, antidiuretic hormone, epinephrine, and testosterone (Brashers, Jones, & Huether, 2014). These hormones are released into the bloodstream and bind to cells that possess the appropriate hormone receptors. Cells with the appropriate receptors can increase the number of receptors when the concentration of the hormones in the blood is low. Conversely, when the blood concentration of the hormone is high, the receptors on the cells decrease. In this way, cells can continually adjust to changing metabolic needs within the body and maintain homeostasis (Brashers et al., 2014).

When disorders of the endocrine system occur, patients may be initially asymptomatic or may report vague symptoms. Endocrine disorders may be primary or may result as a complication of another disease process. The two most commonly encountered endocrine disorders in seriously ill patients are diabetes and thyroid disease.

Thyroid Disease

The thyroid gland is located inferior to the thyroid cartilage and has two lobes that lie on either side of the trachea. The two lobes are connected by the isthmus, which crosses over the center of the trachea (Brashers et al., 2014; Levesque, 2012). The thyroid is involved in the regulation of thyroid hormone (TH), thyroid-stimulating hormone (TSH), thyroxine(T_4), triiodothyronine (T_3), calcitonin, and iodine. The functioning of the thyroid is primarily controlled by the pituitary gland. Dysfunction of the pituitary gland or of the thyroid itself can result in hypothyroidism or hyperthyroidism (Brashers et al., 2014; Levesque, 2012; Sargis, 2018).

Hypothyroidism

Hypothyroidism is a common disorder affecting almost 4% of the population in the United States. Hypothyroidism is defined as TSH levels greater than 4.5 mIU/L (Orlander, Varghese, & Freeman, 2018). According to Levesque (2012), symptoms of hypothyroidism include the following:

> **Key Point**
>
> Roughly 20 million Americans have thyroid disease, but up to 60% are not aware of their condition (American Thyroid Association, 2019).

- Cold intolerance
- Fluid retention
- Dry, coarse skin and increased perspiration
- Nerve entrapment and paresthesia
- Blurred vision
- Impaired hearing
- Feelings of fullness in the neck and throat
- Neck pain
- Sore throat
- Low-grade fever
- Galactorrhea
- Constipation
- Depression and emotional lability
- Irregular menses and infertility

- Fatigue

- Muscle and joint pain

Clinical signs of hypothyroidism often include weight gain, dry skin, jaundice, pallor, periorbital puffiness, goiter, hoarseness, decreased systolic blood pressure, increased diastolic blood pressure, pericardial effusion, bradycardia, nonpitting edema, pitting edema of

> **Key Point**
>
> Myxedema coma, sometimes called myxedema crisis, describes an acute medical emergency resulting from severe hypothyroidism. This rare but life-threatening condition often results in the need for intubation and mechanical ventilation (Eledrisi, 2018; Levesque, 2012).

the lower extremities, and painless thyroid enlargement (Levesque, 2012; Mayo Clinic, 2019). Hypothyroidism can be medically managed with levothyroxine 1 to 2 mg/kg/d.

Hyperthyroidism

Hyperthyroidism results from overproduction of T_4 and/or T_3. Most (60%–80%) of patients who have hyperthyroidism have Graves' disease. Graves' disease is an autoimmune disorder that causes destruction of the TSH receptors on thyroid follicular cells. Patients who have hyperthyroidism may experience nervousness, irritability, fine tremor, and muscle weakness. Examination may reveal goiter, bruit over the thyroid, hyperactivity, heat intolerance, sweating, hair loss, and palmer erythema (DeLeo, Lee, & Braverman, 2016; Levesque, 2012).

Diagnosis of hyperthyroidism is suspected when the TSH level is low. T_3 and T_4 levels must be reviewed to distinguish subclinical hyperthyroidism from overt hyperthyroidism. Medical treatment involves antithyroid medications such as methimazole or propylthiouracil. Beta-blockers are used to control adrenergic

> **Key Point**
>
> Thyroid storm is an acute manifestation of thyrotoxicosis. It is a medical emergency that is associated with hyperthyroidism. Symptoms include sweating, fever, tachycardia, hypertension, agitation, confusion, and diarrhea. It must be promptly treated with antithyroid drugs, inorganic iodine, bile acid sequestrants, beta-blockers, and glucocorticoids (DeLeo, et al., 2016; Levesque, 2012).

symptoms. Radioactive iodine therapy or thyroidectomy are treatment options if antithyroid medications fail to induce remission of symptoms (DeLeo et al., 2016; Kravets, 2016).

Diabetes

In the United States, over 30 million people have diabetes, seven million of which have not been formally diagnosed (Centers for Disease

Control and Prevention, 2018b). Diabetes is a metabolic disorder characterized by abnormal insulin production or action. Diabetes is categorized as either type 1 (T1DM) or type 2 (T2DM). T1DM occurs most frequently in children and adolescents and has a genetic component. However, genetic predisposition does not account for most cases. In fact, 80% of those with T1DM do not have a family history of the disease. One possible explanation for the onset of T1DM in those without a family history is destruction of pancreatic beta cells via an autoimmune response (Levesque, 2012); the key feature of T1DM is the inability to produce insulin.

T2DM is primarily characterized by insulin resistance rather than the absence of insulin production. Risk factors for T2DM include the following:

- Increased age
- Hypertension
- Hypercholesterolemia
- Overweight and obesity
- Smoking
- Physical inactivity
- Hyperglycemia (Centers for Disease Control and Prevention, 2018a; Levesque, 2012).

Patients who have diabetes incur twice the medical costs of those without the disease due to the increased need for emergency care and treatment of diabetes-related complica-

> **Key Point**
>
> Wound healing is often delayed in patients who have diabetes due to inflammation and altered glucose levels (Salazar, Ennis, & Koh, 2016).

tions such as retinopathy, neuropathy, and macrovascular problems that increase the risk of stroke and cardiac events (Centers for Disease Control and Prevention, 2018a; Leontis & Hess-Fischl, 2019).

Medical management of diabetes involves maintaining blood glucose levels within normal range (A1C <5.7% or fasting plasma glucose <100 mg/dL; American Diabetes Association, 2019). Episodes of hypo- or hyperglycemia should be appropriately managed (see Chapter 16, Symptom Management) and systemic complications minimized. However, in patients who have active and incurable comorbidities, care plans must be individualized to prioritize comfort and quality of life. Invasive and painful interventions such as blood glucose monitoring should be discontinued when they no longer contribute to the patient's quality of life. The administration of insulin and oral antihyperglycemics should be adjusted according to the patient's nutritional intake and symptoms (Dunning, Savage, Duggan, & Martin, 2014).

CONCLUSION

Endocrine disorders are commonly encountered in hospice and palliative care settings and must be managed in a way that promotes the patient's quality of life. When interventions are discontinued, extensive teaching and family support are needed. The nurse should frequently review the goals of care with the patient and family and ensure that interventions to promote comfort are undertaken.

Chapter Summary

- Endocrine disorders stem from dysfunction of one or more of the organs in the endocrine system.

- Dysfunction of the pituitary gland or of the thyroid itself can result in hypothyroidism or hyperthyroidism. Hypothyroidism is defined as TSH levels greater than 4.5 mIU/L. Hyperthyroidism results from overproduction of T_4 and/or T_3. Most (60%–80%) of patients who have hyperthyroidism have Graves' disease. Medical treatment involves antithyroid medications such as methimazole or propylthiouracil. Beta-blockers are used to control adrenergic symptoms.

- Diabetes is a metabolic disorder characterized by abnormal insulin production or action. Diabetes is categorized as either type 1 (T1DM) or type 2 (T2DM). T1DM occurs most frequently in children and adolescents and is characterized by lack of insulin production. T2DM is primarily characterized by insulin resistance rather than the absence of insulin production.

- At the end of life, interventions that are painful or invasive should be discontinued. Patient and family teaching are necessary to alleviate fear and anxiety related to discontinuation of interventions.

PRACTICE QUESTIONS

1. A hospice patient who has a long-standing history of hypothyroidism is actively dying from complications of cardiac disease. The patient is no longer able to take oral medications. The nurse should

   a. Obtain liquid levothyroxine

   b. Administer the levothyroxine topically

   c. Hold the levothyroxine

   d. Maintain open intravenous (IV) access

2. Hyperthyroidism is associated with

   a. Graves' disease

   b. Myxedema coma

   c. Infertility

   d. Hearing loss

3. Beta-blockers may be used to treat symptoms of

   a. Diabetes

   b. Hypothyroidism

   c. Hyperthyroidism

   d. b and c

4. Most patients who have type 1 diabetes have

   a. Obesity

   b. Childhood onset

   c. Family history of diabetes

   d. Insulin resistance

5. Which of the following is an expected finding in a terminally ill patient with a lengthy history of type 2 diabetes?

   a. Obesity

   b. Jaundice

   c. Delayed wound healing

   d. Altered levels of consciousness

■ REFERENCES

American Diabetes Association. (2019). *Diagnosing diabetes and learning about prediabetes*. Retrieved from http://www.diabetes.org/diabetes-basics/diagnosis/

American Thyroid Association. (2019). *General information*. Retrieved from https://www.thyroid.org/media-main/press-room/

Brashers, V. L., Jones, R. E., & Huether, S. E. (2014). Mechanisms of hormonal regulation. In K. L. McCance & S. E. Huether (Eds.), *Pathophysiology: The biologic basis for disease in adults and children* (7th ed., pp. 689–714). St. Louis, MO: Elsevier.

Centers for Disease Control and Prevention. (2018a). *Coexisting conditions and complications*. Retrieved from https://www.cdc.gov/diabetes/data/statistics-report/coexisting.html

Centers for Disease Control and Prevention. (2018b). *Risk factors for complications*. Retrieved from https://www.cdc.gov/diabetes/data/statistics-report/risks-complications.html

DeLeo, S., Lee, S. Y., & Braverman, L. E. (2016). Hyperthyroidism. *Lancet, 388*(10047), 906–918. doi:10.1016/S0140-6736(16)00278-6

Dunning, T., Savage, S., Duggan, N., & Martin, P. (2014). Palliative and end of life care for people with diabetes: A topical issue. *Diabetes Management, 4*(5), 449–460. Retrieved from https://www.openaccessjournals.com/articles/palliative-and-end-of-life-care-for-people-with-diabetes-a-topical-issue.pdf

Eledrisi, M. S. (2018). *Myxedema coma or crisis*. Retrieved from https://emedicine.medscape.com/article/123577-overview

Kravets, I. (2016). Hyperthyroidism: Diagnosis and treatment. *American Family Physician, 93*(5), 363–370. Retrieved from https://pdfs.semanticscholar.org/8000/d629a10dbf38665d073a5091c35fc202995f.pdf

Leontis, L. M., & Hess-Fischl, A. (2019). *Type 2 diabetes complications*. Retrieved from https://www.endocrineweb.com/conditions/type-2-diabetes/type-2-diabetes-complications

Levesque, C. (2012). Endocrine problems. In J. G. W. Foster & S. S. Prevost (Eds.), *Advanced practice nursing of adults in acute care* (pp. 444–524). Philadelphia, PA: F.A. Davis.

Mayo Clinic. (2019). *Hypothyroidism (Underactive thyroid)*. Retrieved from https://www.mayoclinic.org/diseases-conditions/hypothyroidism/symptoms-causes/syc-20350284

Orlander, P. R., Varghese, J. V., & Freeman, L. M. (2018). *Hypothyroidism*. Retrieved from https://emedicine.medscape.com/article/122393-overview#a5

Salazar, J. J., Ennis, W. J., & Koh, T. (2016). Diabetes medications: Impact on inflammation and wound healing. *Journal of Diabetic Complications, 30*(4), 746–752. doi:10.1016/j.jdiacomp.2015.12.017

Sargis, R. M. (2018). *How your thyroid works*. Retrieved from https://www.endocrineweb.com/conditions/thyroid/how-your-thyroid-works

12 Immunologic Disorders

You can't be involved in healthcare without being involved in the battle against AIDS.
—Wolfowitz (2006)

LEARNING OBJECTIVES

After completing this section, the nurse will be able to

1. Identify signs of decline in HIV-positive patients
2. Discuss symptom management for patients who have HIV
3. Relate hospice admission criteria to a terminal diagnosis of HIV/AIDS

THE IMMUNE SYSTEM

The sole purpose of the immune system is to protect the individual from potentially harmful antigens. Generally, immune responses involve the production and/or mobilization of lymphocytes (T cells, B cells, and natural killer [NK] cells), neutrophils, and monocytes/macrophages. Alterations in the proper functioning of the immune system result in exaggerated immune response (allergy), immune response toward one's own cells (autoimmunity), immune response to tissues that are intended to be helpful such as transfusions or organ or tissue transplants (alloimmunity), or breakdown of the immune system (immune deficiency; Rote & McCance, 2014).

Any alteration in the functioning of the immune system can cause serious harm to the host, and some can be fatal. Terminality is a consideration when a systematic immunological disease is severe and refractory. The HIV specifically attacks and devastates the immune system. It is the only immunological disease cited as a primary terminal diagnosis for admission to hospice. Thus, the remainder of this chapter will focus on HIV.

HIV

HIV-positive status was once considered a death sentence. But, due to the advanced treatments that have been developed in recent decades, HIV is now considered a serious chronic illness.

> **Key Point**
>
> Roughly 20% to 25% of individuals who are HIV-positive are unaware of their status (U.S. Department of Health and Human Services, 2018b).

The hallmark characteristic of HIV, as with other immune deficiency disorders, is the patient's tendency to present with infections that are normally not pathogenic, such as *Pneumocystis jirovecii* (formerly called *Pneumocystis carinii*), widespread and recurrent candida infections, cytomegalovirus, and others.

Symptoms of HIV

When a patient initially contracts HIV, flu-like symptoms such as fever, fatigue, anorexia, insomnia, headache, dyspnea, diarrhea, lymphedema, and sore throat appear (Gorman, 2015; Kirton & Sherman, 2015). In addition to succumbing to opportunistic infections, the patient who has immune deficiency

> **Key Point**
>
> Comorbidities often seen in patients who have HIV include the following:
>
> - Hepatitis A, B, and/or C
> - Bone disorders like osteoporosis
> - Anemia
> - Altered fat distribution (Gorman, 2015)

is also at risk for recurrent bronchitis, otitis, cystitis, or sepsis, despite treatment (Rote & McCance, 2014). In some cases, the patient may experience no symptoms or symptoms so mild that they do not seek medical treatment until the condition worsens. HIV is suspected when the patient is aware of exposure, has recurrent or multiple opportunistic infections, or has an unexpected decrease in T cells.

Those at highest risk for contracting HIV are those who

- Have unprotected sex
- Exchange sex for money
- Use injection drugs
- Have partners who use injection drugs or are HIV positive

Screening of at-risk individuals is possible using rapid blood or sputum testing. The results from these tests are available within 5 to 40 minutes. Although rapid testing is useful for screening, positive results from these tests must be confirmed through conventional methods (U.S. Preventative Task Force, 2016) because "one-third of acute viral infections give false negative results" (Zulfiqar et al., 2017, p. 6) in rapid testing. Early diagnosis and treatment of HIV can prolong the patient's life and decrease the possibility of transmission to another person (U.S. Preventative Task Force, 2016).

Diagnosing HIV

When symptoms of HIV are suspected, the first diagnostic test of choice is the enzyme-linked immunosorbent assay (ELISA) test. The ELISA test is not considered to be definitive, so the Western blot test is used to confirm a positive ELISA test. If the Western blot test is positive, the treatment plan will include antiretroviral therapy (ART; see Table 12.1) and sometimes prophylactic antibiotics.

A diagnosis of HIV simply means that the patient has contracted the virus and must strictly adhere to an antiviral medication regimen. In some cases, especially in patients with multiple comorbidities, CD4 counts can drop even with adherence to the antiviral regimen.

Table 12.1 Antiretroviral Therapy

Category	Action	Examples
NRTIs	Block the action of reverse transcriptase, which prevents replication of the virus	Zidovudine (Retrovir), tenofovir (Viread), lamivudine (Epivir), emtricitabine (Emtriva), abacavir (Ziagen)
NNRTIs	Bind to reverse transcriptase and alter it, which prevents replication of the virus	Efavirenz (Sustiva), etravirine (Intelence), nevirapine (Viramune/Viramun XR [extended release]), rilpivine (Edurant)
Fusion inhibitors	Block HIV from entering the host's CD4 cells	Enfuviritide (Fuzeon)
CCR5 antagonists	Block CCR5 coreceptors on immune cells, which prevents the virus from entering the cell	Maraviroc (Selzentry)
Integrase inhibitors	Block the action of integrase, an enzyme that is important in the process of HIV replication	Dolutegravir (Tivicay), raltegravir (Isentress)
Postattachment inhibitors	Block CD4 receptors on certain immune cells, which prevents HIV from entering the cell	Ibakizumab (Trogarzo)

NNRTIs, nonnucleoside reverse transcriptase inhibitors; NRTIs, nucleoside reverse transcriptase inhibitors.
Sources: U.S. Department of Health and Human Services. (2018a). FDA-approved HIV medicines. Retrieved from https://aidsinfo.nih.gov/understanding-hiv-aids/fact-sheets/21/58/fda-approved-hiv-medicines; U.S. Food & Drug Administration. (2018). Antiretroviral drugs used in the treatment of HIV infection. Retrieved from https://www.fda.gov/ForPatients/Illness/HIVAIDS/Treatment/ucm118915.htm

Patients who are diagnosed with HIV are at risk for

- Opportunistic infections
- Specific cancers
- Neurological manifestations of HIV
- Numerous side effects of ARTs
- Depression and anxiety
  (Gorman, 2015; Kirton & Sherman, 2015)

Stages of HIV

According to the U.S. Department of Health and Human Services (2018b), there are three stages of HIV infection. These stages are acute HIV, chronic HIV, and AIDS. Each of these stages are described as follows:

Acute HIV is the earliest stage of infection and occurs within 2 to 4 weeks of exposure. In this stage, the patient may experience flu-like symptoms as the virus rapidly multiplies and begins to destroy CD4 cells. In acute HIV, the viral load is very high and the infection is easily spread. In the absence of early diagnosis and treatment, the infection will worsen dramatically and will progress rapidly.

Chronic HIV infection ensues after initial contraction of the virus. The virus continues to replicate, but at a slower pace than during the acute phase. The patient may be asymptomatic but can still transmit the virus to others. Without treatment, the disease will progress to AIDS within 10 years.

AIDS is the most severe stage of HIV infection. AIDS is diagnosed when the CD4 count drops below $200/mm^3$. When this occurs, it indicates that the immune system is failing and the patient is vulnerable to numerous and potentially deadly infections (Gorman, 2015). Because the patient is immunologically compromised, even a seemingly minor infection can be physically overwhelming. Opportunistic infections may emerge as immunity decreases. Without treatment, the prognosis is roughly 3 years from the onset of this stage.

Treatment

In order to reap the full benefit of pharmacological treatment (see Table 12.1), the patient must strictly adhere to the prescribed treatment regimen or risk viral devastation of the immune system. In fact, adherence to antiviral medications is so important that it is considered the most significant predictor of positive long-term prognosis (Gorman, 2015). Compliance is related to the complexity of the drug regimen, the severity of the patient's symptoms, younger age of the patient, presence of mental illness, and the availability of a support network (Gorman, 2015).

The chronicity and incurability of HIV contributes to anxiety and depression. Many antidepressants and anxiolytics are available that can be used in conjunction with ART. Goals of care in the early stages of HIV should center on maximizing function and longevity within the limits of the disease process and preventing transmission of the virus (Centers for Disease Control and Prevention, 2017). Because "patients with AIDS . . . experience bouts of severe illness and debilitation alternating with periods of symptom stabilization" (Kirton & Sherman, 2015, p. 630), palliative care should be incorporated into the treatment plan as early as possible.

The interdisciplinary team should focus on

- Prevention of potentially life-threatening infections
- Preventing transmission of HIV
- Health promotion (diet, exercise, stress management, emotional support, immunizations)
- Managing side effects of treatment
- Managing exacerbations
- Provision of spiritual support for patient and family
- Formulation of an advance care plan
- Routine clinical examinations and laboratory testing
- Teaching regarding the importance of adherence to treatment regimen
  (Gorman, 2015; Kirton & Sherman, 2015)

End-of-Life Considerations

As HIV/AIDS progresses, common symptoms include pain, fatigue, anemia, weight loss, cough, fever, dyspnea, diarrhea, skin lesions, opportunistic infections, arthritis, arthralgia, and stomatitis (Gorman, 2015).

Nursing care for patients who have HIV or AIDS entails

- Monitoring for signs of worsening condition
- Reviewing medication list for potential drug–drug interactions
- Promoting compliance with the drug regimen
- Addressing sequelae of the HIV infection as they arise

The nurse must also monitor for opportunistic infections and malignancies such as

- Lymphoma
- Kaposi's sarcoma
- Tuberculosis

- Thrush
- Candida esophagitis
- Herpes simplex esophagitis
- Idiopathic esophageal ulcer
- Microsporidiosis
- Cryptosporidiosis
- Mycobacterium avium complex
- Cytomegalovirus
  (Kirton & Sherman, 2015).

Disease Trajectory

The terminal phase of HIV/AIDS is usually preceded by marked weight loss and noticeable physical and mental decline. In the final stages, the patient may be bedbound with physical wasting, dyspnea at rest, decubitus, fever, and changes in mentation. Care should be focused on the treatment of symptoms such as pain, dyspnea, and fever. The actual cause of death may be related to overwhelming infection, cancer, neurological disease, malnutrition, or multisystem organ failure (Kirton & Sherman, 2015).

Hospice Criteria

When signs of disease progression become apparent and the patient's goals are consistent with foregoing curative care, hospice care should be considered when the patient has either

1A: CD4+ less than 25 cells/mcL

or

1B: Persistent viral load greater than 100,000

and at least one of the following:

- Central nervous system (CNS) lymphoma
- Untreated or refractory wasting (loss of more than 33% lean body mass)
- Mycobacterium avium complex bacteremia (untreated)
- Progressive multifocal leukoencephalopathy
- Systemic lymphoma
- Visceral Kaposi's sarcoma
- Renal failure with no dialysis
- Cryptosporidium infection
- Refractory toxoplasmosis
  and
- Palliative Performance Scale (PPS) score of less than 50%

▪ CONCLUSION

HIV is a chronic but life-threatening disease that affects all aspects of an individual's life. Rapid screening tests can be used for at-risk individuals, but positive results should be confirmed with conventional methods. Treatment includes the use of antiretroviral agents as well as adjuvants to treat anxiety, depression, pain, and other symptoms that may arise. Spiritual, emotional, and psychological care and support should be provided by an interdisciplinary team from the time of diagnosis. When the disease progresses to the terminal phase, discussions regarding end-of-life wishes, including hospice eligibility, should take place.

Chapter Summary

- The immune system provides protection from potentially harmful antigens. Immunological diseases can affect multiple body systems and can be fatal.

- HIV is cited as a primary terminal diagnosis for hospice admission.

- Risk factors for HIV include having unprotected sex, exchanging sex for money, using injection drugs, and having partners who use injection drugs or are HIV positive.

- The hallmark characteristic of HIV is the tendency to succumb to unusual infections on a regular basis.

- At the time of infection with HIV, the patient may experience flu-like symptoms. HIV is suspected when the patient is aware of exposure, has recurrent opportunistic infections, or has a sudden drop in T cells.

- Rapid HIV screening involves blood or sputum testing and results are usually available within 5 to 40 minutes. However, rapid screening has a high potential for false negative results.

- The Western blot test should be used to confirm a positive ELISA test. If the Western blot test is positive, then ART should be initiated.

- The stages of HIV infection are acute HIV, chronic HIV, and AIDS. Acute HIV occurs in the first 1 to 2 weeks after exposure and involves the onset of flu-like symptoms, which later subside. Chronic HIV sets in after the acute phase. The rate of viral replication slows, but the patient can still transmit the virus. Without treatment, the disease will progress to AIDS. AIDS is the most severe form of HIV infection and is diagnosed when CD4 counts drop below $200/mm^3$. Without treatment, the predicted mortality is roughly 3 years.

- The most significant predictor of mortality is adherence to the drug regimen.

- As HIV/AIDS progresses, common symptoms include pain, fatigue, anemia, weight loss, cough, fever, dyspnea, diarrhea, skin lesions, opportunistic infections, arthritis, arthralgia, and stomatitis.

- Treatment includes the use of antiretroviral agents as well as adjuvants to treat anxiety, depression, pain, and other symptoms that may arise. Spiritual, emotional, and psychological care and support should be provided by an interdisciplinary team from the time of diagnosis.

- The terminal phase of HIV/AIDS is usually preceded by marked weight loss and noticeable physical and mental decline. In the final stages, the patient may be bedbound with physical wasting, dyspnea at rest, decubti, fever, and changes in mentation.

- Palliative care should be initiated early in the disease process to minimize symptomatology.

- End-of-life care should be discussed when the burden of treatment outweighs the benefit or when it is consistent with the patient's goals.

▪ PRACTICE QUESTIONS

1. A palliative care nurse is assessing a patient who has HIV for depression. Which of the following statements, if made by the patient, would alert the nurse to the need for further evaluation and treatment?

   a. "My medication regimen is overwhelming."

   b. "Two of my closest friends died recently of AIDS and I'm afraid I'm next."

   c. "I find it very hard to sleep because I just keep thinking about my illness."

   d. "Sometimes I wonder if I'd just be better off dead."

2. Which of the following nursing diagnoses is the highest priority for a patient with chronic HIV?

   a. Risk for infection

   b. Noncompliance with medication regimen

   c. Knowledge deficit regarding needle safety

   d. Potential for altered nutrition

3. A patient who has a primary diagnosis of hepatitis C tells the palliative care nurse that he may have been exposed to HIV recently. The nurse's best response is

   a. "If you are taking antiviral medications for hepatitis C, you won't manifest HIV."

   b. "Tell me more about your potential exposure."

   c. "You should begin antiviral therapy right away."

   d. "We can screen you for HIV now using a rapid test."

4. A patient who has chronic HIV is overheard telling the hospice chaplain that "my CD4 count is up so I'm not contagious now." The nurse should

   a. Inform the chaplain that the patient can still transmit the virus

   b. Ask the patient what her last CD4 count was

   c. Provide patient education regarding disease transmission

   d. Assure the patient that her assessment of her condition is correct

5. Which if the following infections would alert the palliative care nurse to the need for HIV screening of a patient?

   a. Chronic sinusitis

   b. Recurrent strep throat

   c. *Pneumocystis jirovecii*

   d. Hepatitis A

6. Which of the following statements, if made by the spouse of a hospice patient with a primary diagnosis of HIV, would alert the nurse to a need for further education?

    a. "I will call you right away if I see signs of infection."

    b. "I don't need to wear gloves when changing his bed."

    c. "I'm glad I can still kiss him goodnight."

    d. "We share insulin needles to save money, but I clean them with alcohol before I use them."

7. A 73-year-old hospice patient with AIDS asks the nurse if any of his daily activities should be stopped. Which of the following should the nurse recommend stopping?

    a. Grocery shopping

    b. Picking up his grandchild from day care

    c. Going to church

    d. Walking his dog

8. On an initial visit with a patient who has been newly diagnosed with HIV, the highest priority of the palliative care team is

    a. Reinforcing the need for medication compliance

    b. Developing an advance directive

    c. Managing treatment side effects

    d. Encouraging health-promoting activities

9. A patient who has AIDS recently began taking an opioid medication for pain. The patient reported fatigue and dry mouth after taking the opioid. The nurse knows that the symptoms are

    a. Related to the antiviral medications

    b. An interaction between the opioid and the antiviral medications

    c. Side effects of the opioid

    d. Signs of a decrease in CD4 cells

10. The family of an actively dying patient who has a primary diagnosis of AIDS informs the nurse that the patient is disoriented to time and place. The nurse should

    a. Request inpatient care for the patient

    b. Start supplemental oxygen

    c. Arrange a family meeting with the hospice team

    d. Assure the family that these changes are expected at this stage of the disease process

▪ REFERENCES

Centers for Disease Control and Prevention. (2017). *Recommendations for HIV screening of gay, bisexual, and other men who have sex with men – United States, 2017.* Retrieved from https://www.cdc.gov/mmwr/volumes/66/wr/mm6631a3.htm

Gorman, L. M. (2015). The palliative advanced practice registered nurse in the specialty outpatient setting. In C. Dahlin, P. J. Coyne, & B. R. Ferrell (Eds.), *Advanced practice palliative nursing* (pp. 151–158). New York, NY: Oxford University Press.

Kirton, C. A., & Sherman, D. W. (2015). Patients with acquired immunodeficiency syndrome. In B. R. Ferrell, N. Coyle, & J. A. Paice (Eds.), *Oxford textbook of palliative nursing* (4th ed., pp. 628–649). New York, NY: Oxford University Press.

Rote, N. S., & McCance, K. L. (2014). Alterations in immunity and inflammation. In K. L. McCance & S. E. Huether (Eds.), *Pathophysiology: The biologic basis for disease in adults and children* (7th ed., pp. 262–297). St. Louis, MO: Elsevier.

U.S. Department of Health and Human Services. (2018a). *FDA approved HIV medicines.* Retrieved from https://aidsinfo.nih.gov/understanding-hiv-aids/fact-sheets/21/58/fda-approved-hiv-medicines

U.S. Department of Health and Human Services. (2018b). *The stages of HIV infection.* Retrieved from https://aidsinfo.nih.gov/understanding-hiv-aids/fact-sheets/19/46/the-stages-of-hiv-infection

U.S. Food and Drug Administration. (2018). *Antiretroviral drugs used in the treatment of HIV infection.* Retrieved from https://www.fda.gov/ForPatients/Illness/HIVAIDS/Treatment/ucm118915.htm

U.S. Preventive Task Force. (2016). *Human immunodeficiency virus (HIV) infection: Screening.* Retrieved from https://www.uspreventiveservicestaskforce.org/Page/Document/RecommendationStatementFinal/human-immunodeficiency-virus-hiv-infection-screening

Wolfowitz, P. (2006, October 29). Interview with Paul Wolfowitz – full transcript/Interviewers: F. Grouigneau & R. Hiault. *Financial Times.* Retrieved from https://www.ft.com/content/3836c4c4-6787-11db-8ea5-0000779e2340

Zulfiqar, H. F., Javed, A., Sumbal, Afroze, B., Ali, Q., Akbar, K., . . . Husnain, T (2017). HIV diagnosis and treatment through advanced technologies. *Frontiers in Public Health, 5*(32), 1–16. doi:10.3389/fpubh.2017.00032

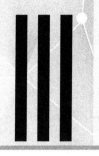

13

Pain Assessment

Pain is whatever the experiencing person says it is,
existing whenever he says it does.
—McCaffery (1968, p. 95)

LEARNING OBJECTIVES

After completing this section, the nurse will be able to

1. Distinguish between acute and chronic pain
2. Identify types of pain according to the description (i.e., somatic, visceral, neuropathic)
3. Discuss how chronic pain affects the whole person
4. Choose tools to determine a patient's risk for opioid misuse

PAIN OVERVIEW

Pain is "an unpleasant sensory and emotional experience associated with actual or potential tissue damage, or described in terms of such damage" (International Association for the Study of Pain, 2017). Physiologically, pain signals travel through the nervous system and are then interpreted through the following process (see Figure 13.1):

- The afferent pathways send pain signals to the spinal gate in the dorsal horn of the peripheral nervous system and then to the central nervous system (CNS)
- Pain signals travel to the brainstem, mid-brain, diencephalon, and the cerebral cortex, where they are interpreted
- Pain is modulated within the efferent pathways of the CNS (Huether, Rodway, & DeFriez, 2014).

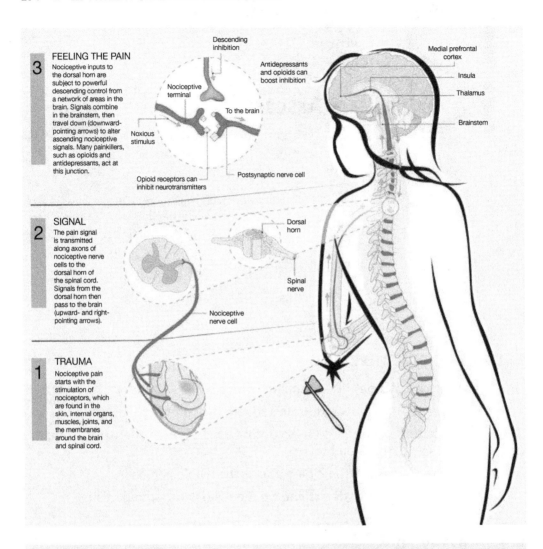

FEELING THE PAIN

Nociceptive inputs to the dorsal horn are subject to powerful descending control from a network of areas in the brain. Signals combine in the brainstem, then travel down (downward-pointing arrows) to alter ascending nociceptive signals. Many painkillers, such as opioids and antidepressants, act at this junction.

Descending inhibition

Nociceptive terminal

Noxious stimulus

To the brain

Opioid receptors can inhibit neurotransmitters

Postsynaptic nerve cell

Antidepressants and opioids can boost inhibition

Medial prefrontal cortex

Insula

Thalamus

Brainstem

SIGNAL

The pain signal is transmitted along axons of nociceptive nerve cells to the dorsal horn of the spinal cord. Signals from the dorsal horn then pass to the brain (upward- and right-pointing arrows).

Dorsal horn

Spinal nerve

Nociceptive nerve cell

TRAUMA

Nociceptive pain starts with the stimulation of nociceptors, which are found in the skin, internal organs, muscles, joints, and the membranes around the brain and spinal cord.

FIGURE 13.1 Pain pathway.

Source: Holmes, D. (2016). The pain drain. *Nature, 535,* S2–S3. Retrieved from https://www.nature.com/articles/535S2a#rightslink

In clinical practice, pain is categorized by the length of time it lasts. Acute pain is related to immediate harm; it is a signal to withdraw from the source of the pain. Acute pain has a sudden onset and lasts for only a few seconds to minutes. The pain usually diminishes when the noxious stimulus is removed. However, there are several autonomic symptoms that are associated with acute pain including tachycardia, hypertension, diaphoresis, and pupillary dilation (Huether et al., 2014). Acute pain is most often related to cutaneous and deep somatic tissue injury or visceral organ insult. Thus, acute pain can be more specifically described as somatic or visceral (see Figure 13.2).

In contrast to acute pain, chronic pain lasts at least 3 months, which is beyond the expected healing time for most injuries. Unlike acute pain,

Acute pain

Somatic pain
Arises from injured connective tissue, muscle, skin, or bone injury. Often described as sharp and well-localized but can also be dull, achy, throbbing, and poorly localized.

Visceral pain
Arises from internal organs and/or viscera. Usually dull, achy, gnawing, or crampy. Sometimes associated with nausea, vomiting, hypotension, restlessness, and/or shock. Often radiates away from site of injury.

FIGURE 13.2 Acute pain.

chronic pain serves no useful purpose (Huether et al., 2014). Symptoms that are sometimes associated with chronic pain include the following:

- Depression
- Poor appetite
- Insomnia
- Preoccupation with the pain
- Avoidance of activities that provoke the pain (Huether et al., 2014)

Because of the multidimensional sources of suffering associated with chronic pain, patients can develop one or more manifestations of chronic pain or chronic pain syndromes. According to Huether et al. (2014), these may include the following:

Specific and nonspecific low back pain is usually recurrent, refractory, and causes impaired mobility and, in some cases, complete debilitation.

Myofascial pain syndrome (MPS) is related to injury to the muscles, fascia, and/or tendons. Diagnoses related to MPS are myositis, fibrositis, myofibrositis, myalgias, or muscle strain. In the early stages of MPS, the pain is generally sharp and localized but becomes dull, achy, and diffuse over time.

Neuropathic pain originates in the central or peripheral nervous system and is usually described as shooting, burning, stabbing, tingling, or as pins and needles. There are two types of neuropathic pain: peripheral and central. Peripheral neuropathic pain is typically caused by trauma to the peripheral nerves and can result from diabetic neuropathy, nutritional deficiencies, HIV, or carcinoma. This type of pain can be evoked by activity and allodynia may be present. Central neuropathic pain is caused by dysfunction of the CNS (brain or spinal cord), which primarily results from spinal cord trauma, tumors, vascular lesions, multiple sclerosis, Parkinson's disease, postherpetic neuralgia, phantom limb pain, and/or reflex sympathetic dystrophy.

Radicular pain results from compression of the nerve root(s) in the neck or spine. This type of pain is usually related to sciatica, injury, compression, herniated disk, foraminal stenosis, or inflammation. It is often described as sharp, stabbing, and radiating from the spine or neck to the arms or legs.

Complex regional pain syndrome (CRPS) can result from major or minor injury and presents primarily as neuropathic pain; it often involves allodynia. Associated symptoms are diaphoresis, vascular changes, asthenia, and in advanced cases, disuse of the affected limb. If diagnosed early, physical therapy and nerve blocks help to prolong functionality.

Key Point
Pain that is felt in an area other than where it originates is called referred pain. Both acute and chronic pain can be referred.

Chronic postoperative pain is a CRPS that may involve phantom limb pain, chronic donor site pain, postthoracotomy pain syndrome, postmastectomy pain syndrome, and joint arthroplasty pain. Treatment of this type of pain must be multimodal to ameliorate both the acute and chronic aspects.

Cancer pain is chronic and associated with neuropathies and/or paresthesias. Cancer pain can be related to tumor growth, treatments, or coexisting diseases. Frequent assessment of the source, severity, and character of the pain is necessary as these can change rapidly depending on disease progression. Management of this type of pain requires both long-acting and short-acting interventions.

Pain Assessment

Although pain clearly has a physiologic basis, McCaffery's (1968) well-accepted definition of pain emphasizes the primacy of the patient's experience and personal description of his or her pain. McCaffery's definition states that "pain is whatever the experiencing person says it is, existing whenever he says it does" (p. 95). Thus, the cornerstone of good pain management is masterful assessment, which is predicated on gathering both subjective and objective data.

Subjective data include the patient's perception of pain in terms of intensity, temporality, radiating nature, and character. Objective data that lends clarity to the pain assessment includes the patient's medical history. For example, a long-standing diagnosis of type 2 diabetes increases the likelihood of neuropathic pain. Similarly, an athlete may be more prone to somatic pain related to muscle injury.

Other objective data include physical manifestations of pain such as tachypnea, tachycardia, diaphoresis, guarding, grimacing, and/or rebound tenderness. Objective assessment data are secondary to the patient's report because pain is wholly a subjective experience. Objective assessment data, however, is used to support the patient's reports and to draw conclusions about the source and nature of the pain.

Gathering data about the patient's pain is best done in a methodical way. One common way of assessing pain is through the P-Q-R-S-T mnemonic, which provides an organized approach to pain assessment (see Figure 13.3).

P: Palliative and provocative factors

Ask: What makes the pain better or worse?

• The patient's response to this question helps the nurse to determine whether the pain regimen is effective or needs to be modified according to the patient's report.

Q: Quality of the pain

Ask: Please describe what the pain feels like to you.

• The words the patient uses to describe the pain help the nurse to differentiate what type of pain the patient is experiencing.
• **Neuropathic pain** is generally described as burning, tingling, shocking, shooting, radiating, numbness, 'pins and needles'.
• **Visceral pain** is generally described as gnawing, stretching, pressure, crampy, deep, poorly localized.
• **Somatic pain** is generally described as dull, sore, throbbing.

R: Radiation

Ask: Is the pain in one area? Can you point to it? Does it travel or radiate?

• The response to this question helps to differentiate neuropathic from somatic pain or visceral pain.
• Pain that is well-localized is generally somatic. Pain that radiates is usually neuropathic. Visceral pain is often poorly localized.

S: Severity

Ask: Can you tell me how bad the pain is on a scale of 1 to 10? One means the pain is barely noticeable and 10 means it is the worst pain you have ever felt.

• The patient's response to this question provides a snapshot of how intense the pain is for the patient right now. It also helps the patient and nurse determine if goals are met after intervention.

T: Timing

Ask: Does the pain seem to be better or worse at a certain time of the day? When did it start? How long does it last? Does it ever wake you up?

• The patient's response to this question helps determine whether the pain is due to muscle fatigue, arthritis, or immobility. It is also useful in planning the timing of interventions to alleviate the pain.

FIGURE 13.3 Pain assessment.

The P-Q-R-S-T assessment relies heavily on the patient's self-report of the pain experience. Yet some patients are not able to express their feelings or to answer assessment questions appropriately. For patients who are unable to speak, such as those very near death, or those who have dysarthria or dysphasia, an appropriate scale should be used to routinely and uniformly assess and document the patient's level of comfort. One such tool is the Face, Legs, Activity, Cry, Consolability (FLACC) scale (see Figure 13.4). The FLACC scale was originally developed for use in children (Merkel, Voepel-Lewis, Shayevitz, & Malviya, 1997), but has been used in many other settings with nonverbal patients.

Another tool used for nonverbal patients is the Wong–Baker FACES Scale (Wong & Baker, 1988). Although the scale was originally developed for uniform pain assessment in children, it has been used in numerous settings and has been translated in several languages. The translation of the tool that matches the patient's preferred language should be used to avoid cultural misinterpretation of the facial expressions.

A similar tool, the Faces Pain Scale-Revised (FPS-R) was also developed for use in children. The facial expressions differ from the Wong–Baker FACES Scale in that they do not include smiles or tears (International Association for the Study of Pain, 2018), which may be interpreted as happiness or sadness rather than the absence or presence of pain (Figure 13.5). The FPS-R is recommended for children under the age of 8 because after this age most children can report pain using a traditional 0 to 10 scale (International Association for the Study of Pain, 2018). However, the FPS-R has been used in many aggregates who cannot adequately express their pain verbally, including adults who have physical or cognitive deficits (cf., Kim & Buschmann, 2006; Ware, Epps, Herr, & Packard, 2006).

A pain scale that was developed specifically for patients who have dementia is the Pain Assessment in Advanced Dementia (PAINAD) scale (see Figure 13.6; Warden, Hurley, & Volicer, 2003). In addition to dementia, the patients who were part of the original validation study for this tool were aphasic or otherwise lacked the ability to communicate their level of pain verbally. The PAINAD includes only five items, so it is a quick assessment for nonverbal patients that is easy to use in the clinical setting (Ware et al., 2006).

Factors That Influence the Pain Experience and the Expression of Pain

Pain, especially chronic or intractable pain, permeates every aspect of a patient's life. Ferrell and Rhiner (1991) have offered a comprehensive depiction of how pain impacts not only the patient's physical well-being but also diminishes the patient's psychological, psychosocial, and spiritual well-being (see Figure 13.7).

FLACC Behavioral Pain Assessment Scale			
CATEGORIES	SCORING		
	0	1	2
Face	No particular expression or smile	Occasional grimace or frown; withdrawn, disinterested	Frequent to constant frown, clenched jaw, quivering chin
Legs	Normal position or relaxed	Uneasy, restless, tense	Kicking or legs drawn up
Activity	Lying quietly, normal position, moves easily	Squirming, shifting back and forth, tense	Arched, rigid, or jerking
Cry	No cry (awake or asleep)	Moans or whimpers, occasional complaint	Crying steadily, screams or sobs; frequent complaints
Consolability	Content, relaxed	Reassured by occasional touching, hugging, or being talked to; distractable	Difficult to console or comfort

How to Use the FLACC

In patients who are awake: observe for 1 to 5 minutes or longer. Observe legs and body uncovered. Reposition patient or observe activity. Assess body for tenseness and tone. Initiate consoling interventions if needed.

In patients who are asleep: observe for 5 minutes or longer. Observe body and legs uncovered. If possible, reposition the patient. Touch the body and assess for tenseness and tone.

Face
> Score 0 if the patient has a relaxed face, makes eye contact, shows interest in surroundings.
> Score 1 if the patient has a worried facial expression, with eyebrows lowered, eyes partially closed, cheeks raised, mouth pursed.
> Score 2 if the patient has deep furrows in the forehead, closed eyes, an open mouth, deep lines around nose and lips.

Legs
> Score 0 if the muscle tone and motion in the limbs are normal.
> Score 1 if patient has increased tone, rigidity, or tension; if there is intermittent flexion or extension of the limbs.
> Score 2 if patient has hypertonicity, the legs are pulled tight, there is exaggerated flexion or extension of the limbs, tremors.

Activity
> Score 0 if the patient moves easily and freely, normal activity or restrictions.
> Score 1 if the patient shifts positions, appears hesitant to move, demonstrates guarding, a tense torso, pressure on a body part.
> Score 2 if the patient is in a fixed position, rocking; demonstrates side-to-side head movement or rubbing of a body part.

Cry
> Score 0 if the patient has no cry or moan, awake or asleep.
> Score 1 if the patient has occasional moans, cries, whimpers, sighs.
> Score 2 if the patient has frequent or continuous moans, cries, grunts.

Consolability
> Score 0 if the patient is calm and does not require consoling.
> Score 1 if the patient responds to comfort by touching or talking in 30 seconds to 1 minute.
> Score 2 if the patient requires constant comforting or is inconsolable.

Whenever feasible, behavioral measurement of pain should be used in conjunction with self-report. When self-report is not possible, interpretation of pain behaviors and decisions regarding treatment of pain require careful consideration of the context in which the pain behaviors are observed.

Interpreting the Behavioral Score
Each category is scored on the 0–2 scale, which results in a total score of 0–10.

0 = Relaxed and comfortable	**4–6** = Moderate pain
1–3 = Mild discomfort	**7–10** = Severe discomfort or pain or both

FIGURE 13.4 FLACC scale.

Source: Merkel, S. I., Voepel-Lewis, T., Shayevitz, J. R., & Malviya, S. (1997). The FLACC: A behavioral scale for scoring postoperative pain in young children. *Pediatric Nursing, 23*(3), 293–297. The FLACC scale was developed by Sandra Merkel, MS, RN, Terri Voepel-Lewis, MS, RN, and Shobha Malviya, MD, at C. S. Mott Children's Hospital, University of Michigan Health System, Ann Arbor, MI. Used with permission.

Suffering in any of the identified areas decreases the patient's quality of life, as discussed as follows:

- The *physical dimension* of the pain experience involves the patient's perception of the pain in terms of the quality and severity of the pain. It also entails any related symptoms such as nausea, anxiety, depression, or sleep disturbance. Pain can also limit physical activity leading to immobility or weight gain, which further exacerbates the patient's physical limitations. Physical manifestations of pain may

Faces Pain Scale—Revised (FPS-R)

Instructions:
"The faces show how much pain or discomfort someone is feeling. The face on the left shows no pain. Each face shows more and more pain and the last face shows the worst pain possible. Point to the face that shows how bad your pain is right NOW."

Scoring: The score the chosen face as 0, 2, 4, 6, 8 or 10, counting left to right so 0 = "no pain" and 10 = "worst pain possible"

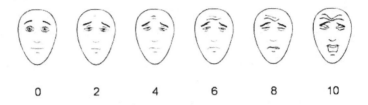

| 0 | 2 | 4 | 6 | 8 | 10 |

FIGURE 13.5 Faces Pain Scale–Revised.

Source: Used with permission from IASP; this figure may not be used or modified without express written consent from IASP. http://www.iasp-pain.org/Education/Content.aspx?ItemNumber= 1519&navItemNumber=577

also be related to activity or a particular time of day, which give clues to the source of the pain.

- *Psychological* well-being is inextricably intertwined with pain. Patients who experience pain, particularly on a long-term basis, are more apt to experience anxiety, depression, and hopelessness. Patients who have chronic pain must focus their attention on planning activities around their pain medications and how they feel on a day-to-day basis, which significantly impacts their quality of life. Reliable and valid measures such as the Patient Health Questionnaire (PHQ-9) depression screening tool (Kroenke, Spitzer, & Williams, 2001) and/or the General Anxiety Disorder (GAD-10) tool (Spitzer, Kroenke, Williams, & Lowe, 2006) should be used to screen patients for depression or anxiety that can result from unrelenting pain.

- In terms of the patient's social well-being, pain limits the patient's ability to engage in social and community activities without limitation. When the patient's ability to participate in daily activities is impacted by the pain and a caregiver is needed, the family dynamic is altered. Social dimensions impacted by severe or chronic pain include work, church attendance, shopping, and family or community activities. Withdrawal from such activities can lead to isolation, which furthers the patient's suffering.

  Social consequences of pain and the reporting of pain are also influenced by cultural norms and expectations. Acceptance and expression of pain are learned cultural responses (Peacock & Patel, 2008). The hospice nurse must be aware of cultural norms related to pain expression, while also avoiding stereotypes. To do this, it is recommended that the nurse ask the patient or caregiver whether there are

Pain Assessment in Advanced Dementia Scale (PAINAD)

Instructions: Observe the patient for five minutes before scoring his or her behaviors. Score the behaviors according to the following chart. Definitions of each item are provided on the following page. The patient can be observed under different conditions (e.g., at rest, during a pleasant activity, during caregiving, after the administration of pain medication).

Behavior	0	1	2	Score
Breathing Independent of vocalization	• Normal	• Occasional labored breathing • Short period of hyperventilation	• Noisy labored breathing • Long period of hyperventilation • Cheyne-Stokes respirations	
Negative vocalization	• None	• Occasional moan or groan • Low-level speech with a negative or disapproving quality	• Repeated troubled calling out • Loud moaning or groaning • Crying	
Facial expression	• Smiling or inexpressive	• Sad • Frightened • Frown	• Facial grimacing	
Body language	• Relaxed	• Tense • Distressed pacing • Fidgeting	• Rigid • Fists clenched • Knees pulled up • Pulling or pushing away • Striking out	
Consolability	• No need to console	• Distracted or reassured by voice or touch	• Unable to console, distract, or reassure	
			TOTAL SCORE	

(Warden et al., 2003)

Scoring:

The total score ranges from 0–10 points. A possible interpretation of the scores is: 1–3 = mild pain; 4–6 = moderate pain; 7–10 = severe pain. These ranges are based on a standard 0–10 scale of pain, but have not been substantiated in the literature for this tool.

Source:

Warden V, Hurley AC, Volicer L. Development and psychometric evaluation of the Pain Assessment in Advanced Dementia (PAINAD) scale. *J Am Med Dir Assoc.* 2003;4(1):9-15.

PAINAD Item Definitions

(Warden et al., 2003)

Breathing

1. *Normal breathing* is characterized by effortless, quiet, rhythmic (smooth) respirations.
2. *Occasional labored breathing* is characterized by episodic bursts of harsh, difficult, or wearing respirations.
3. *Short period of hyperventilation* is characterized by intervals of rapid, deep breaths lasting a short period of time.
4. *Noisy labored breathing* is characterized by negative-sounding respirations on inspiration or expiration. They may be loud, gurgling, wheezing. They appear strenuous or wearing.
5. *Long period of hyperventilation* is characterized by an excessive rate and depth of respirations lasting a considerable time.
6. *Cheyne-Stokes respirations* are characterized by rhythmic waxing and waning of breathing from very deep to shallow respirations with periods of apnea (cessation of breathing).

Negative Vocalization

1. *None* is characterized by speech or vocalization that has a neutral or pleasant quality.
2. *Occasional moan or groan* is characterized by mournful or murmuring sounds, wails, or laments. Groaning is characterized by louder than usual inarticulate involuntary sounds, often abruptly beginning and ending.
3. *Low level speech with a negative or disapproving quality* is characterized by muttering, mumbling, whining, grumbling, or swearing in a low volume with a complaining, sarcastic, or caustic tone.

FIGURE 13.6 PAINAD Tool.

Source: Warden, V., Hurley, A. C., & Volicer, L. (2003). Development and psychometric evaluation of the Pain Assessment in Advanced Dementia (PAINAD) scale. *Journal of the American Medical Directors Association,* 4(1), 9–15.

4. *Repeated troubled calling out* is characterized by phrases or words being used over and over in a tone that suggests anxiety, uneasiness, or distress.
5. *Loud moaning or groaning* is characterized by mournful or murmuring sounds, wails, or laments in much louder than usual volume. Loud groaning is characterized by louder than usual inarticulate involuntary sounds, often abruptly beginning and ending.
6. *Crying* is characterized by an utterance of emotion accompanied by tears. There may be sobbing or quiet weeping.

Facial Expression

1. *Smiling or inexpressive*. Smiling is characterized by upturned corners of the mouth, brightening of the eyes, and a look of pleasure or contentment. Inexpressive refers to a neutral, at ease, relaxed, or blank look.
2. *Sad* is characterized by an unhappy, lonesome, sorrowful, or dejected look. There may be tears in the eyes.
3. *Frightened* is characterized by a look of fear, alarm, or heightened anxiety. Eyes appear wide open.
4. *Frown* is characterized by a downward turn of the corners of the mouth. Increased facial wrinkling in the forehead and around the mouth may appear.
5. *Facial grimacing* is characterized by a distorted, distressed look. The brow is more wrinkled, as is the area around the mouth. Eyes may be squeezed shut.

Body Language

1. *Relaxed* is characterized by a calm, restful, mellow appearance. The person seems to be taking it easy.
2. *Tense* is characterized by a strained, apprehensive, or worried appearance. The jaw may be clenched. (Exclude any contractures.)
3. *Distressed pacing* is characterized by activity that seems unsettled. There may be a fearful, worried, or disturbed element present. The rate may be faster or slower.
4. *Fidgeting* is characterized by restless movement. Squirming about or wiggling in the chair may occur. The person might be hitching a chair across the room. Repetitive touching, tugging, or rubbing body parts can also be observed.
5. *Rigid* is characterized by stiffening of the body. The arms and/or legs are tight and inflexible. The trunk may appear straight and unyielding. (Exclude any contractures.)
6. *Fists clenched* is characterized by tightly closed hands. They may be opened and closed repeatedly or held tightly shut.
7. *Knees pulled up* is characterized by flexing the legs and drawing the knees up toward the chest. An overall troubled appearance. (Exclude any contractures.)
8. *Pulling or pushing away* is characterized by resistiveness upon approach or to care. The person is trying to escape by yanking or wrenching him- or herself free or shoving you away.
9. *Striking out* is characterized by hitting, kicking, grabbing, punching, biting, or other form of personal assault.

Consolability

1. *No need to console* is characterized by a sense of well-being. The person appears content.
2. *Distracted or reassured by voice or touch* is characterized by a disruption in the behavior when the person is spoken to or touched. The behavior stops during the period of interaction, with no indication that the person is at all distressed.
3. *Unable to console, distract, or reassure* is characterized by the inability to soothe the person or stop a behavior with words or actions. No amount of comforting, verbal or physical, will alleviate the behavior.

FIGURE 13.6 PAINAD Tool *(continued)*.

any culturally bound interventions that should be implemented to support the patient through her or his pain. Ways to promote "culturally comfortable" care include viewing each patient as a unique person and respecting the patient's perspective on his or her pain, promoting shared decision-making regarding interventions for pain, and adapting care to the patient's unique needs (Narayam, 2010).

- *Spiritual* well-being is impacted by severe or chronic pain as the patient tries to find deeper meaning in her or his suffering. Besides medicine, spirituality is a common source of solace for patients in pain (Kiser-Larson, 2017). Patient's may turn to her or his faith for strength to get through the difficulties related to pain, or alternatively, may lose faith due to suffering. The hospice nurse can use a brief screening tool, such as the FICA Spiritual History Tool (Pulchalski & Romer, 2000), to assess for spiritual distress, and should also work closely with the members of the interdisciplinary team, particularly the hospice chaplain, to address the patient's spiritual needs.

Pain Impacts the Dimensions of Quantity of Life

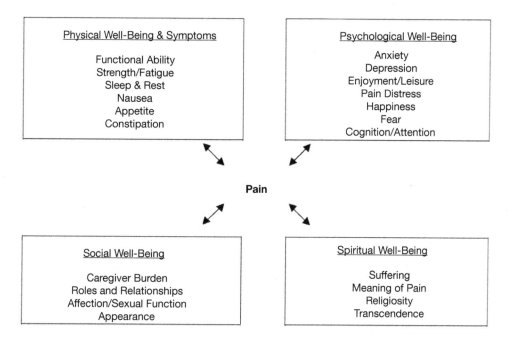

FIGURE 13.7 Effects of pain on quality of life.

Source: Ferrell, B. R., & Rhiner, M. (1991). High tech comfort: Ethical issues in cancer pain management for the 1990's. *Journal of Clinical Ethics, 2,* 108–112; copyright by *The Journal of Clinical Ethics;* all rights reserved.

Pain is a personal experience and is interpreted through the patient's unique personal, cultural, socioeconomic, gender-specific, and racial lenses. Healthcare providers must strive to conduct a comprehensive pain assessment for every patient and to work collaboratively with patients to individualize the plan of care. For some patients, such as those patients who have a history of opioid addiction, a more in-depth, comprehensive pain assessment is required.

Key Point

Questions to elicit cultural information about the patient's perception of pain include the following:

- Is touching acceptable to you?

- What words do you use to describe pain?

- How do people in your family usually react to pain?

- How do you usually cope with pain?

- What types of treatment(s) would you find acceptable to treat your pain?

- Do you seek advice from any nonmedical healers when you are sick? (Fink & Gates, 1995)

Pain Assessment and Substance Abuse

Roughly 17% of patients who have advanced cancer have alcohol dependence and about 8% of have opioid addiction. Patients who have current or past substance abuse disorder (SUD) require special care and attention because they usually have a more severe pain experience and may require a higher dose of opioid medications to manage their pain (Compton & Chang, 2017). Importantly, about 40% of patients who have SUD have a concomitant mental, behavioral, or emotional disorder. Thus an integrated approach to the care of seriously ill patients who have SUD is necessary. The plan of care should include interventions such as cognitive behavioral therapy, complementary approaches to care, counseling, family and individual support, and assessment for the risk of recovery setback (Compton & Chang, 2017).

A patient's social history may give clues to their risk for substance abuse or to past SUD, which is critical information to obtain because serious illness may be a trigger for substance abuse (Gorski, 2013; Kirsh & Passik, 2006) and an obstacle to promoting safety and sobriety. Tools that are used to screen for risk of drug or alcohol misuse are the AUDIT-C (Bush, Kivlahan, McDonell, Fihn, & Bradley, 1998; see Figure 13.8) and the Opioid Risk Tool (Webster & Webster, 2005; see Figure 13.9).

> **Key Point**
>
> The healthcare provider should use objective data such as medical records, urine toxicology, and information from the state monitoring program to determine if pain medication diversion or misuse has occurred (U.S. Department of Health & Human Services, Substance Abuse and Mental Health Services Administration, 2011).

▪ CONCLUSION

Pain assessment is a complex undertaking that relies on both subjective and objective findings. A thorough pain assessment is the cornerstone to excellent pain management. Further, symptoms associated with pain should be carefully considered by the clinician to determine the source and nature of the pain. Patients who have chronic pain should also be assessed for depression, anxiety, and immobility that can be related to their pain. Patients should also be screened for SUD or for the risk of relapse if they have a history of SUD. In addition to skillful pain assessment, patient and family support is crucial throughout the patient's illness.

AUDIT-C - Overview

The AUDIT-C is a 3-item alcohol screen that can help identify persons who are hazardous drinkers or have active alcohol use disorders (including alcohol abuse or dependence). The AUDIT-C is a modified version of the 10 question AUDIT instrument.

Clinical Utility

The AUDIT-C is a brief alcohol screen that reliably identifies patients who are hazardous drinkers or have active alcohol use disorders.

Scoring

The AUDIT-C is scored on a scale of 0–12.

Each AUDIT-C question has 5 answer choices. Points allotted are:

a = 0 points, b = 1 point, c = 2 points, d = 3 points, e = 4 points

▩ **In men**, a score of 4 or more is considered positive, optimal for identifying hazardous drinking or active alcohol use disorders.

▩ **In women**, a score of 3 or more is considered positive (same as above).

▩ However, when the points are all from Question #1 alone (#2 & #3 are zero), it can be assumed that the patient is drinking below recommended limits and it is suggested that the provider review the patient's alcohol intake over the past few months to confirm accuracy.[3]

▩ Generally, the higher the score, the more likely it is that the patient's drinking is affecting his or her safety.

Psychometric Properties

For identifying patients with heavy/hazardous drinking and/or Active-DSM alcohol abuse or dependence

	Men[1]	Women[2]
≥3	Sens: 0.95 / Spec. 0.60	Sens: 0.66 / Spec. 0.94
≥4	Sens: 0.86 / Spec. 0.72	Sens: 0.48 / Spec. 0.99

For identifying patients with active alcohol abuse or dependence

≥3	Sens: 0.90 / Spec. 0.45	Sens: 0.80 / Spec. 0.87
≥4	Sens: 0.79 / Spec. 0.56	Sens: 0.67 / Spec. 0.94

1. Bush K, Kivlahan DR, McDonell MB, et al. The AUDIT Alcohol Consumption Questions (AUDIT-C): An effective brief screening test for problem drinking. Arch Internal Med. 1998 (3): 1789–1795.
2. Bradley KA, Bush KR, Epler AJ, et al. Two brief alcohol–screening tests from the Alcohol Use Disorders Identification Test (AUDIT): Validation in a female veterans affairs patient population. Arch Internal Med Vol 163, April 2003: 821–829.
3. Frequently Asked Questions guide to using the AUDIT-C can be found via the website: www.oqp.med.va.gov/general/uploads/FAQ%20AUDIT-C

FIGURE 13.8 AUDIT-C Tool.

Source: Audit-C Overview. https://www.integration.samhsa.gov/images/res/tool_auditc.pdf.

AUDIT-C Questionnaire

Patient Name _____   Date of Visit _____

1. **How often do you have a drink containing alcohol?**
   - ☐ a. Never
   - ☐ b. Monthly or less
   - ☐ c. 2-4 times a month
   - ☐ d. 2-3 times a week
   - ☐ e. 4 or more times a week

2. **How many standard drinks containing alcohol do you have on a typical day?**
   - ☐ a. 1 or 2
   - ☐ b. 3 or 4
   - ☐ c. 5 or 6
   - ☐ d. 7 to 9
   - ☐ e. 10 or more

3. **How often do you have six or more drinks on one occasion?**
   - ☐ a. Never
   - ☐ b. Less than monthly
   - ☐ c. Monthly
   - ☐ d. Weekly
   - ☐ e. Daily or almost daily

AUDIT-C is available for use in the public domain.

FIGURE 13.8 AUDIT-C Tool *(continued)*.

Chapter Summary

- Pain is an unpleasant sensation primarily associated with tissue damage.
- Pain signals are carried on afferent pathways to the peripheral nervous system and CNS.
- Pain signals are interpreted in the brainstem, diencephalon, and the cerebral cortex, and are then modulated within the efferent pathways of the CNS.
- Acute pain has a sudden onset and lasts only seconds to minutes.
- Chronic pain lasts more than 3 months and serves no useful purpose.

(continued)

Opioid Risk Tool

This tool should be administered to patients upon an initial visit prior to beginning opioid therapy for pain management. A score of 3 or lower indicates low risk for future opioid abuse, a score of 4 to 7 indicates moderate risk for opioid abuse, and a score of 8 or higher indicates a high risk for opioid abuse.

Mark each box that applies	Female	Male
Family history of substance abuse		
Alcohol	1	3
Illegal drugs	2	3
Rx drugs	4	4
Personal history of substance abuse		
Alcohol	3	3
Illegal drugs	4	4
Rx drugs	5	5
Age between 16 – 45 years	1	1
History of preadolescent sexual abuse	3	0
Psychological disease		
ADD, OCD, bipolar, schizophrenia	2	2
Depression	1	1
Scoring totals		

Questionnaire developed by Lynn R. Webster, MD to assess risk of opioid addiction.

FIGURE 13.9 Opioid Risk Tool.

Source: Webster, L. R., & Webster, R. M. (2005). Predicting aberrant behaviors in opioid-treated patients: Preliminary validation of the Opioid Risk Tool. *Pain Medicine,* 6(6), 432–442. doi: https://doi.org/10.1111/j.1526-4637.2005.00072.x

---

Chapter Summary (*continued*)

- Somatic pain is associated with connective tissue, muscle, skin, or bone injury. It is usually described as localized and sharp, but can be diffuse and dull.

- Visceral pain is related to injury to an organ or the viscera. It is usually described as achy, dull, or crampy and often radiates away from the site of injury.

- Neuropathic pain originates in the peripheral or CNS and is usually shooting, burning, stabbing, or tingling.

- Pain assessment includes both subjective and objective data.

- The P-Q-R-S-T model is commonly used to assess pain.

(continued)

Chapter Summary (*continued*)
• Several tools can be used to assess pain in patients who are not able to verbalize their discomfort (cf., FLACC scale, PAINAD tool, FACES Scale).
• Pain expression can be influenced by cultural norms and religious beliefs.
• Pain a ffects multiple dimensions of the patient's life.
• Patients who have a history of SUD require focused support throughout their illness to help prevent recovery setback.

▪ PRACTICE QUESTIONS

1. Mrs. Alvarez is a 67-year-old patient who has stage 4 chronic obstructive pulmonary disease (COPD) as well as hypertension, hypercholesterolemia, and type 2 diabetes mellitus. She is seen today in the palliative care clinic for a follow-up visit. Through a translator, she states that she is having dull pain in her chest that is a 6 out of 10 and radiates through her right shoulder blade. The nurse knows that the type of pain Mrs. Alvarez is describing is

    a. Chronic

    b. Somatic

    c. Visceral

    d. Neuropathic

2. Which of the following should the nurse ask Mrs. Alvarez first?

    a. How long have you have had the pain?

    b. Have you had your gall bladder removed?

    c. Have you taken anything for the pain?

    d. Do you have any other symptoms with the pain?

3. Which of the following should the nurse do for Mrs. Alvarez at this time?

    a. Administer an albuterol inhaler

    b. Administer 5 mg of morphine sulfate

    c. Advise the patient to be seen in the emergency department

    d. Coach the patient in taking several deep breaths

4. A 90-year-old hospice patient tells the nurse that he has trouble walking in his house because he sometimes has numbness in his feet along with tingling in his toes. The nurse should first

    a. Ask the patient if he has diabetes

    b. Administer 5 mg of morphine now

    c. Develop a safety plan with the patient

    d. Tell the patient to inspect his feet daily

5. The pain described in the previous question is
   a. Neuropathic
   b. Visceral
   c. Somatic
   d. Acute

6. Arlene DeJune is a 48-year-old hospice patient who has end-stage ovarian cancer. She tells the nurse that she does not feel like eating and wants to sleep all the time. The nurse should
   a. Review the patient's pain regimen
   b. Determine if the patient is misusing prescribed pain medications
   c. Conduct a depression screening for the patient
   d. Consult with the hospice social worker immediately

7. A patient who has bladder cancer denies pain even though he is grimacing and clenching his teeth. The nurse knows that his pain expression is
   a. Likely influenced by his culture
   b. Incongruent with pain expression norms
   c. Poorly controlled and should be treated now
   d. Impeding the nurse's assessment

8. Mr. Wentz is a 76-year-old patient who has terminal cancer. He states that he is no longer able to attend religious services due to chronic pain. The most appropriate nursing diagnosis for the patient is
   a. Interrupted family processes
   b. Social isolation
   c. Activity intolerance
   d. Ineffective coping

9. A tool that is used to specifically assess pain in patients who have dementia is the
   a. FLACC scale
   b. P-Q-R-S-T
   c. FACES scale
   d. PAINAD scale

10. Patients who have a history of substance abuse disorder usually have
    a. Higher pain tolerance
    b. Stoic pain expression
    c. A more intense pain experience
    d. A need for lower doses of opioids

■ REFERENCES

Bradley, K. A., Bush, K. R., Epler, A. J., Dobie, D. J., Davis, T. M., Sporleder, J. L., . . . Maynard, C. (2003, April). Two brief alcohol-screening tests from the Alcohol use Disorders Identification Test (AUDIT): Validation in a female Veterans Affairs patient population. *JAMA Internal Medicine, 163*, 821–829.

Bush, K., Kivlahan, D. R., McDonell, M. B., Fihn, S. D., & Bradley, K. A. (1998). The AUDIT alcohol consumption questions (AUDIT-C): An effective brief screening test for problem drinking. *Archives of Internal Medicine, 158*(16), 1789–1795. doi:10.1001/archinte.158.16.1789

Compton, P., & Chang, Y. P. (2017). Substance abuse and addiction: Implications for pain management in patients with cancer. *Clinical Journal of Oncology Nursing, 21*(2), 203–209. doi:10.1188/17.CJON.203-209

Ferrell, B. R., & Rhiner, M. (1991). High tech comfort: Ethical issues in cancer pain management for the 1990's. *Journal of Clinical Ethics, 2*, 108–112.

Fink, R. S., & Gates, R. (1995). Cultural diversity and cancer pain. In D. B. McGuire, C. H. Yarbro, & B. R. Ferrell (Eds.), *Cancer pain management* (2nd ed., pp. 19–36). Boston, MA: Jones & Bartlett.

Gorski, T. T. (2013). *Terminal illness & relapse: Why stay sober if you're dying?* Retrieved from https://terrygorski.com/2013/11/22/terminal-illness-and-relapse-why-stay-sober-if-youre-dying/

Huether, S. E., Rodway, G., & DeFriez, C. (2014). Pain, temperature regulation, sleep, and sensory function. In K. L. McCance, S. E. Huether, V. L. Brashers, & N. S. Rote (Eds.), *Pathophysiology: The biologic basis for diseases in adults and children* (7th ed., pp. 484–526). St .Louis, MO: Elsevier Mosby.

International Association for the Study of Pain. (2017). *IASP terminology*. Retrieved from http://www.iasp-pain.org/Education/Content.aspx?ItemNumber=1698#Pain

International Association for the Study of Pain. (2018). *Faces pain scale – Revised home*. Retrieved from http://www.iasp-pain.org/Education/Content.aspx?ItemNumber=1519

Kim, E. J., & Buschmann, M. T. (2006). Reliability and validity of the Faces pain scale with older adults. *International Journal of Nursing Studies, 43*(4), 447–456. doi:10.1016/S1474-4422(14)70103-6

Kirsh, K., & Passik, S. D. (2006). Palliative care of the terminally ill drug addict. *Cancer Investigation, 24*, 425–431. doi:10.1080/07357900600705565

Kiser-Larson, N. (2017). The experience of intense pain: Nursing management and intervention. *Journal of Christian Nursing, 34*(2), 89–96. doi:10.10.1097/CJN. 0000000000000362

Kroenke, K., Spitzer, R. L., & Williams, J. B. (2001). The PHQ-9: Validity of a brief depression severity measure. *Journal of General Internal Medicine, 16*, 606–613. Retrieved from http://www.jgim.org/

McCaffery, M. (1968). *Nursing practice theories related to cognition, bodily pain, and man- environment interactions*. Los Angeles: University of California at Los Angeles Students' Store.

Merkel, S. I., Voepel-Lewis, T., Shayevitz, J. R., & Malviya, S. (1997). The FLACC: A behavioral scale for scoring postoperative pain in young children. *Pediatric Nursing, 23*(3), 293–297.

Narayam, M. C. (2010). Culture's effect on pain assessment and management. *American Journal of Nursing, 111*(4), 38–47. doi:10.1097/01.NAJ.0000370157.33223.6d

Peacock, S., & Patel, S. (2008). Cultural influences on pain. *Reviews in Pain, 1*(2), 609. doi:10.1177/204946370800100203

Pulchalski, C., & Romer, A. (2000). Taking a spiritual history allows clinicians to understand patients more fully. *Journal of Palliative Medicine, 3*(1), 129–137. doi:10.1089/jpm.2000.3.129

Spitzer, R. L., Kroenke, K., Williams, J. B. W., & Lowe, B. (2006). A brief measure for assessing generalized anxiety disorder. *Archives of Internal Medicine, 166*(10), 1092–1097. doi:10.1001/archinte.166.10.1092

U.S. Department of Health & Human Services, Substance Abuse and Mental Health Services Administration. (2011). *A treatment improvement protocol: Managing chronic pain in adults with or in recovery from substance use disorders*. Retrieved from https://store.samhsa.gov/shin/content/SMA12-4671/TIP54.pdf

Warden, V., Hurley, A. C., & Volicer, L. (2003). Development and psychometric evaluation of the Pain Assessment in Advanced Dementia (PAINAD) scale. *Journal of the American Medical Directors Association, 4*(1), 9–15.

Ware, L. J., Epps, C. D., Herr, K., & Packard, A. (2006). Evaluation of the revised Faces pain scale, verbal descriptor scale, numeric rating scale, and Iowa pain thermometer in older minority adults. *Pain Management Nursing, 7*(3), 117–125. doi:10.1097/01.JAM.0000043422.31640.F7

Webster, L. R., & Webster, R. M. (2005). Predicting aberrant behaviors in opioid-treated patients: Preliminary validation of the opioid risk tool. *Pain Medicine, 6*(6), 432–442. doi:10.1111/j.1526-4637.2005.00072.x

Wong, D., & Baker, C. (1988). Pain in children: Comparison of assessment scales. *Pediatric Nursing, 14*(1), 9–17. Retrieved from http://www.pediatricnursing.net/interestarticles/1401_Wong.pdf

14 Pain Management Interventions

For death or pain is not formidable, but the fear of pain or death.
—Epictetus (1890, p. 98)

LEARNING OBJECTIVES

After completing this section, the nurse will be able to

1. Differentiate among various types of pain according to the patient's symptoms
2. Identify complex pain syndromes
3. Explain the risks and benefits of pharmacological and nonpharmacological pain interventions

PAIN MANAGEMENT OVERVIEW

Effective pain management is predicated on excellent pain assessment. The primary barrier to effective pain control is incomplete pain assessment. Systemic or organizational barriers include limitations on the types of medications that can be used in certain healthcare settings, reimbursement issues, and lack of availability of needed medications. Individual factors that limit proper pain management include lack of knowledge on the part of the provider, patient or family fears regarding addiction or somnolence, and concerns about side effects (Gunnarsdottir et al., 2017; Zuccaro et al., 2012).

Patients, families, and sometimes healthcare providers have beliefs about addiction that prevent proper pain management. However, addiction in terminally ill patients who have no prior history of opioid addiction is rare. Patients are more likely to develop a tolerance to opioid medications over time, which is not generally a concern (American Hospice Foundation, 2014). Patients and families must receive information on the differences between addiction and tolerance as well as other aspects of physical responses to pain management interventions. Key terms are defined as follows:

- *Addiction:* Compulsive use of a substance that occurs when it is used in a way other than intended. Patients have cravings when the substance is withdrawn, with an overriding inability to control their perceived need for the substance, even though there may be an awareness that the substance, or overuse of the substance, is harmful

- *Dependence:* A state in which the person feels that they can only function normally when using a specific substance. Abrupt withdrawal of the substance causes withdrawal symptoms

- *Pseudoaddiction:* The mistaken assumption that a patient who is seeking pain relief is addicted to a substance

- *Tolerance:* Occurs when the patient no longer has a therapeutic response to the drug and a higher dose is required to achieve the prior effectiveness
  (National Institute on Drug Abuse, 2017; Paice, 2015; Reynolds, Drew, & Dunwoody, 2013)

Sources of Pain in Terminally Ill Patients

Pain is one of the most common and most feared symptoms at the end of life (Paice, 2015). Patients who have terminal conditions may experience pain from multiple sources, including chronic conditions, wounds, malignancies, and immobility. The type of pain that the patient experiences is specifically related to the source of the pain.

Nociceptive pain originates in the peripheral and nociceptive fibers and may involve both physical and psychological dimensions (Zaki, Wagner, Singer, Keysers, & Gazzola, 2016). Nociceptive pain is generally categorized as either somatic or visceral. One common source of somatic pain in adults is arthritis pain (Arthritis Foundation, 2018). Other sources of somatic pain in terminally ill patients may include skin or connective tissue damage, such as may occur with a fall or from decubiti. Somatic pain is generally experienced as sharp and localized but can also manifest as dull and diffuse, depending on the source of the pain.

Visceral pain is related to pain in the organs or viscera. It is experienced as gnawing and achy and usually requires a multimodal approach to pain management. Visceral pain is also common at the end of life and is often related to "metastases, biliary obstruction, and pancreatitis, as well as pancreatic tumors and small bowel or colon obstruction" (Groninger & Vijayan, 2014, p. 30).

Neuropathic pain is often described as burning or shooting and can be related to nerve damage or pressure on nerves due to tumor growth (Gilron, Baron, & Jensen, 2014). Neurological pain is caused by injury or disease of the nervous system. It can result from diagnoses such as multiple sclerosis, HIV and AIDS, multiple myeloma, spinal cord surgery or herniated disc, amyotrophic lateral sclerosis, and others. Treatment of neuropathic pain involves a multimodal approach, which may include "nonopioids, gabapentinoids, tricyclic antidepressants, and serotonin–norepinephrine reuptake inhibitors (all first-line therapies), as well as anticonvulsants and sodium channel blocking antiarrhythmics" (Groninger & Vijayan, 2014, p. 30). The use of opioids for the treatment of neuropathic pain should be considered a second-, or even third-line, intervention (Smith, 2012). When opioids are used to treat neuropathic pain, methadone is a good choice (Abrahm, 2014). Clinicians should be aware, however, that if opioids are used in the treatment of neuropathic pain, higher doses of opioids are usually needed for effective treatment (Paice, 2015).

Approaches to Pain Management

Skilled pain management is the cornerstone of excellent end-of-life care. The World Health Organization (WHO) developed the WHO pain ladder to help guide interventions for patients experiencing cancer pain (see Figure 14.1). The stepwise approach indicates that the first step in the management of cancer pain is nonopioid medication with or without adjuvant therapies. Adjuvant therapies may include nonsteroidal anti-inflammatory drugs (NSAIDs), COX-2 inhibitors, muscle relaxants, psychotropic medications, antidepressants, antiepileptic drugs, anxiolytics, sedative/hypnotics, amphetamines, antiarrhythmics, calcium channel blockers, ketamine, lidocaine, capsaicin, tramadol, botulinum toxin, and other miscellaneous drugs (Shanti, Tan, & Shanti, 2012).

If the patient's pain is not responsive to the interventions initiated in step 1, then step 2 involves the use of opioid medications with or without adjuvants. Nonopioids may also be used with opioids, if indicated. If the pain persists or worsens, then step 3 involves the use of opioids for moderate to severe pain, which may involve the use of both long-acting and short-acting pain medications as well as adjuvants.

The WHO pain ladder is a useful visual cue for providers to choose interventions that are appropriate for the severity of pain that the patient experiences. However, healthcare providers must also be aware of specific pharmacological and nonpharmacological interventions used to treat various types of pain.

Pharmacological Pain Interventions

There are three basic categories of analgesics that are used to ameliorate the suffering associated with acute or chronic pain. These include nonopioids, opioids, and adjuvants, which are also called coanalgesics (Paice, 2015).

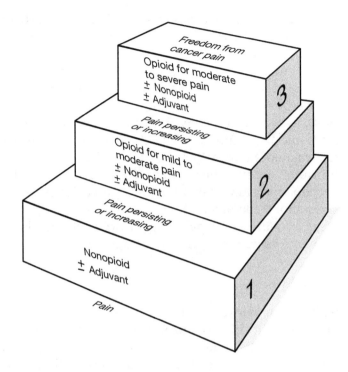

FIGURE 14.1 WHO pain ladder.

WHO, World Health Organization.
Source: World Health Organization. (2018). WHO's cancer pain ladder for adults. Retrieved from http://www.who.int/cancer/palliative/painladder/en/

Nonopioid Drugs

Nonopioid drugs should be used to treat chronic pain whenever possible (Dowell, Haegerich, & Chou, 2016). Nonopioid medications used to alleviate pain are acetaminophen and NSAIDs (see Table 14.1).

- Acetaminophen is an effective analgesic and antipyretic but it has no effect on inflammation. Acetaminophen can be administered orally, rectally, and intravenously. The maximum daily dose of acetaminophen for adults is 4,000 mg. However, the manufacturer of Tylenol (McNeil) recommends a maximum daily dose of 3,000 mg, based on the U.S. Food and Drug Administration (FDA) Center for Drug Evaluation and Research (CDER) recommendation, but this is not an FDA mandate (Krenzelok & Royal, 2012). The FDA has, however, limited the amount of acetaminophen per tablet or capsule to 325 mg and has issued labeling requirements concerning potential allergic reactions, the maximum daily dose of acetaminophen, and a warning against the consumption of three or more alcoholic drinks daily while taking acetaminophen (FDA, 2018).

- NSAIDs have analgesic, antipyretic, and anti-inflammatory properties. They are categorized as nonselective COX-2 inhibitors and selective COX-2 inhibitors. The most commonly used NSAIDs are aspirin,
ibuprofen, naproxen, and celecoxib. The maximum daily doses for
NSAIDs vary by the drug. Some potential adverse effects of NSAID
use include the following:

  ▪ Platelet dysfunction, which can lead to bleeding

  ▪ Cardiovascular risks, including myocardial infarction and stroke

  ▪ Hepatotoxicity

  ▪ Nephrotoxicity

  ▪ Gastric upset or gastric bleeding
  (Paice, 2015; Smith & Castor, 2015)

Table 14.1 Selected Nonsteroidal Anti-inflammatory Drugs and Acetaminophen

Drug	Dose and Schedule (Patients Over 50 kg)	Dose and Schedule (Patients Under 50 kg)	Key Points
Acetamino-phen	Orally: 500–1,000 mg q4h Rectally: 325–650 mg q4–6h IV: 1,000 mg over 15 minutes	Orally: 10–15 mg/kg q4h Rectally: 15–20 mg/kg q4 h IV: 15 mg/kg q6h	Maximum daily dose of 4,000 mg. In patients under 50 kg, maximum daily dose of IV acetaminophen is 75 mg Reduce dose by 50% for patients who have impaired liver function
Aspirin	Oral: 325–650 mg q4 h for pain or fever Rectally: 300–600 mg q4h	Orally: 10–15 mg/kg q4h Rectally: 15–20 mg/kg q4h	Maximum daily dose of 4,000 mg Nonselective COX-2 inhibitor Robust antiplatelet properties May cause gastric, renal, and CNS toxicity Nausea, vomiting, diaphoresis, and tinnitus occur at toxic doses
Celecoxib	Orally: 100–200 mg daily; may be increased to BID	No data available	Selective COX-2 inhibitor Risk for renal and cardiac toxicities No effect on platelets

(continued)

Table 14.1 Selected Nonsteroidal Anti-inflammatory Drugs and Acetaminophen *(continued)*

Drug	Dose and Schedule (Patients Over 50 kg)	Dose and Schedule (Patients Under 50 kg)	Key Points
Choline magnesium trisalicylate	Orally: 500–750 mg q8h	Orally: 25 mg/kg q8h	Maximum daily dose of 3,000 mg Less antiplatelet action than other NSAIDs Minimal GI toxicity
Ibuprofen	Orally: 200–400 mg q6h	Orally: 10 mg/kg q6–8h	Maximum daily dose of 1,200 mg (OTC), 3,200 mg (prescription) Potential toxicities similar to aspirin Patients taking aspirin for cardiac protection should not use ibuprofen Use with caution in geriatric patients Patients who have peptic ulcer disease, chronic kidney disease, or congestive heart failure should not use ibuprofen
Indomethicin	Orally: 25–50 mg BID; may increase to TID	0.5–1 mg/kg q8h	Maximum daily dose of 150–200 mg Risk for serious renal and cardiac toxicities
Ketorolac	IV/IM: 30–60 mg initial dose Bolus of 15–30 mg may be given IV or SQ q6h Continuous IV/SQ infusion may be used for only 3–5 days, then discontinued	IV/IM: 0.25–1 mg/kg q6hs Use for only 3–5 days, then discontinue	Significant GI and renal toxicities May precipitate renal failure in severely dehydrated patients May prolong bleeding time

(continued)

Table 14.1 Selected Nonsteroidal Anti-inflammatory Drugs and Acetaminophen *(continued)*			
Drug	Dose and Schedule (Patients Over 50 kg)	Dose and Schedule (Patients Under 50 kg)	Key Points
Naproxen	Orally or rectally: 500–750 mg q8h	Orally or rectally: 5 mg/kg q8h	Maximum daily dose 650 mg (OTC); 1,500 mg (prescription) Lowest risk for cardiac toxicity

CNS, central nervous system; GI, gastrointestinal; IM, intramuscular; IV, intravenous; NSAIDs, nonsteroidal anti-inflammatory drugs; SQ, subcutaneous.
Sources: Coyle, N., & Layman-Goldstein, M. (2007). Pharmacologic management of adult cancer pain. *Cancer Network, 21*(2). Retrieved from http://www.cancernetwork.com/palliative-and-supportive-care/pharmacologic-management-adult-cancer-pain; Paice, J. A. (2015). Pain at the end of life. In B. R. Ferrell, N. Coyle, & J. A. Paice (Eds.), *Oxford textbook of palliative nursing* (pp. 135–153). New York, NY: Oxford University Press; Smith, E. L., & Castor, T. (2015). Pain management in geriatric patients. In K. A. Sackheim (Ed.), *Pain management and palliative care* (pp. 245–263). New York, NY: Springer Publishing Company; U.S. Food and Drug Administration. (2016). Indomethacin capsules, USP. Retrieved from https://www.accessdata.fda.gov/drugsatfda_docs/label/2016/018829s022lbl.pdf.

Opioid Drugs

Opioid drugs are categorized as such because they are naturally derived from the opium poppy plant. Even synthetic narcotics are chemically manufactured to mimic the chemical structure of opium. All opioid analgesics are used to treat moderate to severe pain and/or dyspnea. Common opioid medications include morphine, codeine, fentanyl, hydrocodone, hydromorphone, levorphanol, methadone, oxycodone, and tramadol (see Table 14.2).

For most patients, oral administration of an opioid is the most effective and least invasive route. Buccal, transdermal, sublingual, subcutaneous, or rectal routes are possibilities when the oral route is not an option. Administration routes that are invasive or painful, such as IM or peripheral IV, should be avoided (Paice, 2015). However, if a patient already has a peripherally inserted central catheter (PICC line) or another type of central venous catheter (CVC) in place, it can be used if parenteral medications are needed, such as when pain is severe and/or escalating.

Administration of opioids should be undertaken carefully and titrated steadily and slowly, particularly in opioid-naïve patients (Dalal, 2016). Clinical responses to opioids may vary greatly due to individual factors. Thus a dose-titration approach is recommended to achieve optimum pain control with the fewest adverse effects (Paice, 2015). Adverse effects of opioids are related to the binding sites of the drugs (Pathan & Williams, 2012) and can include the following:

• Respiratory depression

• Nausea and/or vomiting

Table 14.2 Commonly Used Opioids

Drug	Drug Action	Approximate Equianalgesic Oral Dose	Approximate Equianalgesic Parenteral Dose	Recommended Starting Dose (Patient >50 kg)	Recommended Starting Dose (Patient <50 kg)	Key Points
Morphine	Mu receptor agonist, weak kappa receptor agonist	30 mg	10 mg	Oral: 15 mg q3–4h Parenteral: 5 mg q3–4h	Oral: 0.3 mg/kg q3–4h Parenteral: 5 mg q3–4h	Morphine is the standard by which all opioids are measured. Constipation, nausea, and sedation are the most common side effects. Risk for respiratory depression. Common side effects such as nausea and sedation usually dissipate within a few days. Patients do not build a tolerance to the constipating effects of morphine (or other opioids). Availability: parenteral, oral, supp. Long-acting and short-acting forms available
Codeine	Mu and kappa receptor agonist	150 mg	50 mg	Oral: 30 mg q3–4h Parenteral: 30 mg q2h (IM/IV)	Oral: 0.5 mg/kg q3–4h Parenteral: not recommended	Roughly 10% of the Caucasian population lacks the enzyme that converts codeine to morphine, making it ineffective for them. Often combined with acetaminophen or guaifenesin Availability: parenteral, oral, supp.

(continued)

Table 14.2 Commonly Used Opioids (*continued*)

Drug	Drug Action	Approximate Equianalgesic Oral Dose	Approximate Equianalgesic Parenteral Dose	Recommended Starting Dose (Patient >50 kg)	Recommended Starting Dose (Patient <50 kg)	Key Points
Fentanyl	Mu receptor agonist, weak kappa and delta agonist	Noninjectable fentanyl products are for opioid-tolerant patients only. Do not convert mcg for mcg among fentanyl products (i.e., transdermal patch, transmucosal lozenge, and nasal spray)				Fentanyl 100 mcg patch ≈ 4 mg IV morphine per hour Fentanyl is lipid soluble; absorption is decreased in cachexic patients Breakthrough pain medication should be used in conjunction with long-acting transdermal patch Availability: parenteral, oral, transdermal, nebulized, transmucosal
Hydrocodone	Mu and kappa receptor agonist	30 mg	Not available	Oral: 5 mg q3–4h Parenteral: not available	Oral: 0.1 mg/kg q3–4h Parenteral: not available	Only available in combination with other drugs such as acetaminophen, which limits usefulness in end-of-life and palliative care settings Hydrocodone is a synthesized form of codeine Used to treat moderate to severe pain and as a cough suppressant Equipotent to codeine Availability: oral

(*continued*)

Table 14.2 Commonly Used Opioids (continued)

Drug	Drug Action	Approximate Equianal-gesic Oral Dose	Approximate Equianal-gesic Par-enteral Dose	Recommended Starting Dose (Patient >50 kg)	Recommended Starting Dose (Patient <50 kg)	Key Points
Hydromor-phone	Mu receptor agonist, weak kappa and delta agonist	6 mg	1.5 mg	Oral: 2 mg q3–4h Parenteral: 0.5 mg q3–4h	Oral: 0.03 mg/kg q3–4h Parenteral: 0.005 mg/kg q3–4h	Faster onset than morphine and more potent Increased blood plasma levels with renal disease. Removed with dialysis Availability: parenteral, oral, supp. Long-acting formulation available
Levorphanol	Mu-opioid receptor agonist with some effect at kappa and delta receptors	4 mg	2 mg	Oral: 4 mg q6–8h Parenteral: 2 mg q6–8h	Oral: 0.04 mg/kg q6–8h Parenteral: 0.02 mg/kg q6–8h	Causes less nausea and vomiting than morphine; longer half-life than morphine; may lead to accumulation with repeated administration Availability: parenteral and oral
Methadone	Mu-opioid receptor agonist with some effect at kappa and delta receptors; NMDA-receptor antagonist	10 mg	10 mg	Oral: 5 mg q12h Parenteral: not recommended	Oral: 0.1 mg/kg q12h Parenteral: not recommended	Risk for toxicity due to accumulation, including respiratory depression and sedation related to long half-life of drug Less costly than many other opioid medications Myoclonus may occur with parenteral use PRN dosing not recommended. Should not be used for breakthrough pain

(continued)

Table 14.2 Commonly Used Opioids (continued)

Drug	Drug Action	Approximate Equianalgesic Oral Dose	Approximate Equianalgesic Parenteral Dose	Recommended Starting Dose (Patient >50 kg)	Recommended Starting Dose (Patient <50 kg)	Key Points
Oxycodone	Mu-opioid receptor agonist, strong effect at kappa agonist and some effect at delta receptors	20 mg	Not available	Oral: 5 mg q3–4h Parenteral: not available	Oral: 1 mg/kg q3–4h Parenteral: not available	Onset of action 5–10 minutes Less nausea and vomiting than morphine Extensively metabolized by the liver; use caution in patients with hepatic disease Often combined with acetaminophen Availability: oral, supp. Extended-release form available
Tramadol	Partial mu receptor agonist	100 mg	Not recommended	Oral: 50–100 mg q3–4h Parenteral: 50–100 mg q3–4h	Not recommended	Synthetic codeine analogue; less effective for severe or chronic pain Adverse effects are nausea, vomiting, dizziness, and constipation. *Lowers seizure threshold* Availability: parenteral, oral, supp. Extended-release form available

IM, intramuscular; IV, intravenous; NMDA, N-methyl-D-aspartate.

Sources: Detail-Document, P. L. (2012). Equianalgesic dosing of opioids for pain management. Pharmacist's letter/prescriber's letter. Retrieved from https://www.nhms.org/sites/default/files/Pdfs/Opioid-Comparison-Chart-Prescriber-Letter-2012.pdf; Paice, J. A. (2015). Pain at the end of life. In B. R. Ferrell, N. Coyle, & J. A. Paice (Eds.). Oxford textbook of palliative nursing (pp. 135–153). New York, NY: Oxford University Press; Yaksh, T., & Wallace, M. (2018). Opioids, analgesia, and pain management. In L. L. Brunton, R. Hilal-Dandan, & B. C. Knollman (Eds.), Goodman & Gillman's: The pharmacological basis of therapeutics (13th ed., pp. 355–420). New York, NY: McGraw-Hill Education.

- Dizziness
- Decreased mental acuity
- Pruritus
- Diaphoresis
- Noncardiogenic pulmonary edema
- Constipation
- Dysphoria
- Increased pressure in the biliary tract
- Urinary retention
- Hypotension
- Delirium
  (Dalal, 2016; Yaksh & Wallace, 2018)

Although mild side effects are somewhat common, patients generally develop a tolerance to most side effects of opioids, except constipation. Constipation must, therefore, be aggressively managed using both pharmacological and nonpharmacologic interventions (Rogers, Mehta, Shengelia, & Reid, 2013). Some patients will experience a pseudoallergy, which manifests as an allergic reaction to the opioid, such as pruritus (Zhang, Li, Shi, & Zhang, 2018). However, true allergic reactions to opioids are rare. If an allergic reaction does occur, it is usually to a morphine derivative. In such cases, a test dose of a synthetic opioid, such as fentanyl, may be attempted (Paice, 2015; Wahler, Smith, & Mulcahy, 2017). If the patient has a true allergy to morphine drugs, as well as to fentanyl and meperidine, methadone may be used (Abrahm, 2014).

Management of the adverse effects of opioids may involve reducing the dose, rotating to another opioid, changing the administration route, or managing side effects pharmacologically. Adverse effects of opioids are sometimes related to the accumulation of toxic metabolites. This accumulation is especially concerning in patients whose drug metabolism and elimination are impaired due to hepatic or renal disease, so close monitoring of patients with organ failure is warranted (Paice, 2015). When toxicity occurs, opioid rotation becomes necessary. Other reasons for opioid rotation include lack of analgesic efficacy, drug–drug interactions, change in the patient's clinical status, and practical issues such as cost or lack of availability of a drug (Smith & Peppin, 2014).

Opioid Rotation and Opioid Conversion

The terms opioid rotation and opioid conversion are often used interchangeably, but they are not exactly the same. Opioid conversion is a calculation to determine the equivalent dose of an opioid when compared to another opioid. Opioid conversion calculations are done when changing the route of an opioid or when rotating from one opioid to another due to side effects, lack of efficacy, or other reasons.

Oral to Parenteral or Parenteral to Oral Conversions

The route of an opioid medication may need to be changed when a patient is no longer able to swallow oral medications. In such cases, the drug may remain the same, but the route will change. The conversion guideline for converting an opioid from the oral to parenteral route is roughly 3:1 (see Box 14.1).

Box 14.1 Changing Routes—Same Drug

Example

    Mrs. Smith has been taking 30 mg of morphine immediate release for pain orally every 6 hours, but is no longer able to swallow. When converting the morphine dose for the parenteral route, the dose would be one-third of the oral dose, or 10 mg.

Another Example

    A 30-year-old patient in a palliative care unit has been receiving 30 mg of morphine via IV daily for pain. The patient is now ready to be discharged and the parenteral dose will be converted to oral. The oral dose is three times the IV dose, so the patient would need to take 90 mg of oral morphine daily as an equivalent dose.

One More

    Juan is taking 3 mg of hydromorphone orally for pain about three times every day. He is now admitted to the hospice inpatient unit due to marked deterioration in his condition. Since his pain regimen was effective, the nurse will administer the same drug, but will use a subcutaneous button. The dose will be one-third of the oral dose, so Juan will receive 1 mg of hydrocodone SC three times a day.

Calculating a Long-Acting Dose

When pain is intermittent, an opioid taken on an as-needed basis may bring effective relief. However, in cases where pain is chronic and severe, such as in cases of serious or terminal illness, pain may not be well controlled with a medication taken only on an as-needed basis. To address this problem, the patient should keep a record of the number of doses of the PRN medication taken daily, and then, the total daily dose of the medication should be converted to a long-acting form (see Box 14.2).

Box 14.2 Calculating a Long-Acting Dose—Same Drug

Example

    James LaDier is a 90-year-old patient who is taking immediate-release morphine, 10 mg PO PRN q2h for pain related to prostate cancer. Each day for the past 5 days, he has taken 7 to 8 doses of the medication. When converting to a long-acting dose, the total daily dose would be calculated as follows:

    8 doses of 10 mg in 24 hours = 8 doses × 10 mg = 80 mg (total daily dose)

    Then, the long-acting dose would be calculated as:

    80 mg divided into two doses per day = 40 mg long-acting morphine every 12 hours

---

(continued)

Box 14.2 Calculating a Long-Acting Dose—Same Drug (*continued*)

Another Example

A. J. Rush has been taking 5 mg of oxycodone immediate release for pain related to colon cancer. The patient reported that he was taking only 1 to 2 doses daily in previous months, but now the pain has become severe and over the past several days, 10 to 12 doses were needed daily for comfort. To convert to a long-acting formulation of the same drug, the total daily dose of the medication should be calculated as follows:

5 mg of oxycodone × 12 doses in 24 hours = 5 mg × 12 doses = 60 mg (total daily dose)

then, the long-acting dose would be calculated as:

60 mg divided into two doses to be given every 12 hours = 30 mg of long-acting oxycodone every 12 hours

One More

Sam is taking 6 doses of immediate-release morphine (20 mg each) for pain each day. She asks the nurse in the palliative care clinic if she can use a long-acting medication because she wants to travel without always thinking of her pain. The long-acting dose would be calculated as follows:

6 doses of 20 mg in 24 hours = 6 doses × 20 mg = 120 mg (total daily dose)

then, the long-acting dose would be calculated as:

120 mg divided into two doses to be given every 12 hours = 60 mg long-acting morphine every 12 hours

---

Calculating the Breakthrough (Rescue) Dose for Oral Opioids

When patients are using long-acting pain medications, there is a possibility that they will still experience pain from time to time throughout the day. Therefore, a short-acting (immediate-release) opioid should be prescribed along with the long-acting opioid. When possible, the breakthrough medication should be from the same class of opioid analgesics as the long-acting opioid (Kishner, 2018). To calculate the correct dose of the breakthrough medication, 10% to 20% of the total daily dose of the long-acting opioid should be prescribed for use every 1 to 2 hours for pain (Bodtke & Ligon, 2016). The actual amount of the breakthrough dose prescribed will depend on several factors, but as with all opioid prescribing decisions, a lower dose should be used and then it can be titrated upward if necessary (see Box 14.3).

Box 14.3 Calculating Breakthrough Doses—Oral Medications

Example

A patient is taking 60 mg of long-acting morphine every 24 hours (30 mg q12h): 10% of this total daily dose is 6 mg (prescribed as 5 mg PO q1–2h as needed for breakthrough pain).

(continued)

> **Box 14.3 Calculating Breakthrough Doses—Oral Medications (*continued*)**
>
> **Another Example**
>
> A patient is taking 60 mg of long-acting oxycodone every 12 hours. To calculate the correct dose of immediate-release oxycodone to be used for breakthrough pain, the total daily dose should be calculated as 60 mg long-acting oxycodone twice daily = 120 mg each day. Multiply this amount by 10% for a breakthrough dose of 12 mg (prescribed as 10 mg PO q1–2h as needed for breakthrough pain).
>
> **One More**
>
> A patient in the ICU is prescribed 50 mg of extended-release morphine every 12 hours for pain. The correct breakthrough dose for this patient would be calculated by determining the total daily dose (50 mg × 2 doses in 24 hours = 100 mg/d) and then calculating 10% of that total to obtain 10 mg of immediate-release morphine to be taken q1–2h for breakthrough pain.

Calculating the Breakthrough (Rescue) Dose for Parenteral Opioids

Patients who are receiving parenteral opioids for pain management may experience breakthrough pain, just as patients taking oral opioids do. The correct dose of a parenteral breakthrough medication is roughly 50% to 100% of the hourly rate given every 15 minutes as needed (Bodtke & Ligon, 2016; see Box 14.4).

> **Box 14.4 Calculating Breakthrough Doses—Parenteral Medications**
>
> **Example**
>
> A patient who is receiving 10 mg of IV morphine per hour would need a breakthrough dose of at least 50% of the hourly dose, or 5 mg q15 minutes.
>
> **Another Example**
>
> A patient receiving 2 mg of hydromorphone IV hourly would need a breakthrough dose of at least 50% of the hourly dose, or 1 mg q15 minutes.
>
> **One More**
>
> A patient receiving 30 mg of morphine hourly would need a breakthrough dose of at least 50% of the hourly dose, or 15 mg every 15 minutes.

Note: If a patient requires more than 3 to 4 doses of breakthrough medication daily, the long-acting opioid should be increased. When the long-acting opioid is increased, the dose of the breakthrough medication must also be recalculated.

Converting From One Opioid to Another

When changing from one opioid to another, an equianalgesic table should be used as a guide to avoid errors (see Table 14.3).

Table 14.3 Opioid Equianalgesic Dosing Guideline

Opioid	Approximate Equianalgesic Dose (Oral and Transdermal)
Morphine (reference)	30 mg
Codeine	200 mg
Fentanyl transdermal	12.5 mcg/hr
Hydrocodone	30 mg
Hydromorphone	7.5 mg
Oxycodone	20 mg
Oxymorphone	10 mg

Source: Indian Health Service, U.S. Department of Health and Human Services. (n.d.). Retrieved from https://www.ihs.gov/painmanagement/treatmentplanning/safeopioidprescribing/

When changing the patient's opioid, but not changing the route of administration, use the equianalgesic table to calculate the equivalent dose of the new drug using the following steps:

1. Calculate the 24-hour current dose
2. Use the conversion table to determine the equianalgesic ratio
3. Calculate new dose using ratios
4. Reduce the dose to account for cross-tolerance

Incomplete cross-tolerance occurs when the newly-introduced drug causes unexpected hyperalgesia. When changing opioids, incomplete cross-tolerance is thought to be due to the individual's response to the new opioid or the molecular differences between opioids (Bodtke & Ligon, 2016). To account for cross-tolerance, the equianalgesic dose of the newly introduced drug should be reduced by 50% to avoid overdose and/or hyperalgesia (Prescriber's Letter, 2012). The newly introduced drug can be slowly titrated upward to achieve effective pain management. Throughout the titration process, the patient should be carefully monitored and breakthrough medication should be available (Kishner, 2018). For conversion examples, see Box 14.5.

Box 14.5 Converting From One Opioid to Another

Example

Mrs. Edwards is taking 60 mg of extended-release morphine every 12 hours orally and is using two doses of 10 mg immediate-release morphine daily for breakthrough pain. She is experiencing myoclonus and reports marked fatigue. In addition to adding lorazepam to her drug regimen, her opioid will be changed to oxycodone. The correct dose of the new drug will be calculated as follows:

1. Calculate the 24-hour dose of the morphine: 60 mg + 60 mg + 10 mg + 10 mg = 140 mg/24 hr

---

(continued)

> **Box 14.5 Converting From One Opioid to Another (*continued*)**
>
> 2. Use the conversion table to determine the equianalgesic ratio: 15 mg of PO morphine = 10 mg of PO oxycodone
>
> 3. Calculate the new dose using the ratios: 140 mg of morphine/15 × 10 = 93.33 mg of oxycodone in 24 hours
>
> 4. Reduce the dose to account for cross-tolerance: 93 × 0.5 = 46.5/24 hr
>
> **Another Example**
>
> A patient is prescribed 60 mg of extended-release morphine every 12 hours and does not use any breakthrough doses of the immediate-release morphine. The patient is no longer able to swallow and a fentanyl transdermal patch will be prescribed. To calculate the correct dose:
>
> 1. Calculate the 24-hour dose of the morphine: 60 mg + 60 mg = 120 mg/24 hr
>
> 2. Use the conversion table to determine the equianalgesic ratio: 45 to 135 mg of PO morphine in 24 hours = fentanyl transdermal (TD) 50 mcg/hr
>
> 3. Calculate the new dose using the ratios: N/A
>
> 4. Reduce the dose to account for cross-tolerance: Important! The equianalgesic dose is not reduced to account for incomplete cross-tolerance when converting from morphine to fentanyl TD. So, the patient would be converted to a 50 mcg fentanyl patch, changed q72h.
>
> Converting to fentanyl TD is a bit different from converting to one oral opioid to another. The 24-hour opioid equivalent must always be converted to the morphine 24-hour equivalent first. To determine whether your calculation is roughly accurate, a good rule of thumb is that the number of mcg per hour of TD Fentanyl should be about half the number of milligrams of oral morphine per day (McPherson, 2009).
>
> **One More**
>
> A patient is currently taking hydrocodone with APAP (7.5/300 mg), two tablets eight times daily, for severe back pain related to a trauma. The patient's condition is chronic and a long-acting pain medication is needed. To convert to a long-acting morphine product:
>
> 1. Calculate the 24-hour dose of the hydrocodone: (7.5 mg + 7.5 mg) × 8 doses/24 hr = 120 mg/24hr
>
> 2. Use the conversion table to determine the equianalgesic ratio: 15 mg of hydrocodone = 15 mg of PO morphine.
>
> 3. Calculate the new dose using the ratios: 120 mg of hydromorphone/15 mg × 15 mg = 120 mg of morphine in 24 hours
>
> 4. Reduce the dose to account for cross-tolerance: 120 mg × 0.5 = 60 mg/24 hr. Thus, the patient would be prescribed one 30 mg extended-release morphine tablet every 12 hours. The calculation for breakthrough dosing (above) would be used to determine the amount of medication that should be prescribed.

Sometimes, the patient's opioid *and* route of administration must be changed. As an example, if converting from an oral preparation of one drug to an intravenous preparation of another drug, the following method should be used to determine the correct dose (Box 14.6):

1. Calculate the 24-hour current dose.

2. Use the equianalgesic ratio of PO to IV form of the previous drug.

3. Calculate new dose using ratios for the previous drug.

4. Use the equianalgesic ratio of the form of the previous drug to the IV form of the new drug.

5. Calculate new dose using ratios.

6. Reduce dose by 50% to account for cross-tolerance.

Box 14.6 Converting From One Opioid to Another *AND* Changing the Route of Administration

Example

   A patient is to be admitted from home to the hospice inpatient unit for severe pain. The patient is currently taking 60 mg of extended-release morphine every 12 hours and is using 20 mg of immediate-release morphine every 2 hours for breakthrough pain as needed. She has taken 9 doses of the breakthrough medication daily for the past 2 days. Her pain medication will be changed to IV hydromorphone (via previously placed PICC line). The correct amount will be calculated as follows:

1. Calculate the 24-hour current dose: 60 mg of morphine daily $\times$ 2 + 20 mg of morphine $\times$ 9 = 120 mg PO + 180 mg PO = 300 mg PO Morphine/24 hr

2. Use the equianalgesic 3:1 ratio of PO to IV morphine: 15 mg PO Morphine = 5 mg IV morphine

3. Calculate new dose using ratios: 300/15 $\times$ 5 = 100 mg IV morphine/24 hr

4. Use the equianalgesic 5:1 ratio of IV morphine to IV hydromorphone: 5 mg morphine = 1 mg hydromorphone

5. Calculate new dose using ratios: 100/5 $\times$ 1 = 20 mg IV hydromorphone/24 hr

6. Reduce dose 50% for cross-tolerance: 20 $\times$ 0.5 = 10 mg/24 hr = 0.4 mg IV continuous infusion

---

When using opioid medications for the treatment of moderate to severe pain, around-the-clock dosing or long-acting preparations should be used to ensure proper pain control. A breakthrough medication should always be prescribed with a long-acting medication for optimum pain management. Patients should also be taught to take their prescribed pain medications exactly as directed and to never crush or break long-acting formulations. When using pain medication as needed, or when using medication for breakthrough pain, the patient should take the medication at the onset of the pain and not wait until the pain is severe. In some cases, even expertly designed opioid pain regimes may not address all of the patient's symptoms. In such cases, adjuvant medications may be used to treat multiple dimensions of the patient's pain.

Use of Adjuvant Drugs (Coanalgesics)

Adjuvants are also called coanalgesics and are used to reduce pain either in conjunction with opioids or alone (Paice, 2015). The purpose of adding adjuvants is to enhance the patient's comfort, especially patients experiencing neuropathic pain or mixed pain syndromes that require multimodal approaches. Examples of adjuvant therapies include antidepressants, corticosteroids, calcium channel blockers, and topical anesthetics, to name a few. Some specific adjuvants are very effective in the treatment of certain types of pain, such as bone pain, somatic pain, and so on (see Table 14.4).

In addition to adjuvant medications, palliative chemotherapy is useful for reducing the size of tumors that cause pressure and pain. Palliative radiation can also be incorporated into the end-of-life or palliative plan of care to reduce metastasis and alleviate bone pain. Palliative radiation is especially useful for treating the pain associated with spinal compression when combined with steroids. It is also used to alleviate the symptoms associated with superior vena cava syndrome, with about 70% of patients responding to the treatment (Abrahm, 2014). In addition to adjuvant medications, nonpharmacological interventions are often used to diminish pain in addition to other therapies.

Nonpharmacological Pain Interventions

Nonpharmacological interventions may be used concurrently with pharmacological interventions to reduce pain and alleviate symptoms associated with suffering in not only the physical dimension but also the psychological, spiritual, and social dimensions. Some nonpharmacological interventions are targeted to a specific symptom; others are used to enhance general well-being and promote a sense of peacefulness. Nonallopathic interventions, when combined with allopathic interventions, are referred to as complementary modalities. When nonallopathic methods are used *instead of* allopathic interventions, they are referred to alternative methods. Together, complementary and alternative medicines are referred to as Complimentary and Alternative Medicine (CAM).

CAM therapies are often rooted in traditional Chinese medicine (TCM), which promotes health through reestablishing balance. In TCM, body, mind, and spirit are viewed as an integrated whole and various interventions are used to restore health in a holistic manner. Acupuncture is a TCM intervention intended to promote inner harmony and balance by restoring the flow of energy through the meridians. Needles, pressure, or electrical currents are used to open the channels between the patient's internal and external environment, allowing energy to move freely. Acupuncture has been used to treat pain in cancer patients with mixed results. It has been found to be effective for dyspnea, fatigue, hot flashes, and xerostomia (Abrahm, 2014). Yet, it is often underutilized in hospice and palliative care (Standish, Kozak, & Congdon, 2008). Another energy-based intervention that has been used in palliative and end-of-life care is reiki.

Reiki involves the movement of energy to the patient through the reiki practitioner for the purpose of balancing the patient's energy and chakras. Reiki is often done with a specific intention, tailored to the patient's needs. Palliative care patients who received reiki reported that

Table 14.4 Adjuvant Analgesic Medications

Type of Pain	Drug Class	Drug Examples and Starting Doses	Key Points
Bone pain or pain from bony metastasis Vertebral compression fractures Arthritis pain Joint pain	Biphosphanates	Pamidrinate 60–90 mg IV over 2 hours every 2–4 weeks	May also consider radiofrequency ablation or radiopharmaceuticals (i.e., strontium chloride-89, samariaum-153) for metastatic bone pain. Monitor for dyspepsia and "steroid psychosis" and glucose intolerance if using corticosteroids.
	Corticosteroids	Dexamethasone 2–20 mg PO/SC daily; may give up to 100 mg IV bolus for pain crisis Prednisone 15–30 mg PO TID	
	NSAIDs	Diclofenac 1.3% patch BID Ibuprofen 400–800 mg PO q6h (with food) Ketolorac 30 mg PO/SC/IV q6h	
Somatic pain (described as sharp and well localized—the patient can point to the source of the pain)	Antispasmotics	Baclofen 10–20 mg q6h Tizanidine 2 mg PO TID Dantrolene 25 mg PO qd × 7 days, then 25 mg PO TID × 7 days, then 50 mg PO TID × 7 days, then 100 mg PO qid (max). D/C if no response after 45 days	For patients experiencing proximal muscle weakness, consider hydrotherapy or physical therapy (at home), if patient is able to tolerate this therapy. Provide assistive devices in home for safety and to promote independence. Baclofen is FDA-approved for muscle spasticity. Baclofen may cause muscle weakness and/or cognitive changes. Skeletal muscle relaxants and antispasmotics enhance the efficacy of NSAIDs for treating muscle injury or spasm. Skeletal muscle relaxants are relatively contraindicated in patients who have liver or renal disease.

(continued)

Table 14.4 Adjuvant Analgesic Medications (*continued*)

Type of Pain	Drug Class	Drug Examples and Starting Doses	Key Points
Somatic pain (*continued*)	NSAIDs	Diclofenac 1.3% patch BID Ibuprofen 400–800 mg PO q6h (with food) Ketolorac 30 mg PO/SC/IV q6h	Benzodiazapines are FDA-approved for spasticity, but the somnolence caused by combining these drugs with opioids prohibits injudicious use.
	Skeletal muscle relaxants	Carisoprodol 250–350 mg TID and at HS Metaxolone 800 mg PO TID to QID (on empty stomach) Chlorzoxazone 250–500 mg PO TID to QID (max 750/dose) Cyclobenzaprine 5–10 mg PO TID up to 3 weeks Ophenadrine 100 mg PO BID for musculoskeletal pain; 100 mg PO at HS for leg cramps Methocarbamol starting with 1,500 mg PO QID × 2–3 days, then reduce to 1,000 mg PO QID; 1,000 mg IV × 1 for muscle spasm	
Neuropathic pain (described as shooting, burning, tingling, or as pins and needles)	Anticonvulsants	Gabapentin 100–300 mg PO TID Carbamezapine 200 mg PO q12h (monitor blood levels) Clonazepine 0.5 mg PO BID Lamotrigine 100–200 mg PO q12h Phenytoin 300–400 mg PO QD (monitor blood levels) 50 mg PO q8h	Monitor patients for side effects of medications such as nausea, vomiting, sedation, dizziness, or anticholinergic effects (antidepressants and anticonvulsants). Neuropathic pain often requires a multimodal approach to pain management. If pain is severe and refractory at the end of life, sedation may be considered.

(continued)

Table 14.4 Adjuvant Analgesic Medications (*continued*)

Type of Pain	Drug Class	Drug Examples and Starting Doses	Key Points
Neuropathic pain (*continued*)	Antidepressants	Pregabalin 25–50 mg PO q8h Toprimate 100–200 mg PO q12h Desipramine 10–25 mg PO at HS Duloxetine 30–60 mg mg PO daily Nortriptyline 10–50 mg PO at HS Trazodone 25–150 mg PO at HS Venlafaxine XR 37.5 mg PO daily	Use of topical lidocaine should be considered when even light touch or clothing is painful on the skin. Neuropathic pain related to post-herpetic neuralgia may be treated using a lidocaine patch. The patch should not be used on broken skin. Importantly, antiviral medications should be used during active herpes zoster or simplex outbreaks in conjunction with analgesics and co-analgesics.
	Anesthetics	Ketamine 10–15 mg PO q6h or IV dose of 5–10 mg × 1, which may be repeated in 15–30 minutes. Starting infusion dose is 0.2 mg/kg/hr. May increase by 0.1 mg/kg/hr q6h Lidocaine 1–5 mg/kg hourly IV or SC Mexiletine 150 mg BID to TID	
Visceral pain (described as achy, dull, spasmic, crampy, or gnawing. This type of pain often radiates away from the site of injury). This type of pain may be related to ischemia, organ damage, obstruction, or bladder spasms, among other causes.	Anticholinergics	B and O (belladonna and opium) suppositories 30 or 60 mg up to QID Dicyclomine 10–20 mg PO up to TID PRN Glycopyrrolate 0.2–0.4 mg PO/SC every 2–4 hours and titrate Hyoscyamine 0.125 mg PO/SL q4-8h Scopalamine 1–2 TD patch(es) q3 days. For acute bowel obstruction: 10 mcg/hr SC/IV continuous infusion or 0.1 mg SC every 6 hr. Titrate every 24 hr.	Anticholinergics are used to reduce secretions in cases of painful bowel obstruction. Ocreotide has been found to be effective and to have minimal adverse effects, but may be cost-prohibitive. B and O suppositories are useful for patients who have bladder or rectal spasms. Consider pretreating rectal area with lidocaine or hydrocortisone prior to administration in patients with rectal cancer. Use of benzodiazepines with opioids increases the risk of opioid side effects, particularly respiratory depression.

(*continued*)

Table 14.4 Adjuvant Analgesic Medications *(continued)*

Type of Pain	Drug Class	Drug Examples and Starting Doses	Key Points
Visceral pain *(continued)*	Antisecretory agent	Ocreotide 100 mcg SC/IV q8h	Metoclopramide may decrease the risk for aspiration in patients fed via NG tube. However, it should be used cautiously in patients who have CHF due to increased risk for fluid overload.
	Benzodiazapines	Lorazepam 0.5–1 mg PO/SC q4h	
	Prokinetic agent	Metoclopramide 5–10 mg PO/SC q4h	
	Corticosteroids	Dexamethasone 2–20 mg PO/SC daily. May give up to 100 mg IV bolus for pain crisis Prednisone 15–30 mg PO TID	

CHF, congestive heart failure; D/C, discharge; FDA, Food and Drug Administration; IV, intravenous; NG, nasogastric; NSAIDs, nonsteroidal anti-inflammatory drugs; SC, subcutaneous; TD, transdermal.

Sources: Abrahm, J. L. (2014). *A physician's guide to pain and symptom management in cancer patients* (3rd ed.). Balitimore, MD: Johns Hopkins University Press; Bodtke, S., & Ligon, K. (2016). *Hospice and palliative medicine handbook: A clinical guide.* Retrieved from http://www.hpmhandbook.com/; Milgrom, D. P., Lad, N. L., Koniaris, L. G., & Zimmers, T. A. (2017). Bone pain and muscle weakness in cancer patients. *Current Osteoporosis Reports, 15*(2), 76–87. doi:10.1007/s11914-017-0354-3; Paice, J. A. (2015). Pain at the end of life. In B. R. Ferrell, N. Coyle, & J. A. Paice (Eds.), *Oxford textbook of palliative nursing* (pp. 135–153). New York, NY: Oxford University Press; Peng, X., Wang, P., Li, S., Zhang, G., & Hu, S. (2015). Randomized clinical trial comparing octreotide and scopolamine butylbromide in symptom control of patients with inoperable bowel obstruction due to advanced ovarian cancer. *Journal of Surgical Oncology. 13*(5), 1–6. doi:10.1186/s12957-015-0455-3; Roland, E., & von Gunten, C. F. (2009). Current concepts in malignant bowel obstruction management. *Current Oncology Reports, 11*(4), 298–303. Retrieved from https://link.springer.com/journal/11912; Saulino, M., Anderson, D. J., Doble, J., Farid, R., Gul, F., Konrad, P., . . . Boster, A. L. (2016). Best practices for intrathecal baclofen therapy: Troubleshooting. *Neuromodulation: Technology at the Neural Interface, 19*(6), 632–641. doi:10.1111/ner.12467; Warusevitane, A., Karunatilake, D., Sim, J., Lally, F., & Roffe, C. (2015). Safety and effect of metoclopramide to prevent pneumonia in patients with stroke fed via nasogastric tubes trial. *Stroke, 46*(2), 454–460. doi:10.1161/STROKEAHA.114.006639

their self-identified concerns were ameliorated through the session and they felt calmer, more relaxed, and more focused afterward (Nyatanga, Cook, & Goddard, 2018). It has also been found to be beneficial for improving overall quality of life and perceived well-being at the end of life (Henneghan & Schnyer, 2015). Another practice intended to promote harmony and balance is yoga.

Yoga involves specific motions and poses that are intended to bring together the body, mind, and spirit. Yoga has been found to increase exercise tolerance, decrease fear and anxiety, and improve relaxation. It also has beneficial effects on flexibility, balance, and mobility (Abrahm, 2014; Selman, Williams, & Simms, 2012).

Not all palliative care or hospice patients possess the strength or stamina to participate in yoga. In such instances, home-based physical therapy can help to preserve physical function, manage functional decline, promote independence, decrease pain, and promote overall quality of life (Wilson & Barnes, 2018). In addition to physical therapy, application of heat and/or cold to painful or injured muscles, the use of a transcutaneous electrical nerve stimulation (TENS) unit, or massage can bring relief (Abrahm, 2014; Malanga, Yan, & Stark, 2015).

Beyond physical suffering, serious illness can bring spiritual, psychological, and social distress. Interventions that have been effective for addressing these nonphysical aspects of illness include individual and family counseling, prayer and spiritual rituals, hypnosis, music therapy, art therapy, guided meditation, pet therapy, and relaxation techniques (c.f., Beng et al., 2015; Montgomery, Sucala, Baum, & Schnur, 2017; Warth, Keßler, Hillecke, & Bardenheuer, 2015).

■ CONCLUSION

Pain is one of the most feared symptoms in times of serious or terminal illness. Effective pain management in hospice and palliative care requires the integrated expertise of the interdisciplinary hospice team. Both pharmacological and nonpharmacological interventions are important for addressing not only the physical aspects of serious illness but also the social, psychological, and spiritual dimensions. Patient and family support and education are crucial to promoting an understanding of pain assessment and pain management techniques.

Chapter Summary

- Effective pain management is predicated on excellent pain assessment. The primary barrier to effective pain control is incomplete pain assessment.

- Key terms in pain management include addiction, drug dependence, pseudoaddiction, and tolerance. Healthcare providers, as well as patients and families, should understand the differences among these terms when planning pain management interventions.

- The type of pain that the patient experiences is specifically related to the source of the pain.

(continued)

Chapter Summary (*continued*)

- Patients can experience somatic, visceral, and/or neuropathic pain at the end of life due to their terminal illness, concomitant illnesses, or injury.
- Nonopioid medications are used to treat mild to moderate pain and fever. NSAIDs also have anti-inflammatory properties.
- Opioid drugs are derived from the opium poppy plant. They are used to treat moderate to severe pain.
- The oral route of administration should always be used first. If this is not possible, then other routes can be used, with the least invasive routes prioritized. The IM route is discouraged.
- True morphine allergies are rare, but other drugs may be used to control pain in the case of morphine allergy.
- Although mild side effects are somewhat common. Patients generally develop a tolerance to most side effects of opioids, except constipation.
- Changes to the opioid drug regimen must be carefully undertaken. Opioid drug conversion calculations specific to the patient's needs should be used.
- Adjuvant medications can and should be used to alleviate pain or symptoms associated with the underlying illness. Adjuvant medications should be chosen based on the patient's specific symptoms.
- Nonpharmacological interventions such as acupuncture, reiki, yoga, physical therapy, application of heat or cold or a TENS unit, massage, counseling, and hypnosis, among others, are effective ways to address physical and nonphysical pain.
- Although most episodes of acute pain can be managed effectively, sedation may be considered if pain is intractable and severe.

▦ PRACTICE QUESTIONS

1. A patient who has multiple sclerosis reports burning pain in her hands. This type of pain is
   a. Somatic
   b. Neuropathic
   c. Visceral
   d. Nociceptive

2. In treating the patient in the previous question, which of the following would not be a first choice for pain management?
   a. Antidepressants
   b. Sodium channel blockers
   c. Gabapentinoids
   d. Opioids

3. According to the World Health Organization's pain ladder, which of the following would be an appropriate intervention for mild pain?
   a. A non-opioid with an adjuvant
   b. Acetaminophen with an opioid

    c. Short-acting opioid only

    d. Long-acting opioid with a breakthrough dose

4. Which is the best choice for a palliative care patient who has an acute somatic injury?

    a. Morphine 5 mg PO q2h

    b. Acetaminophen 650 mg q4h PRN

    c. Ibuprofen 400 mg PO QID × 4 days

    d. Lidocaine patch to affected area every 48 hours

5. A patient who is actively dying is no longer able to swallow oral medications. Which is the best choice for administering necessary medications now?

    a. Rectal

    b. Intravenous (IV)

    c. Transdermal

    d. Aerosol

6. An opioid-naïve patient taking morphine for cancer pain reports pruritus on his arms shortly after the first dose. The nurse should

    a. Administer naloxone immediately

    b. Monitor the patient closely

    c. Give activated charcoal

    d. Apply lotion to the arms

7. When changing an opioid from the oral to the parenteral route, the conversion ratio is generally

    a. 5:1

    b. 10:1

    c. 1:1

    d. 3:1

8. The breakthrough dose of an oral opioid should be what percentage of the total daily dose?

    a. 50%

    b. 5%

    c. 10%

    d. 75%

9. A patient taking 100 mg of long-acting morphine q12h has needed 6 to 8 doses of 10 mg immediate-release morphine in the past 24 hours. The nurse knows that

    a. The breakthrough dose should be increased

    b. The long-acting dose should be increased

   c. Both the long-acting and short-acting medication doses should be increased

   d. The opioid should be rotated

10. A patient receiving intravenous (IV) hydromorphone at a rate of 4 mg/hr should have a breakthrough dose of

   a. 2 mg of hydromorphone q1h PRN

   b. 1 mg of hydromorphone q30 minutes PRN

   c. 8 mg of hydromorphone q14 minutes PRN

   d. 2 mg of hydromorphone q15 minutes PRN

▪ REFERENCES

Abrahm, J. L. (2014). *A physician's guide to pain and symptom management in cancer patients* (3rd ed.). Baltimore, MD: Johns Hopkins University Press.

American Hospice Foundation. (2014). *Use of opiates to manage pain in the seriously and terminally Ill patient.* Retrieved from https://americanhospice.org/caregiving/use-of-opiates-to-manage-pain -in-the-seriously-and-terminally-ill-patient/

Arthritis Foundation. (2018). *Arthritis facts.* Retrieved from https://www.arthritis.org/about -arthritis/understanding-arthritis/arthritis-statistics-facts.php

Beng, T. S., Chin, L. E., Guan, N. C., Yee, A., Wu, C., Jane, L. E., . . . Meng, C. B. C. (2015). Mindfulness-based supportive therapy (MBST) proposing a palliative psychotherapy from a conceptual perspective to address suffering in palliative care. *American Journal of Hospice and Palliative Medicine, 32*(2), 144–160. doi:10.1177/1049909113508640

Bodtke, S., & Ligon, K. (2016). *Hospice and palliative medicine handbook: A clinical guide.* Retrieved from www.hpmhandbook.com

Coyle, N., & Layman-Goldstein, M. (2007). Pharmacologic management of adult cancer pain. *Cancer Network, 21*(2). Retrieved from http://www.cancernetwork.com/palliative-and-supportive -care/pharmacologic-management-adult-cancer-pain

Dalal, S. (2016). Assessment and management of opioid side effects. In E. Bruera, I. Higginson, C. F. von Gunten, & T. Morita (Eds.), *Textbook of palliative medicine and supportive care* (2nd ed., pp. 409–422). Boca Raton, FL: Taylor & Francis.

Detail-Document, P. L. (2012). *Equianalgesic dosing of opioids for pain management. Pharmacist's letter/prescriber's letter.* Retrieved from https://www.nhms.org/sites/default/files/Pdfs/Opioid-Comparison-Chart-Prescriber-Letter-2012.pdf

Dowell, D., Haegerich, T. M., & Chou, R. (2016). CDC guideline for prescribing opioids for chronic pain— United States, 2016. *JAMA, 315*(15), 1624–1645. doi:10.1001/jama.2016.1464

Epictetus. (1890). *The works of Epictetus: Consisting of his discourses, in four books, the enchiridion, and fragments.* Boston: Little, Brown, and Company.

Gilron, I., Baron, R., & Jensen, T. (2014). Neuropathic pain: Principles of diagnosis and treatment. *Mayo Clinic Proceedings, 90*(4), 532–545. doi:10.1016/j.mayocp.2015.01.018

Groninger, H., & Vijayan, J. (2014). Pharmacologic pain management at end of life. *American Family Physician, 90*(1), 26–32. Retrieved from https://www.aafp.org/afp/2014/0701/p26.pdf

Gunnarsdottir, S., Sigurdardottir, V., Kloke, M., Radbruch, L., Sabatowski, R., Kaasa, S., . . . Klepstad, P. (2017). A multicenter study of attitudinal barriers to cancer pain management. *Supportive Care in Cancer, 25*(11), 3595–3602. doi:10.1007/s00520-017-3791-8

Henneghan, A. M., & Schnyer, R. N. (2015). Biofield therapies for symptom management in palliative and end-of-life care. *American Journal of Hospice & Palliative Medicine, 32*(1), 90–100. doi:10.1177/1049909113509400

Indian Health Service, The Federal Health Program for American Indians and Alaska Natives. (n.d.). *Safe opioid prescribing.* Retrieved from https://www.ihs.gov/ painmanagement/treatmentplanning/safeopioidprescribing/

Kishner, S. (2018). *Opioid equivalents and conversions.* Retrieved from https://emedicine.medscape .com/article/2138678-overview

Krenzelok, E. P., & Royal, M. A. (2012). Confusion: Acetaminophen dosing changes based on no evidence in adults. *Drugs in R & D, 12*(2), 45–48. Retrieved from https://link.springer.com/article/ 10.2165/11633010-000000000-00000

Malanga, G. A., Yan, N., & Stark, J. (2015). Mechanisms and efficacy of heat and cold therapies for musculoskeletal injury. *Postgraduate Medicine, 127*(1), 57–65. doi:10.1080/00325481.2015.992719

McPherson, M. L. M. (2009). *Demystifying opioid conversion calculations: A guide for effective dosing.* Bethesda, MD: American Society of Health-System Pharmacists.

Milgrom, D. P., Lad, N. L., Koniaris, L. G., & Zimmers, T. A. (2017). Bone pain and muscle weakness in cancer patients. *Current Osteoporosis Reports, 15*(2), 76–87. doi:10.1007/s11914-017-0354-3

Montgomery, G. H., Sucala, M., Baum, T., & Schnur, J. B. (2017). Hypnosis for symptom control in cancer patients at the end-of-life: A systematic review. *International Journal of Clinical and Experimental Hypnosis, 65*(3), 296–307. doi:10.1080/00207144.2017.1314728

National Institute on Drug Abuse. (2017). *The neurobiology of drug addiction.* https://www.drugabuse.gov/neurobiology-drug-addiction

Nyatanga, B., Cook, D., & Goddard, A. (2018). A prospective research study to investigate the impact of complementary therapies on patient well-being in palliative care. *Complementary Therapies in Clinical Practice, 31*, 111–125. doi:10.1016/j.ctcp.2018.02.006

Paice, J. A. (2015). Pain at the end of life. In B. R. Ferrell, N. Coyle, & J. A. Paice (Eds.), *Oxford textbook of palliative nursing* (pp. 135–153). New York, NY: Oxford University Press.

Pathan, H., & Williams, J. (2012). Basic opioid pharmacology: An update. *British Journal of Pain, 6*(1), 11–16. doi:10.1177/2049463712438493

Peng, X., Wang, P., Li, S., Zhang, G., & Hu, S. (2015). Randomized clinical trial comparing octreotide and scopolamine butylbromide in symptom control of patients with inoperable bowel obstruction due to advanced ovarian cancer. *Journal of Surgical Oncology, 13*(5), 1–6. doi:10.1186/s12957-015-0455-3

Prescriber's Letter. (2012). *Equianalgesic dosing of opioids for pain management.* Retrieved from https://www.nhms.org/sites/default/files/Pdfs/Opioid-Comparison-Chart-Prescriber-Letter-2012.pdf

Reynolds, J., Drew, D., & Dunwoody, C. (2013). *American Society for Pain Management Nursing position statement: Pain management at the end of life.* Retrieved from http://www.aspmn.org/documents/PainManagementattheEndofLife_August2013.pdf

Rogers, E., Mehta, S., Shengelia, R., & Reid, M. C. (2013). Four strategies for managing opioid-induced side effects in older adults. *Clinical Geriatrics, 21*(4), 1–15. Retrieved from https://www.ncbi.nlm.nih.gov/pmc/articles/PMC4418642/

Roland, E., & von Gunten, C. F. (2009). Current concepts in malignant bowel obstruction management. *Current Oncology Reports, 11*(4), 298–303. Retrieved from https://link.springer.com/journal/11912

Saulino, M., Anderson, D. J., Doble, J., Farid, R., Gul, F., Konrad, P., . . . Boster, A. L. (2016). Best practices for intrathecal baclofen therapy: Troubleshooting. *Neuromodulation: Technology at the Neural Interface, 19*(6), 632–641. doi:10.1111/ner.12467

Selman, L. E., Williams, J., & Simms, V. (2012). A mixed-methods evaluation of complementary therapy services in palliative care: Yoga and dance therapy. *European Journal of Cancer Care, 21*, 87–97. doi:10.1111/j.1365-2354.2011.01285.x

Shanti, B. F., Tan, G., & Shanti, I. F. (2012). Adjuvant analgesia for management of chronic pain. *Practical Pain Management, 6*(3), 1–5. Retrieved from https://www.practicalpainmanagement.com/treatments/pharmacological/adjuvant-analgesia-management-chronic-pain

Smith, E. L., & Castor, T. (2015). Pain management in geriatric patients. In K. A. Sackheim (Ed.), *Pain management and palliative care* (pp. 245–263). New York, NY: Springer Publishing Company.

Smith, H. S. (2012). Opioids and neuropathic pain. *Pain Physician, 15*, ES93–ES110. Retrieved from http://painphysicianjournal.com/2012/july/2012; 15; ES93-ES110.pdf

Smith, H. S., & Peppin, J. F. (2014). Toward a systematic approach to opioid rotation. *Journal of Pain Research, 14*(7), 589–608. Retrieved from https://www.ncbi.nlm.nih.gov/pmc/articles/PMC4207581/pdf/jpr-7-589.pdf

Standish, L. J., Kozak, L., & Congdon, S. (2008). Acupuncture is underutilized in hospice and palliative medicine. *American Journal of Hospice and Palliative Medicine, 25*(4), 298–308. doi:10.1177/1049909108315916

U.S. Food and Drug Administration. (2016). *Indomethacin capsules, USP.* Retrieved from https://www.accessdata.fda.gov/drugsatfda_docs/label/2016/018829s022lbl.pdf

U.S. Food and Drug Administration. (2018). *FDA drug safety communication: Prescription acetaminophen products to be limited to 325 mg per dosage unit; Boxed warning will highlight potential for severe liver failure.* Retrieved from https://www.fda.gov

Wahler, R. G., Smith, D. B., & Mulcahy, K. B. (2017). Nebulized fentanyl for dyspnea in a hospice patient with true allergy to morphine and hydromorphone. *Journal of Pain & Palliative Care Pharmacotherapy, 31*(1), 38–42. doi:10.1080/15360288.2017.1279499

Warth, M., Keßler, J., Hillecke, T. K., & Bardenheuer, H. J. (2015). Music therapy in palliative care: A randomized controlled trial to evaluate effects on relaxation. *Deutsches Ärzteblatt International, 112*(46), 788. doi:10.3238/arztebl.2015.0788

Warusevitane, A., Karunatilake, D., Sim, J., Lally, F., & Roffe, C. (2015). Safety and effect of metoclopramide to prevent pneumonia in patients with stroke fed via nasogastric tubes trial. *Stroke, 46*(2), 454–460. doi:10.1161/STROKEAHA.114.006639

Wilson, C. M., & Barnes, C. (2018). Physical therapy in interdisciplinary palliative care and hospice teams. *Rehabilitation Oncology, 36*(2), 143–145. doi:10.1097/01.REO.0000000000000109

World Health Organization. (2018). *WHO's cancer pain ladder for adults.* Retrieved from http://www.who.int/cancer/palliative/painladder/en/

Yaksh, T., & Wallace, M. (2018). Opioids, analgesia, and pain management. In L. L. Brunton, R. Hilal-Dandan, & B. C. Knollman (Eds.), *Goodman & Gillman's: The pharmacological basis of therapeutics* (13th ed., pp. 355–420). New York, NY: McGraw-Hill Education.

Zaki, J., Wagner, T. D., Singer, T., Keysers, C., & Gazzola, V. (2016). The anatomy of suffering: Understanding the relationship between nociceptive and empathic pain. *Trends in Cognitive Science, 20*(4), 249–259. doi:10.1016/j.tics.2016.02.003

Zhang, B., Li, Q., Shi, C., & Zhang, X. (2018). Drug-induced pseudoallergy: A review of the causes and mechanisms. *Pharmacology, 101,* 104–110. doi:10.1159/000479878

Zuccaro, S. M., Vellucci, R., Sarzi-Puttini, P., Cherubino, P., Labianca, R., & Fornasari, D. (2012). Barriers to pain management. *Clinical Drug Investigation, 32*(1), 11–19. doi:10.2165/11630040-000000000-00000

15

Pain Management Evaluation

True genius resides in the capacity for evaluation of uncertain,
hazardous, and conflicting information.
—Winston Churchill

LEARNING OBJECTIVES

After completing this section, the nurse will be able to

1. Identify common side effects of opioid therapy
2. Describe signs of opioid-induced toxicity
3. Recognize and respond to signs of opioid overdose

PAIN MANAGEMENT EVALUATION

Pain management is an important issue in all healthcare settings. In hospital settings, the Joint Commission recommends that a team leader or leadership team be available for pain management, safe opioid prescribing, and evaluation of pain interventions. It is also recommended that patients take part in developing measurable pain goals and that both pharmacological and nonpharmacological interventions are used to meet those goals (Joint Commission, 2018). Similarly, the American Society for Pain Management Nursing (ASPMN) "holds the position that nurses and other health care providers must advocate for optimal pain and symptom management to alleviate suffering for every patient receiving end-of-life care" (Reynolds, Drew, & Dunwoody, 2013, p. 172).

Each patient's level of pain should be assessed prior to any intervention, and then again approximately 1 hour after the intervention. Even when a patient appears to be relatively comfortable, pain should be evaluated at least every 8 hours using an appropriate pain scale (Song, Eaton, Gordon, Hoyle, & Doorenbos, 2015). Each assessment and intervention should be carefully documented in the patient's record.

When evaluating the patient's pain, it is also important to document the patient's pain goal and the progress made toward that goal. Opioid medications are commonly used to alleviate pain in hospice and palliative care settings, but if the use of opioids does not adequately decrease the patient's pain, then opioid titration, opioid rotation, and other interventions should be implemented. While using pharmacological interventions, however, it is important to assess for and minimize side effects and adverse effects of opioid medications.

Side Effects and Adverse Effects of Opioids

Although opioids are generally safe, some side effects and adverse effects are quite serious. Common side effects include the following:

- Constipation
- Nausea and vomiting
- Pruritus
- Respiratory depression
- Sedation
- Opioid-induced neurotoxicity (OIN)
  (Wirz, 2017)

Constipation

Opioids slow gastric and intestinal motility, which leads to constipation. For some patients, the constipation can be so severe that they discontinue opioid use. Therefore it is necessary to implement a bowel regimen for every patient taking opioids, which should include both a stool softener (to increase water content of the stool) and a laxative (to increase intestinal motility). In some cases, a prescription medication, such as methylnaltrexone (Relistor) may be necessary to alleviate opioid-induced constipation. Methylnaltrexone is an opioid receptor agonist, which means that it blocks the effects of opioids in the intestinal tract but not the pain-relieving effects of the opioid. It can be administered orally or subcutaneously.

Nausea and Vomiting

Nausea and vomiting related to the use of opioids may also occur due to the effects of opioids on gastric motility and stimulation of the chemoreceptor trigger zones (CTZ). Another cause of opioid-induced nausea and vomiting may be stimulation of the mu-opioid or other opioid receptors. The cause of the nausea and vomiting may be difficult to isolate if patients have other therapies or conditions that can contribute to it. Thus, it is important to choose antiemetics that antagonize specific receptors and to keep in mind that certain medications antagonize specific receptors when changing antiemetics (see also, Chapter 16, Symptom Management). For example:

- Haloperidol antagonizes D_2 receptors
- Promethazine antagonizes H_1 receptors
- Naloxone antagonizes DOR receptor
- Ondansetron, tropisetron, dolasetron, and granisetron antagonize $5\text{-}HT_3$ receptors
- Scopalamine antagonizes ACh receptors
- Aprepitant antagonizes NK-1 receptors
- Dronabinol antagonizes DCB_1 receptors
  (Smith, Smith, & Seidner, 2012)

For most patients, nausea and vomiting occurs within the first days to weeks of opioid therapy and then dissipates. But, for others, symptoms may be severe and persistent, and a daily antiemetic may be required for comfort.

Pruritus

Another fairly common side effect of opioid use is pruritus. Pruritus arises from the superficial layers of the skin and can affect the quality of the patient's life. Pruritus occurs with opioid use and results from histamine release, as well as the effects of opioids at mu-opioid, dopamine, and serotonin receptor sites. Pruritus is common with morphine use, but is also associated with the use of other opioids. In palliative care settings, opioid-induced pruritus may necessitate opioid rotation, dose reduction, discontinuance of the opioid, or the addition of other medications (Rashid, Trivedi, Al-Shathir, Moulton, & Baumrucker, 2018).

Antihistamines are generally recommended for the treatment of opioid-induced pruritus. However, in geriatric patients, antihistamines can cause xerostoma, blurred vision, constipation, and confusion. Thus, other strategies such as topical lotions, opioid rotation, or reducing the dose of the opioid might be good choices in this population. As with other common side effects of opioid therapy, patients usually develop a tolerance to pruritus within a few days (Rogers, Mehta, Shengelia, & Reid, 2013).

Opioid-Induced Sedation

Opioid-induced sedation is another common side effect of the use of opioids. Patients who are opioid naïve are at greatest risk for over-sedation, especially when the dose is titrated upward. Caution is also required when using opioids with patients who have difficulty clearing the drug, such as geriatric patients or those who have renal dysfunction. Besides patient-specific factors, the dose of the opioid, the length of treatment, and the desired goals of treatment also contribute to the risk for opioid-induced sedation (Jarzyna et al., 2011). Most patients are usually able to develop a tolerance to opioid-induced sedation, but it is a serious concern because it may lead to respiratory depression.

Respiratory Depression

Respiratory depression is a decrease in respiratory function that can occur after the administration of an opioid. It may be mild, with the patient fully conscious, or it may lead to respiratory arrest (Jarzyna et al., 2011). Opioid-induced respiratory depression is most common among opioid-naïve patients, but other risk factors include the following:

- History of sleep apnea
- Older age
- Anatomic anomalies
- Comorbid conditions
- Psychological state
- Functional status
- Drug–drug interactions
- Cardiac or respiratory disorders
- Obesity
(Jarzyna et al., 2011)

The primary intervention for the reversal of opioid-induced respiratory depression is naloxone (van der Schier, Roozekrans, van Velzen, Dahan, & Niesters, 2014). Thus, naloxone should be readily available in the clinical setting so that interventions can be quickly implemented. Additionally, nurses must be aware of the risk factors associated with opioid-induced respiratory depression, be competent in assessing patients for opioid-induced respiratory depression, and teach patients and families about the risks for opioid-induced depression (Jungquist, Karan, & Perlis, 2011).

Opioid-Induced Neurotoxicity

OIN is a syndrome that results from an accumulation of opioid metabolites. Any opioid drug can induce OIN, but it is most commonly associated with mor-

Key Point
Meperidine should not be used in palliative care or hospice settings because its active metabolite can cause seizures.

phine. Hydromorphone is the second most common cause. The active metabolites in morphine and hydromorphone are excreted by the kidneys so caution is warranted when using these drugs in geriatric patients or those with renal dysfunction. OIN can also occur with use of fentanyl, sufentanil, and meperidine (Bodtke & Lingon, 2016). Myoclonus is one of the first and most common manifestations of OIN. Management of OIN is aimed at reversing the mechanism, so reducing the dose of the opioid or rotating to a different opioid is recommended. Clonazepam, midazolam agents, benzodiazepines, baclofen, or dantrolene can be used for treating myoclonus (Abrahm, 2014; Walker, 2016).

Opioid Overdose

Opioid overdose can occur when the dose of the administered opioid is too high, which leads to toxicity. Often opioid overdose is related to drug–drug interactions, specifically reactions between opioids and benzodiazepines (Park, Saitz, Ganoczy, Ilgen, & Bohnert, 2015). Patient misuse of opioids may also contribute to overdose (Childers, King, & Arnold, 2015). Signs of opioid overdose include the following:

- Confusion and/or delirium
- Vomiting
- Pinpoint pupils
- Lethargy and/or unresponsiveness
- Loss of consciousness
- Cyanosis
- Respiratory distress or respiratory failure (American Addiction Centers, 2018)

Hospice and palliative care nurses must be skilled at recognizing risk for and symptoms of opioid overdose and responding appropriately. Treating opioid overdose involves administration of naloxone intranasally, sublingually, intravenously, or intramuscularly. The onset of action for naloxone is 1 to 2 minutes.

■ CONCLUSION

Although opioid use for moderate to severe pain is generally safe and effective, some side effects are common and the risks associated with opioid use can be deadly. Thus, the risks should be weighed against the benefits when initiating opioid therapy. Patients and families should be taught to use the opioid exactly as prescribed and to report any untoward side effects. Hospice and palliative care nurses should be aware of the signs of opioid-induced side effects, including toxicity, and take measures to combat the patient's symptoms. Further, the nurse must be able to recognize and respond appropriately to opioid overdose.

Chapter Summary

- Pain should be assessed prior to the intervention and then approximately 1 hour after the intervention. All assessments and interventions should be carefully documented in the patient's chart.
- Every patient who is taking opioids should have an effective bowel regimen in place.
- Nausea and vomiting and pruritus are common side effects of opioid use that tend to dissipate after a few days.
- Sedation related to opioid use is common, but is serious because it can lead to respiratory depression. Respiratory depression occurs on a continuum, with the most serious manifestation being respiratory arrest.

(continued)

> **Chapter Summary** (*continued*)
>
> - OIN results from the buildup of opioid metabolites. Generally, one of the first signs of OIN is myoclonus.
> - Opioid overdose is a potentially deadly consequence of opioid use. Hospice and palliative care nurses must expertly recognize and respond to signs of opioid overdose.

■ PRACTICE QUESTIONS

1. The only side effect of opioid use that a patient will not develop a tolerance to is

   a. Constipation

   b. Nausea

   c. Vomiting

   d. Pruritus

2. A patient who is overly sedated from opioid use is at risk for

   a. Myoclonus

   b. Addiction

   c. Respiratory depression

   d. Overdose

3. After increasing the dose of a hospice patient's morphine in response to increasing pain, the nurse notices jerking movements in the patient's arms and legs. The nurse should

   a. Increase the dose of the morphine

   b. Reposition the patient

   c. Administer naloxone

   d. Administer lorazepam

4. The treatment for opioid overdose is

   a. Naloxone

   b. Ondansetron

   c. Lorazepam

   d. Hydromorphone

5. After administering a pain medication to a patient, the nurse should reassess the patient's pain

   a. Every 10 minutes

   b. In 1 hour

   c. Periodically

   d. Within 8 hours

▓ REFERENCES

Abrahm, J. L. (2014). *A physician's guide to pain and symptom management in cancer patients* (3rd ed.). Baltimore, MD: Johns Hopkins University Press.

American Addiction Centers. (2018). *Symptoms of opiate overdose: Vicodin, OxyContin, and Morphine.* Retrieved from https://americanaddictioncenters.org/prescription-drugs/opiate-overdose/

Bodtke, S., & Lingon, K. (2016). *Hospice and palliative medicine handbook: A clinical guide.* Retrieved from www.hpmhandbook.com

Childers, J. W., King, L. A., & Arnold, R. M. (2015). Chronic pain and risk factors for opioid misuse in a palliative care clinic. *American Journal of Hospice and Palliative Medicine, 32*(6), 654–659. doi:10.1177/1049909114531445

Jarzyna, D., Jungquist, C. R., Pasero, C., Willens, J. S., Nisbet, A., Oakes, L., . . . Polomano, R. C. (2011). American Society for Pain Management Nursing guidelines on monitoring for opioid-induced sedation and respiratory depression. *Pain Management Nursing, 12*(3), 118–145. doi:10.1016/j.pmn.2011.06.008

Joint Commission. (2018). *Joint Commission enhances pain assessment and management requirements for accredited hospitals.* Retrieved from https://www.jointcommission.org/assets/1/18/ Joint_Commission_Enhances_Pain_Assessment_and_Management_Requirements_for_Accredited_ Hospitals1.PDF

Jungquist, C. R., Karan, S., & Perlis, M. L. (2011). Risk factors for opioid-induced excessive respiratory depression. *Pain Management Nursing, 12*(3), 180–187. doi:10.1016/j.pmn.2010.02.001

Nightingale, F. (1860). *Notes on nursing.* Retrieved from http://digital.library.upenn.edu/women/ nightingale/nursing/nursing.html

Park, T. W., Saitz, R., Ganoczy, D., Ilgen, M. A., & Bohnert, A. S. (2015). Benzodiazepine prescribing patterns and deaths from drug overdose among US veterans receiving opioid analgesics: Case-cohort study. *BMJ, 350*, h2698. doi:10.1136/bmj.h2698

Rashid, S., Trivedi, D. D., Al-Shathir, M., Moulton, M., & Baumrucker, S. J. (2018). Is there a role for 5-HT3 receptor antagonists in the treatment of opioid-induced pruritus? *American Journal of Hospice and Palliative Medicine, 35*(4), 740–744. doi:10.1177/1049909117736062

Reynolds, J., Drew, D., & Dunwoody, C. (2013). American Society for Pain Management Nursing position statement: Pain management at the end of life. *Pain Management Nursing, 14*(3), 172–175. doi:10.1016/j.pmn.2013.07.002

Rogers, E., Mehta, S., Shengelia, R., & Reid, M. C. (2013). *Clinical Geriatrics, 21*(4), 1–15. Retrieved from http://www.consultant360.com/articles/four-strategies-managing-opioid-induced-side-effects -older-adults

Smith, H. S., Smith, J. M., & Seidner, P. (2012). Opioid-induced nausea and vomiting. *Annals of Palliative Medicine, 1*(2), 121–129. doi:10.3978/j.issn.2224-5820.2012.07.08

Song, W., Eaton, L. H., Gordon, D. B., Hoyle, C., & Doorenbos, A. Z. (2015). Evaluation of evidence-based nursing pain management practice. *Pain Management Nursing, 16*(4), 456–463. doi:10.1016/j.pmn.2014.09.001

van der Schier, R., Roozekrans, M., van Velzen, M., Dahan, A., Niesters, M., & Niesters, M. (2014). Opioid-induced respiratory depression: Reversal by non-opioid drugs. *F1000Prime Reports, 6*, 1–8. doi:10.12703/P6-79. Retrieved from https://www.ncbi.nlm.nih.gov/pmc/articles/PMC4173639/

Walker, P. W. (2016). Other symptoms: Xerostomia, hiccups, pruritus, pressure ulcers and wound care, lymphedema and myoclonus. In S. Yennurajalingam & E. Bruera (Eds.), *Oxford American handbook of hospice and palliative medicine and supportive care* (2nd ed., pp. 195–206). New York, NY: Oxford University Press.

Wirz, S. (2017). Management of adverse effects of opioid therapy. *Zeitschrift fur Gastroenterologie, 55*(4), 394–400. doi:10.1055/s-0043-103348

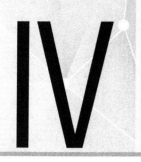

IV

Patient Care: Symptom Management

16

Symptom Management

*In watching diseases, both in private houses and in public hospitals,
the thing which strikes the experienced observer most forcibly is
this, that the symptoms or the sufferings generally considered to be
inevitable and incident to the disease are very often not symptoms
of the disease at all, but of something quite different. . .*
—Nightingale (1860)

■ LEARNING OBJECTIVES

After completing this section, the nurse will be able to

1. Describe symptoms commonly experienced at the end of life
2. Identify the etiologies of common end-of-life symptoms
3. Choose appropriate interventions for end-of-life symptoms

■ SYMPTOM MANAGEMENT AT THE END OF LIFE

Management of distressing symptoms at the end of life requires the specialized skills of the hospice or palliative care team. Most often, end-of-life symptoms are related to the terminal diagnosis. But they may also be related to multisystem organ failure that occurs in the final weeks to days, or they may be iatrogenic.

Once symptoms occur, the primary goal is to alleviate the patient's suffering. In addition to pharmacologic and nonpharmacologic interventions, patient and family education and support are required throughout the end-of-life process. In the following sections, common symptoms will be reviewed according to the associated body system, in accordance with the Hospice and Palliative Nurses Association (HPNA) certification test outline.

Neurological Symptoms

Neurological symptoms at the end of life may be related to the patient's underlying disease or to other causes. Common neurological symptoms that may arise at the end of life include aphasia, dysphagia, altered level of consciousness, myoclonus, paresthesias or neuropathies, seizures, extrapyramidal symptoms (EPS), paralysis, spinal cord compression (SCC), and increased intracranial pressure (ICP). Each of these symptoms will be reviewed.

Aphasia

Aphasia is the inability to understand written or spoken communication (receptive or Wernicke's aphasia), to communicate verbally (expressive or Broca's aphasia), or both (global aphasia). Aphasia may result from tumor growth, neurological or degenerative diseases, head injury, or stroke. Patients who have receptive aphasia are unable to comprehend what is being communicated by others and do not have the ability to repeat what is said to them. Patients who have expressive aphasia may repeat phrases or words that are not appropriate for the situation.

The causes of aphasia may be related to the patient's terminal diagnosis or may be the result of an acute episode. A speech therapist should be consulted to assess the type and extent of aphasia using tests such as the Western Aphasia Test or the Boston Diagnostic Aphasia test. With appropriate and timely interventions, some communication barriers may be overcome through the use of traditional phonetic boards or more advanced eye-tracking or brain-computer interface systems (Hwang, Weng, Wang, Tsai, & Chang, 2014).

Dysphagia

Dysphagia is difficulty swallowing, which increases the patient's risk for aspiration. Patients who have dysphagia may exhibit choking with eating or drinking, drooling, heartburn, pain behind the sternum, and/or hoarseness (American Speech-Language-Hearing Association, 2018). Dysphagia may occur together with odynophagia (painful swallowing) and may result from tumor growth, neurological disease, or overall disease progression. Other factors that may affect swallowing in adults include poor dentition or ill-fitting dentures (Son, Seong, Kim, Chee, & Hwang, 2013).

"Dysphagia is estimated to affect about 8% of the world's population (roughly 590 million people). Texture-modified foods and thickened drinks are commonly used to reduce the risks of choking and aspiration" (Cichero et al., 2017, p. 293). Nurse-initiated interventions such as proper head and neck positioning, slow introduction of foods and liquids, modification of medication administration, and dysphagia screenings are effective in reducing aspiration pneumonia and other adverse outcomes (Hines, Kynoch, & Munday, 2016). Patients who have difficulty swallowing, particularly poststroke, should remain nothing by mouth (NPO) until a formal evaluation by a speech therapist takes place (Fedder, 2017). The patient and family should consider whether formal assessments such as video fluoroscopy, and interventions such as the placement of a feeding tube, are in alignment with the goals of care.

Altered Level of Consciousness

A patient's level of consciousness may change due to disease progression, metabolic changes, or structural issues, such as tumor growth. When a patient's level of consciousness is altered, responses to verbal or tactile stimuli may be delayed or absent. Altered levels of consciousness can be categorized as follows (Boss & Huether, 2014):

- *Confusion*: The patient is unable to think clearly; judgment and decision-making capacity are impaired
- *Disorientation*: The patient first becomes disoriented to time, then to place, and then to person
- *Lethargy*: Decrease in spontaneous speech or movement. The patient responds to verbal or tactile stimuli, but may be disoriented
- *Coma*: The patient has no verbal response to verbal or tactile stimuli. Patient has no motor response to noxious or painful stimuli. Coma can categorized as follows:
  - Light coma: The patient exhibits purposeful movement in response to verbal or tactile stimuli
  - Coma: The patient may respond to verbal or tactile stimuli, but response is not purposeful
  - Deep coma: The patient is unresponsive to any stimuli

The patient's level of consciousness can be assessed using the Glasgow Coma Scale. In palliative care settings, the Consciousness Scale for palliative care may be used (Kovach & Reynolds, 2015). The prognosis for a comatose patient is dependent on the cause and the level of severity of the coma. If possible, the cause of the altered consciousness should be reversed. If the level of consciousness is related to the natural progression of the disease process and curative interventions are not consistent with the plan of care, then supportive nursing interventions should be implemented. Family and caregiver support in the form of active listening, emotional support, and providing space away from the patient for caregivers to unburden their concerns should also be provided (Kovach & Reynolds, 2015).

Myoclonus

Myoclonus is the manifestation of involuntary, jerky muscle movements or twitching of muscles or muscle groups. It is a symptom related to infection, spinal cord injury, stroke, brain tumors, and other disorders (National Institute of Neurological Disorders and Stroke,

2018a). Myoclonus may also result from the accumulation of opioid metabolites, as occurs in opioid-induced neurotoxicity.

Assessment of myoclonus involves carefully determining the time of onset, related symptoms, medication history, current diagnoses, and whether symptoms arise at rest or with movement (Kojovic, Cordivari, & Bhatia, 2011). If possible, the cause(s) of myoclonus should be removed. If the myoclonus is related to opioid-induced neurotoxicity, then the dose of the opioid should be reduced or a different opioid should be used. Pharmacological interventions include clonazepam, midazolam agents, benzodiazepines, baclofen, or dantrolene (Abrahm, 2014; Walker, 2016).

Paresthesias or Neuropathies

Paresthesias are abnormal sensations such as tingling, pins and needles, or burning. Paresthesias can result from nerve impingement or compression, but usually resolve when the pressure is relieved. Chronic paresthesia is often related to neurologic disease or nerve damage. At the end of life, paresthesia may result from neurological disease, tumor growth, or immobility. Alleviation of the symptom is contingent upon identifying and removing the cause, if possible (National Institute of Neurological Disorders and Stroke, 2018b).

Neuropathy, which means nerve damage or disease, can result from high glucose levels, nerve injury, tumor growth, and ischemia (National Institute of Neurological Disorders and Stroke, 2018c). Peripheral neuropathy is particularly common in the lower extremities and can lead to undetected foot infection, injury, or ulceration. Charcot foot, a condition in which the hallmark sign is collapse of the midfoot (sometimes called "rocker foot"), may also result from chronic type 2 diabetes mellitus. The initial symptoms of Charcot foot are pain and inflammation, but these may go undetected in patients who have neuropathy and decreased sensation in their feet (Rogers et al., 2011).

Treatment of neuropathy is the same as the treatment for neuropathic pain. That is, it includes "non-opioids, gabapentinoids, tricyclic antidepressants, and serotonin–norepinephrine reuptake inhibitors (all first-line therapies), as well as anticonvulsants and sodium channel blocking antiarrhythmics" (Groninger & Vijayan, 2014, p. 30). The use of opioids for the treatment of neuropathic pain should be considered a second-, or even third-line, intervention (Smith, 2012). When opioids are used to treat neuropathic pain, methadone is a good choice (Abrahm, 2014). Clinicians should be aware, however, that if opioids are used in the treatment of neuropathic pain, higher doses of opioids are usually needed for effective treatment (Paice, 2015).

Seizures

Seizures are the result of abnormal electrical impulses within the brain. At the end of life, seizures may result from the terminal diagnosis, deterioration of overall condition due to disease progression, drug use or discontinuance, and/or preexisting underlying conditions. Seizures may be of two sorts: focal or generalized. Focal seizures are characterized by an altered level of consciousness during which the patient may have uncontrollable repetitive movements, called automatisms. Focal seizures result from abnormal electrical activity in only one part of the brain. If electrical activity is disorganized throughout the brain tissue, a generalized seizure may occur (National Institute of Neurological Disorders and Stroke, 2018d).

Types of generalized seizures:

- *Absence seizures*, which occur when the patient appears to stare, unfocused, and may or may not have muscle twitching
- *Tonic seizures*, which involve muscle contraction, particularly in the extremities and back
- *Clonic seizures*, which cause repetitive, uncontrollable, bilateral jerking movements
- *Myoclonic seizures*, which manifest with jerking movement of the extremities
- *Atonic seizures*, which involve a loss of muscle tone, and can lead to collapse
- *Tonic–clonic seizures*, which cause a combination of symptoms, including muscle contraction and then relaxation, as well as possible loss of consciousness and autonomic nerve dysfunction
  (National Institute of Neurological Disorders and Stroke, 2018d)

Early detection of generalized seizure activity and prompt intervention optimize recovery. Interventions include the following:

- Protecting the patient's airway
- Ensuring patient safety throughout the seizure
- Suctioning as needed
- Maintaining a calm disposition
- Administering lorazepam 2 mg IV; may repeat up to a total dose of 0.1 mg/kg and infused no faster than 2 mg/min
- Administering phenytoin IV, 15 to 20 mg/kg, not more than 50 mg/min (following the administration of the lorazepam). As an alternative to phenytoin, valproic acid may be used at a rate of 6 mg/kg/min up to a total dose of 30 mg/kg followed by a maintenance dose of 1 to 2 mg/kg/hr.
  (Guide to Care for Patients: Managing Seizures, 2007; Kuriya & Dev, 2016)

Typically, seizures do not last longer than a few minutes. If the cause of the seizure is identified and removed, seizures will not typically reoccur (Bodtke & Lingon, 2016). In all cases, lorazepam is the drug of choice. But midazolam may be used in hospice and palliative care settings, especially because the intranasal route (0.2 mg/kg, q15 minutes, up to three times) is an option (Tradounsky, 2013). In addition to prompt assessment and intervention, patient and family education are needed to ensure safety.

Extrapyramidal Symptoms

EPS are dyskinesias that can be the sequelae of certain neurological disorders or side effects of medications. At the end of life, dopamine antagonists, such as haloperidol, are used to treat delirium and other end-of-life symptoms (Hosker & Bennett, 2016). Patients might exhibit new-onset EPS associated with previously prescribed antipsychotics due to weight loss or interactions with new medications. EPS typically involve akathisia, characterized by restlessness, pacing, parkinsonism, dystonias, and tardive dyskinesia (Bodtke & Lingon, 2016). Prompt intervention for EPS is essential to minimize patient suffering. Upon noting EPS, the patient's medications should be reviewed. If a pharmacological side effect or drug interaction can be identified, then the medication should be discontinued or the dose should be reduced, if possible. Pharmacological interventions include as follows:

- For tardive dyskinesia: lorazepam 0.5 mg PO/SC/IV BID, or propranolol 10 mg PO BID, or clonidine 0.1 to 0.4 mg PO BID
- For parkinsonism or dystonias: benztropine 1 mg PO/SC/IM/IV BID or diphenhydramine 25 to 50 mg PO TID–QID (Bodtke & Ligon, 2016).

Paralysis

Paralysis is characterized by completely or partially blocked transmission of signals from the brain, spinal cord, or nerves to the muscles. Paralysis can be categorized as complete, partial, permanent, temporary, flaccid, or spastic. It may be further described as localized, which often affects the face, hands, feet, or larynx, or generalized. Generalized paralysis is differentiated by the affected areas of the body:

- Monoplegia affects one limb
- Hemiplegia affects the limbs on one side of the body
- Diplegia affects the same area on both sides of the body (e.g., both arms or both sides of the face)
- Paraplegia affects both arms, both legs, and sometimes the muscles of the trunk
- Quadriplegia affects both arms, both legs, and if it is related to a spinal injury, may affect the entire body from the injured vertebrae down, including internal organs
  (Cleveland Clinic Foundation, 2018)

In the United States, over five million people are affected by paralysis, which primarily results from stroke. Other causes include brain or spinal cord injury, multiple sclerosis, and cerebral palsy (Armour, Courtney-Long, Fox, Fredine, & Cahill, 2016). When paralysis is related to brain injury, it may cause locked-in syndrome, which diminishes motor abilities, including speech. Patients who have locked-in syndrome are sometimes able to communicate through eye movements (Demertzi, Jox, Racine, & Laureys, 2014).

Paralysis at the end of life may be related to the terminal illness and irreversible. In such cases, nursing care should focus on preserving function, decreasing risk for injury, and patient and family support. The expertise of the interdisciplinary team is needed to meet the multidimensional needs of the patient and family. If a reversible cause is established, then it should be removed or reduced, if possible.

Spinal Cord Compression

SCC is a medical emergency that occurs when the thecal sac is compressed by surrounding vertebrae at the level of the spinal cord or cauda equina. The compression causes neurological dysfunction and sometimes irreparable damage (Bobb, 2015). SCC often occurs due to malignancy, especially in patients who have breast, prostate, or lung cancer (Kuriya & Dev, 2016). When SCC is related to cancer, the patient's prognosis is generally only about 3 to 6 months (Bobb, 2015). Nonmalignant causes of SCC include benign tumors, degenerative disease, infection, inflammation of the spinal cord related to trauma, herniated disc(s), osteoporosis, or structural anomalies (Bobb, 2015). Hospice and palliative care nurses must identify patients who are at risk for SCC and educate the patient and family on safety with repositioning, signs of SCC, and management options.

SCC typically manifests as sudden back pain that can be localized, referred, or radicular (Kuriya & Dev, 2016). The pain is worse when the patient is lying down and is relieved when the patient stands. If these symptoms are accompanied by bowel or bladder incontinence, SCC should be suspected in patients with cancer until proven otherwise (Bobb, 2015). In patients who have cauda equina syndrome, saddle numbness occurs with decreased urethral or rectal tone (Kuriya & Dev, 2016).

When the symptoms of SCC appear, the patient may be treated empirically, or diagnostic testing may be conducted if it is consistent with the patient's goals of care. x-rays will show bone deformities, tumor, and the overall condition of the spine (Bobb, 2015). Gadolinium-enhanced MRI of the entire spine is an imaging option that reveals the condition of the discs and tissues surrounding the spine. If SCC is suspected and advanced testing is desired, an MRI should be conducted promptly.

Once SCC is diagnosed, high-dose corticosteroid therapy should begin with a 100 mg IV bolus followed by 24 mg dexamethasone PO

QID for 3 days, then tapered doses for 10 days. If a low-dose cortico-steroid regimen is warranted by the patient's condition, a 10 mg IV bolus of dexamethasone followed by 4 mg IV QID for 3 days, then tapered doses for 14 days should be used. Rapid IV bolus doses of corticosteroids may cause perineal burning. If this occurs, the patient should be assured that this is a temporary side effect (Bobb, 2015). If more aggressive interventions are appropriate, decompressive surgery and/or fractionated external-beam radiation therapy are effective in many cases (Abrahm, 2014; Bobb, 2015; Kuriya & Dev, 2016).

Increased ICP

The pressure within the cranium needs to be maintained between 0 and 15 mmHg. Pressure shifts can occur quickly due to the accumulation of blood or cerebral spinal fluid. Other causes of increased ICP include "head trauma, intracranial hemorrhage, embolic stroke, tumors, infections, and alterations in cerebral spinal fluid production and/or absorption" (Schimpf, 2012, p. 161). Early signs of increased ICP include restlessness, altered consciousness, blurred vision, severe headache, nausea and vomiting, behavioral changes, diminished level of consciousness, fever, and lethargy (Johns Hopkins Medicine, 2018; Weaver, 2015).

If interventions are not taken, or are not effective in decreasing increased ICP, hemiplegia or hemiparesis can occur with decorticate and then decerebrate posturing. If the oculomotor nerve becomes compressed, the pupils will stop reacting and will become fixed and dilated. A late sign of increased ICP is Cushing's triad, which involves bradycardia, irregular respirations, and an increase in systolic blood pressure while diastolic blood pressure remains unchanged. If late signs of increased ICP are noted, the patient's prognosis is poor (Weaver, 2015).

Management of increased ICP may involve decompressive surgery or placement of a ventricular drain, if this is consistent with the goals of care (Carney et al., 2016; Weaver, 2015). Hyperosmolar therapy, such as mannitol, may be used intravenously at a rate of 0.25 to 1 mg/kg body weight. If mannitol is used, arterial hypotension, defined as a systolic blood pressure of <90 mmHg should be avoided. Other options include ventilation therapies and high-dose barbiturates if the ICP is refractory. Additionally, infection, deep vein thrombosis (DVT), and seizure prophylaxis are recommended (Carney et al., 2016). If interventions aimed at the cause of the increased ICP are not consistent with the goals of care, nursing care will involve interventions to manage symptoms, such as pain and fever, as well as family education and support (Weaver, 2015).

Cardiovascular Symptoms

At the end of life, cardiovascular symptoms may arise for a variety of reasons. In patients who have a terminal cardiac diagnosis, deteriorating cardiac status is expected. However, cardiovascular symptoms may also manifest as multiorgan system failure ensues. Common end-of-life symptoms related to cardiac status include coagulation issues (bleeding or hemorrhage, thrombi or DVT, pulmonary embolus, and disseminated intravascular coagulation [DIC] syndrome), angina, edema, syncope, and superior vena cava syndrome (SVCS). Each of these symptoms are reviewed in the following sections.

Coagulation Problems

Coagulation disorders are characterized by the inability to regulate clotting or clot formation. Contributing factors include tumor invasion, side effects of treatments, thrombocytopenia, nutritional deficiencies, use of anticoagulants, or inherent coagulation abnormalities (Kuriya & Dev, 2016). Patients who have bleeding disorders or who have internal bleeding may exhibit signs of increased ICP, epistaxis, hemoptysis, hematemesis, melena, hematochezia, hematuria, and/or vaginal bleeding (Kuriya & Dev, 2016).

Bleeding and Hemorrhage

For nonacute bleeding, the nurse should take measures to stop the bleeding and to alleviate the patient's anxiety. Patients and families should be educated regarding the risks for bleeding, especially in relation to liver disease. Interventions to decrease localized bleeding include the following:

- Packing
- Compressive dressings
- Topical hemostatics
- Positioning to decrease blood flow
- Astringents
  (Kuriya & Dev, 2016)

In cases of catastrophic hemorrhage, steps should be taken to stem further bleeding, if consistent with the goals of care. Some interventions include radiation therapy, palliative transcatheter chemoembolization (TACE), endoscopy, vitamin K, vasopressin, antifibrinolytic agents, octreotide (for bleeding esophageal varices), platelet transfusion, or fresh frozen plasma. In some cases, palliative sedation may be considered. If bleeding is excessive and visible, dark-colored towels should be available to reduce the visual impact of the bleeding for the patient and caregivers (Kuriya & Dev, 2016).

Thrombi and DVT

Coagulation problems also contribute to thrombus formation. In patients at risk for clot formation due to immobility, orthopedic trauma, or known circulatory problems, thromboembolic stockings or sequential compression devices may be used prophylactically (Powers & Jones,

2012). Signs of thrombosis depend on the affected organ or vessel. For example, in the case of DVT, the patient may manifest the following symptoms in the affected limb: edema, pain, localized warmth, venous distention, and tenderness when touched (Blevins, 2015; Powers & Jones, 2012).

The "gold standard" for diagnosing DVT is the venogram. However, the test is invasive and may lead to complications. A noninvasive test to detect blood flow is the venous Doppler. The test can be conducted easily and painlessly. Blood flow should be evaluated on both extremities for comparison. Pharmacological treatments for DVT may include heparin, low molecular weight heparin (LMWH), unfractionated heparin, or fondaparinux. Enoxaparin, a LMWH, should not be used in patients who have acute renal failure.

Pulmonary Embolism

Pulmonary embolism (PE) is another consequence of thrombus formation and often results from a deep vein thrombus that migrated to a pulmonary artery (Lavorini et al., 2013). Risk factors for PE include the following:

- Genetic predisposition
- Recent surgery
- Previous DVT or PE
- Immobility
- Hospitalization
- Cancer
- Infection
- Older age
- Heart failure
- Stroke
- Acute respiratory failure
- Rheumatic disease
- Inflammatory bowel disease
  (Lavorini et al., 2013)

The patient may initially be asymptomatic or experience only vague symptoms. In symptomatic patients, unexplained chest pain occurs in about 97% of patients with confirmed PE (Lavorini et al., 2013). Other symptoms may include hypoxemia, pleuritic rub, hypotension, anxiety, diaphoresis, cough, syncope, and/or hemoptysis.

When a thrombus occludes a pulmonary artery, pressure within the right ventricle in the heart increases. On exam, tachycardia, crackles, fever, diaphoresis, pronounced S_2 with closure of the pulmonic and aortic valves, S_3, indicating fluid overload, and possibly an S_4 gallop, indicating thickened ventricular walls secondary to hypertension or aortic stenosis, may be found (Powers & Jones, 2012).

Diagnosing PE may be challenging because laboratory testing is not definitive. Rather, several tests, such as the d-dimer, leukocyte level, erythrocyte sedimentation rate, dehydrogenase, B-type natriuretic peptide, and troponin levels, can all be used to rule out differential diagnoses or to rule in PE. A chest x-ray may be used to rule out some differential diagnoses, but the spiral CT scan with IV contrast can be used to more accurately confirm the presence of a PE. In patients who cannot tolerate IV contrast due to allergy or renal impairment, ventilation/perfusion (V/Q) scanning can be used. The "gold standard" for a diagnosis of PE is confirmation through a pulmonary angiogram, but it is cost-prohibitive and invasive, which limits use in some patients (Morici, 2014; Powers & Jones, 2012).

Treatment of a PE initially focuses on stabilizing the patient. If consistent with the goals of care, invasive measures such as mechanical ventilation or intubation may be initiated to improve ventilation. Alternatively, noninvasive bi-level positive airway pressure ventilation may be used to improve ventilation (Morici, 2014).

Pharmacological interventions center on IV resuscitation and vascular stabilization. Vasopressors, such as norepinephrine, dopamine, or epinephrine may be used for this purpose. Anticoagulation therapy is necessary and several options are available, such as LMWH, unfractionated heparin, fondaparinux, warfarin, and rivaroxaban. In the initial phase of PE, parenteral heparin, LMWH, rivaroxaban, or fondaparinux should be initiated. The patient should be carefully transitioned to an oral agent or another agent such as LMWH, rivaroxaban, or fondaparinux (Morici, 2014).

If aggressive or curative treatments are not in alignment with the goals of care, steps should be taken to alleviate dyspnea and anxiety. Sedation may be required if the patient is severely distressed and symptomatic. Family education is needed throughout the process, as a PE can occur suddenly and the prognosis is poor if interventions are not initiated quickly.

Disseminated Intravascular Coagulation

DIC is a disorder that can be fatal if therapeutic measures are not taken quickly. DIC is characterized by excessive blood clotting. The thrombi formed lead to infarction in multiple vessels and organs, which consequently bring about organ damage. Internal bleeding ensues due to platelet depletion. The hospice and/or palliative care nurse must identify patients who are at risk for DIC due to sepsis, inflammatory disease, cancer, liver disease, trauma, aneurysms, or vascular disorders (Shelton, 2012; Wada, Matsumoto, & Yamashita, 2014).

If DIC occurs, signs of bleeding may be subtle initially and may include bruising, petechiae, purpura, hematuria, hematemesis, hematochezia, and/or hemothorax. Treatment involves replacement of blood and blood products and correction of metabolic shifts. To combat thrombus formation, anticoagulants are used, but cautery or cryoablation may become necessary to control bleeding (Shelton, 2012). Other treatments for DIC include synthetic protease inhibitors and antifibrinolytic therapy. If organ failure occurs due to DIC, natural protease inhibitors are recommended, but antifibrinolytic treatments should be avoided (Wada et al., 2014).

Angina

Angina, also called angina pectoris, is chest pain caused by increased oxygen demands on the cardiac muscle. It can result from exercise, strenuous activity, an obstruction within a cardiac vessel, or myocardial infarction. Angina can be classified as either stable or unstable. Typical manifestations of angina include sudden chest pain, heaviness, tightness, or a squeezing sensation. The pain can sometimes radiate to the jaw, arms, or back. Associated symptoms can include shortness of breath, fatigue, and nausea (McDonald, 2015). When two to three symptoms of angina occur together, it is referred to as atypical angina.

Treatment of angina is directed at relieving the symptoms and ruling out infarction. When angina occurs, the patient should discontinue precipitating activities. Nitroglycerin should be administered sublingually, orally, transdermally, intravenously, or as a lingual spray. When consistent with the goals of care, testing to rule out myocardial infarction or vascular occlusion should take place promptly. Invasive procedures such as angioplasty, stenting, or cardiac bypass graft may be considered when the benefits of such interventions outweigh the risks (McDonald, 2015).

Edema

Edema in the lower extremities is usually due to end-stage organ failure, particularly heart, liver, or kidney failure. Other causes of edema include vascular insufficiency, superior vena cava syndrome (SVCS), and medication side effects (Walker, 2016). In hospice patients, hypoalbuminemia and fluid overload are also potential causes of edema (Bodtke & Ligon, 2016). Edema is categorized as either pitting or nonpitting. Nonpitting edema does not remain indented when pressure placed on the edematous area is removed. Pitting edema, on the other hand, retains an indentation when pressure over the edematous area is released. Pitting edema is graded on a scale of 1 to 4, depending on the depth of the indentation left in the skin when pressure is exerted (see Figure 16.1).

Lower extremity edema can be related to right-sided heart failure or to liver or kidney failure. In severe edema, the weight of the fluid causes

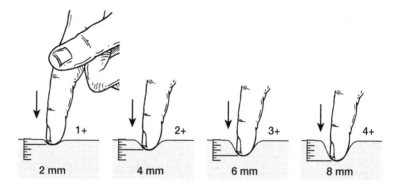

FIGURE 16.1 Pitting edema.

discomfort and decreased mobility. The limb should be elevated, and compression is often helpful in reducing swelling. Diuretics may not be useful, particularly if the edema is refractory. Interventions should be implemented slowly as rapid fluid shifts can increase cardiac symptoms (Bodtke & Ligon, 2016).

Lymphedema is caused by obstruction or removal of the lymph nodes, which is often related to cancer surgeries or other treatments. Lymph accumulation may lead to fibrosis or sclerosis, causing permanent edema. If fibrosis has not yet occurred, elevation and compression may be helpful. Diuretics are generally not effective for lymphedema. However, careful skin care is necessary. Manual lymphatic drainage performed by a trained massage therapist or physical therapist may be helpful in reducing fluid accumulation, promoting mobility, range of motion and quality of life (Bodtke & Ligon, 2016; Walker, 2016).

Syncope

Syncope is a "temporary loss of consciousness usually related to insufficient blood flow to the brain" (American Heart Association, 2018). The most common cause of syncope is hypotension, which can be related to cardiac disease, dehydration, fluid shifts, or postural changes (orthostatic hypotension; American Heart Association, 2018; Dalal, 2016). In hospice and palliative care settings, end-stage cardiac disease and atrial fibrillation are common causes of syncope. Safety is a priority nursing concern for a patient who experiences syncope. The patient and family should be taught to change position slowly and to have assistance available for transfers. Further, the patient should be taught to sit or lie down if warning signs such as nausea, diaphoresis, or lightheadedness occur (American Heart Association, 2018).

Patients who have recurrent episodes of syncope may experience anxiety, somatization, and panic symptoms for which fluoxetine may be helpful (Flevari et al., 2017). If consistent with the plan of care,

testing such as electrocardiogram, laboratory studies to identify dehydration or electrolyte imbalances, or a tilt table test, can be conducted to
identify the cause of the syncope. If the syncope is cardiac-related, pacemaker placement may alleviate cardiac symptoms of fatigue, dyspnea,
and syncope (Spiess, 2017).

Superior Vena Cava Syndrome

SVCS is a condition caused by obstruction of the superior vena cava
and/or nearby lymph nodes or vessels (see Figure 16.2). Most commonly, the obstruction occurs from a primary tumor or metastasis from
lung or breast cancer or lymphoma (Abrahm, 2014; Manthey & Ellis,
2016). The signs of SVCS are consistent with obstructed drainage from
the head, neck, and upper extremities and include the following:

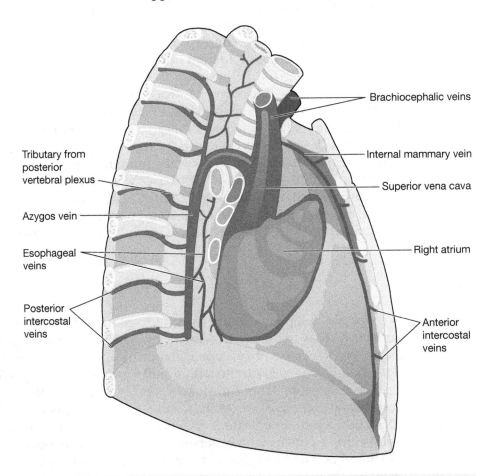

FIGURE 16.2 Superior vena cava.

- Facial swelling, especially after recumbancy
- Jugular vein distension
- Distention of chest veins, upper extremity edema
- Ruddy complexion (facial plethora)

Common symptoms associated with SVCS generally occur over a 2-week period and include the following:

- Cough
- Dyspnea
- Hoarseness
- Blurred vision
- Syncope
- Headache
- Confusion
- Obtundation
  (Abrahm, 2014; Kuriya & Dev, 2016; Manthey & Ellis, 2016)

Diagnosis of SVCS is confirmed through chest x-ray, CT scan, or magnetic resonance angiography (MRA). Once confirmed, treatment options include chemotherapy or radiation, steroid use, diuretics, thrombolytics, and possibly stent placement or bypass. The head of the bed may be raised 45 to 90 degrees to promote drainage from the head and neck. The prognosis for SVCS is fair to poor and ranges from <6 months to 2 years. The prognosis is influenced by the extent of malignancy, patient age (worse prognosis for patients over 50), history of smoking, and use of steroids (Kuriya & Dev, 2016; Manthey & Ellis, 2016). Thus, a discussion regarding goals of care with the interdisciplinary team is essential in discerning how to proceed with therapeutic interventions.

Respiratory Symptoms

At the end of life, respiratory symptoms may arise for a variety of reasons, including chronic lung disease, cancer, or as sequelae of other end-stage disease. Common end-of-life respiratory symptoms and complications include cough, dyspnea and shortness of breath, pleural effusions (PEs), pneumothorax, and increased secretions. Each of these are reviewed in the following secitons.

Cough

Coughing is an innate response to bronchial, laryngeal, or tracheal irritation. In both acute and chronic cough, the reflex is modulated by excitatory and inhibitory pathways in the nervous system (Sharfman & Braun, 2017). Cough can be related to

- Infection
- Bronchitis
- Rhinitis
- Postnasal drip
- Gastroesophageal reflux
- Asthma
- Chronic obstructive pulmonary disease (COPD)
- Pulmonary fibrosis
- Congestive heart failure (CHF)
- Pneumothorax
- Cancer, cancer treatments, and complications of cancer
- Bronchiectasis
- Cystic fibrosis
- Medications that cause cough such as angiotensin-converting enzyme (ACE) inhibitors
  (Dudgeon, 2015).

Acute coughing typically occurs in response to choking or is associated with other self-limiting issues such as acute infection. Chronic cough is defined as coughing that lasts more than 8 weeks. Chronic, forceful coughing can cause pain, fatigue, insomnia, pathological fractures, and hemoptysis. The risk for hemoptysis is increased with the use of anticoagulants or nonsteroidal anti-inflammatory drugs (NSAIDs).

Nursing assessment of cough should include evaluation of the frequency of cough, associated symptoms, the effect on the patient's quality of life, timing of cough (early morning, after meals, evening) and whether the cough is dry or productive. If productive, the color and character of the sputum should also be noted. Patients should be taught to avoid cough triggers such as smoking or other respiratory irritants. If the cough is secondary to gastroesophageal reflux disease (GERD), the head of the bed should be raised when sleeping. Pharmacological interventions for cough are summarized in Table 16.1.

Table 16.1 Pharmacological Interventions for Cough

Drug Class	Drug Action	Examples	Recommended Dose	Key Points
Centrally acting antitussives	Suppress cough by acting on the central cough center	Dextromethorphan	10 mg/5 mL, 10–20 mg PO q4h PRN or 30 mg/5 mL ER, 30–60 mg q12h to a maximum of 120 mg/24 hr	This group of medications decreases the cough stimulus
		Opioids	Codeine 7.5–20 mg PO q4h PRN Morphine 2.5–5 mg PO/SC q4h PRN Nebulized morphine 5 mg in 3–5 mL saline q4h PRN (may need up to 30 mg per treatment to reach therapeutic effect)	Caution: use of dextromethorphan in patients who are taking fluoxetine or paroxetine can cause serotonin syndrome
		Gabapentin	300 mg PO daily. May titrate to 600 PO TID	
Peripherally acting agents	Anesthetize cough receptors in the airways that trigger cough reflex	Benzonatate	100–200 mg PQ q4–8h, maximum of 600 mg in 24 hours	Using guaifenesin in combination with benzonatate improves effectiveness
		Nebulized lidocaine	2% (20 mg/mL) or 4% (40 mg/mL) preservative-free solution; use 5 mL per treatment (100 mg if using 2% solution; 200 mg if using 4% solution)	Nebulized lidocaine improves the effectiveness of each cough and reduces bronchial irritation related to persistent cough Nebulized lidocaine may cause numbness of the throat

(continued)

Table 16.1 Pharmacological Interventions for Cough (continued)

Drug Class	Drug Action	Examples	Recommended Dose	Key Points
Intranasal glucocorticoids	Anti-inflammatory effect	Fluticasone propionate	One to two sprays in each nostril daily	Useful if coughing is related to allergic rhinitis or postnasal drip
		Mometasone	One to two sprays in each nostril daily	May take several days to achieve therapeutic effect
Decongestants	Cause vasoconstriction, which reduces swelling in nasal passages	Phenylephrine hydrochloride	10 mg PO q4 h PRN; maximum of 60 mg in 24 h	Phenylephrine hydrochloride and oxymetazoline may cause anticholinergic side effects
		Oxymetazoline	Two to three sprays in each nostril twice daily	Second-generation oral antihistamines are less sedating and have fewer anticholinergic side effects
		Loratadine	10 mg PO daily	
PPI or H2 blockers	Reduce stomach acid production	Pantoprazole or omeprazole (PPIs)	20–40 mg PO daily	Useful if cough is related to GERD
		Famotidine	20–40 mg PO BID; reduce dose in renal disease	GERD-related cough is often related to tube feedings
Expectorants	Liquefy pulmonary secretions, making it easier to clear the airway of mucus	Guaifenesin	Immediate release: 100 mg/5 mL; 200–400 mg q4h PRN Extended release: 600 mg tablet 600–1,200 mg PO q12h	Do not crush extended-release medications Combination products that include guaifenesin and dextromethorphan are available

GERD, gastroesophageal reflux disease; PIP, proton pump inhibitor.

Sources: Bodtke, S., & Lingon, K. (2016). Hospice and palliative medicine handbook: A clinical guide. Retrieved from www.hpmhandbook.com; Dudgeon, D. (2015). Dyspnea, terminal secretions, and cough. In B. R. Ferrell, N. Coyle, & J. A. Paice (Eds.), Oxford textbook of palliative nursing (4th ed., pp. 246–261). New York, NY: Oxford University Press.

Dyspnea and Shortness of Breath

The most common respiratory symptom is dyspnea. Dyspnea can include features of increased respiratory effort associated with breathing as well as air hunger. Some causes of dyspnea include acute or chronic pulmonary disease, cancer, organ failure, anemia, or deconditioning related to immobility. Although dyspnea is primarily a subjective experience, a 0 to 10 scale or the Modified Borg Scale can be used to assess the severity of the dyspnea (see Chapter 7, Pulmonary Disorders; Sharfman & Braun, 2017).

Management of dyspnea may include the use of supplemental oxygen, but this treatment is mainly effective for hypoxic patients only. If supplemental oxygen is used, a nasal cannula should be used rather than a mask. Other interventions may include noninvasive positive pressure ventilator support, chest wall vibration, neuroelectric muscle stimulation, and breathing training. The use of fans, relaxation techniques, counseling, emotional support, and distraction may also afford the patient some relief.

Pharmacological interventions commonly used to treat dyspnea include opioids and anxiolytics such as

- Morphine 2.5 to 5 mg PO, SC, or IV every 4 hours as needed
- Lorazepam 1 to 2.5 mg sublingually every 4 hours as needed
- Midazolam 1 to 2 mg PO or SC (may produce a synergistic effect when used in combination with morphine for severe dyspnea) (Dudgeon, 2016; Sharfman & Braun, 2017; Walbert, 2016)

Pleural Effusion

PE is the accumulation of fluid between the pulmonary pleurae. Normally, in the pleural space, there are 1 to 15 mL of fluid. In the case of PE, several liters of fluid may be present, which significantly constricts the affected lung. PE is associated with heart, liver, or kidney failure and with infection, inflammation, and lung cancer. PE causes sudden-onset pleuritic pain on the affected side along with dyspnea and tachypnea. On auscultation, a friction rub may be heard over the effusion. Lung sounds may be decreased or absent on the affected side, depending on the extent of the effusion. On percussion, dullness rather than the expected resonance will be heard over the effusion (Hopper, 2015).

The diagnosis of PE can usually be confirmed with chest x-ray. Bedrest is recommended to promote spontaneous resolution (Hopper, 2015). In patients who have advanced disease, palliation of symptoms is the primary goal. The least invasive approach to reducing a PE is pleuroscopy and placement of an indwelling pleural catheter (see Figure 16.3), which should be initiated when the benefits of the intervention outweigh the risks (Engleka, 2016). The appropriateness of

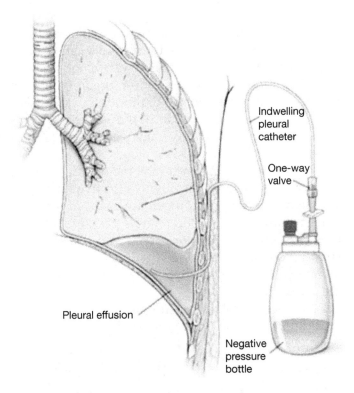

FIGURE 16.3 Indwelling pleural catheter.

Source: https://consultqd.clevelandclinic.org/1-minute-consult-when-should-an-indwelling-pleural-catheter-be-considered-for-malignant-pleural-effusion/

invasive interventions such as chest tube placement and video-assisted thoracic surgery (VATS) is dependent on the patient's overall condition and prognosis (Engleka, 2016).

Pneumothorax

Pneumothorax means that air is present in the pleural space. There are several types of pneumothorax:

- *Spontaneous pneumothorax* occurs primarily in tall, thin patients and smokers. It is also common in those with emphysema or lung cancer.
- *Traumatic pneumothorax* is related to a penetrating injury as can occur from a protruding fractured rib or from an injury such as a knife wound.
- *Open pneumothorax* occurs when air escapes through an opening in the pleural space, such as when a chest tube dislodges.
- *Closed pneumothorax* occurs when air becomes trapped in the pleural space and cannot escape. A tension pneumothorax is a type

of closed pneumothorax. Consequences of a closed pneumothorax include pressure on the heart and great vessels, which leads to a mediastinal shift away from the affected side.

- *Hemothorax* occurs when blood is trapped in the pleural space. (Hopper, 2015)

When pneumothorax occurs, the patient may experience sudden dyspnea, chest pain, tachypnea, restlessness, and anxiety. Asymmetrical chest expansion as well as decreased or absent breath sounds on the affected side may be noted. In the case of tension pneumothorax, hypoxia and hypotension may occur. Heart sounds may be muffled due to pressure on the heart. The diagnosis can be confirmed through chest x-ray and/or ultrasound. The prognosis is poor if interventions are not initiated, although a small pneumothorax may resolve on its own. The treatment for significant pneumothorax may include a chest tube to suction or the placement of a Heimlich valve (see Figure 16.4). Oxygen and proper positioning of the patient may also help to alleviate symptoms associated with pneumothorax (Hopper, 2015).

Terminal Secretions

At the end of life, respiratory secretions may accumulate as the patient becomes unable to clear the airway or to swallow. Terminal secretions are exacerbated by sialorrhea, or excessive oral secretions that can occur at the end of life. The secretions cause a "rattling" noise with each breath that may be distressing to the family or caregivers. However, neither the accumulation of fluid nor the sound produced is thought to be distressing to the patient (Sharfman & Braun, 2017).

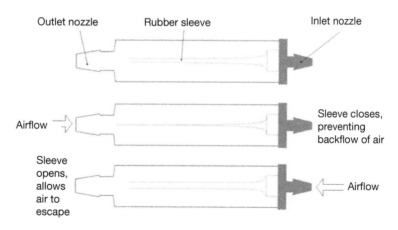

FIGURE 16.4 Heimlich valve.

Source: https://commons.wikimedia.org/wiki/File:Heimlich_valve.GIF

Repositioning the patient as needed and suctioning the oropharynx may help to decrease the sound of secretions moving with respirations. However, deep suctioning is not recommended. If the secretions are causing dyspnea or distress to the patient, the following anticholinergic medications may be used:

- Hyoscyamine 0.4 to 0.6 mg subcutaneously every 4 hours as needed *OR*,

- Atropine eye drops 1%, one to two drops sublingually every 8 hours as needed, *OR*

- Glycopyrrolate 1 mg orally or 0.2 to 0.4 mg subcutaneously or intravenously every 4 to 8 hours as needed
  (Dudgeon, 2015; Twomey & Dowling, 2013)

Gastrointestinal Symptoms

At the end of life, gastrointestinal symptoms may arise for a variety of reasons, including bowel or bladder disease, cancer, medical interventions, or as sequelae of other end-stage diseases. Common end-of-life gastrointestinal symptoms include constipation, diarrhea, bowel incontinence, ascites, hiccups, nausea and vomiting, bowel obstruction, and bleeding. Each of these are reviewed in the following sections.

Constipation

Constipation is a very common symptom in the end-of-life setting, even in the last week of life (Hui, dos Santos, Chisholm, & Bruera, 2015). Signs of constipation include the following:

- Abdominal distention

- Nausea or indigestion

- Fewer than three bowel movements in a week

- Dry, hard stools

- Stools that are difficult to pass or straining with defecation

- Feeling incomplete emptying of the rectum after a bowel movement (National Institute of Diabetes and Digestive and Kidney Diseases, 2018; Nowicki, 2015)

Constipation occurs when stool is retained in the colon or rectum for an extended period of time. This retention may be due to slowed gastrointestinal motility, increased water absorption in the intestines, a bowel obstruction (this may cause obstipation), or some combination of these factors (Nowicki, 2015). Medications used in hospice and palliative care settings, such as antidiarrheals and opioids, may also contribute to constipation. Other factors include immobility, low-fiber diet, and dehydration.

Nursing assessment of constipation involves auscultating bowel sounds, palpation of the abdomen, assessing skin turgor, and taking a detailed patient history to include diet, mobility, usual bowel pattern, any associated issues (i.e., blood in stools, hemorrhoids, pain with defecation), and typical consistency of stools. The extent of constipation may be seen on x-ray. Therapeutic interventions for constipation include encouraging a high-fiber diet, recommending 2 to 3 L of fluid per day (if fluid restriction is not in place), exercise as tolerated, and the use of laxatives (see Table 16.2). If laxatives are used to prevent opioid-induced constipation, the dose of the laxative should be increased if the dose of the opioid is increased.

In some cases, with the use of laxatives, only a small amount of liquid stool may be noted, which is an indication of a fecal impaction. The presence of a fecal impaction may be confirmed through digital exam of the rectum. If an impaction is present, a bisacodyl or glycerin suppository may be given. If digital disimpaction is necessary, 2% lidocaine gel should be applied to the rectum prior to the procedure. However, digital disimpaction should be avoided if perforation or bleeding are possible outcomes, especially in patients who have tumors or open areas in the perianal area (Bodtke & Ligon, 2016; Nowicki, 2015).

Diarrhea

Diarrhea results when fecal matter passes through the intestines too quickly for water to be properly absorbed from the stool. Patients often experience the following symptoms with diarrhea:

- Abdominal pain
- Cramping
- Lethargy
- Weakness
- Nausea and/or vomiting
- Abdominal distention
- Anorexia
- Increased thirst
  (Nowicki, 2015)

Diarrhea can lead to dehydration and nutrient/electrolyte imbalances because of the associated fluid loss. Thus, interventions should be quickly implemented to identify the etiology and treat accordingly. First steps should include the following:

- Discontinuing laxatives
- Assessing for impaction

Table 16.2 Pharmacologic Interventions for Constipation

Laxative	Examples	Onset of Action	Key Points
Bulk-forming laxatives Absorb water, increasing fecal mass and producing colon distention, stimulating peristalsis, and reducing transit time	Psyllium (Metamucil): start at 5–7 g daily Methylcellulose (Citrucel): start at 4–7 g daily	12–72 hours	Requires minimum 300–500 mL fluid with each dose to prevent impaction Should be used prophylactically, not for acute distress due to long onset of action Do not use in patients who have ileus, fecal impaction
Lubricant Coat the surface of the stool and the wall of the intestine, making it easier to pass stool	Glycerin suppository: 1 PR qd Mineral oil: 30–60 mL PO qd	6–8 hours when taken orally; suppository usually effective within 15–30 minutes	Prevents reabsorption of water in stool
Opioid antagonists Block opioid receptors in bowel	Methylnaltrexone (Relistor): For patients with chronic non-cancer pain: 450 mg PO qAM or 12 mg subcutaneously qAM For patient with advanced illness, the dosage is weight-based Naloxegol (Movantik): 12.5–15 mg PO qd	30–60 minutes	Used to treat opioid-induced constipation Prior to beginning therapy opioid antagonists, all maintenance laxatives should be discontinued. Ensure that patient is in close proximity to bathroom prior to administration.
Osmotic laxatives Pull water into stool and increase peristalsis	Lactulose (10 g/15 mL): 15–30 mL daily to a maximum of 60 mL/d in divided doses Polyethylene glycol (Miralax): 17–34 g/d dissolve 1 capful in 8 oz of liquid daily (up to 8 doses daily)	24–48 hours 48–96 hours	Bloating and flatulence may occur

(continued)

Table 16.2 Pharmacologic Interventions for Constipation (*continued*)

Laxative	Examples	Onset of Action	Key Points
Surfactant/detergent laxatives Draw water into colon	Docusate Sodium (Colace): 100 mg qd-BID Mineral oil: 15–45 mL daily	1–3 days Oral: 6–8 hours PR: 2–15 minutes	Liquid is bitter; mix with juice or milk
Bowel stimulants Stimulate submucosal nerve plexus to increase peristalsis	Bisacodyl (Dulcolax): start 5 mg daily to a maximum of 30 mg daily Suppository: 10 mg PR qd Senna (Senokot) Start 15 mg daily to a maximum of 70–100 mg daily	6–10 hours <1 hour 6–12 hours	Avoid in ileus, obstruction Monitor for fluid and electrolyte imbalance Suppository may cause rectal burning Senna may cause cramping, nausea, or vomiting Patients may develop a tolerance

Sources: Arthur, J. A. (2016). Constipation and bowel obstruction. In S. Yennurajalingam & E. Bruera (Eds.) *Oxford American handbook of hospice and palliative medicine and supportive care* (2nd ed., pp.138–152). New York, NY: Oxford University Press; Bodtke, S., & Lingon, K. (2016). *Hospice and palliative medicine handbook: A clinical guide.* Retrieved from www.hpmhandbook.com.

- Identifying signs of infection
- Replacing lost fluids and electrolytes
- Providing proper skin care if incontinence occurs
  (Bodtke & Ligon, 2016; Nowicki, 2015)

If signs of infection, such as fever, are present, antidiarrheal medication should be used cautiously, and for a limited duration. Common antidiarrheals include the following:

- Opioids or opioid-derivatives such as diphenoxylate/atropine (Lomotil) one to two tablets PO BID-QID PRN for loose stools
- Nonopioid antidiarrheal such as loperamide (Immodium) 4 mg PO once at onset of symptoms, then 2 mg PO after each loose stool. Use cautiously in older adults due to anticholinergic side effects. Diphenoxylate/atropine is a better choice for older adults
- Antacids and adsorbents such as bismuth salicylate may be used to treat diarrhea, nausea, and indigestion. Bismuth salicylate also has anti-inflammatory and antibacterial properties; it is available in 262 mg tablets. The usual dose is two tablets hourly as needed to a maximum of 16 tablets in 24 hours
- Bulk-forming or fiber agents may be used to absorb excess water in the stool. For example, psyllium one to two teaspoons may be mixed with liquids up to three times daily
  (Arthur, 2016; Bodtke & Lingon, 2016)

Bowel Incontinence

Bowel incontinence is the uncontrolled passage of stool. It may result from muscle weakness or atrophy, neurological disease, or severe diarrhea. If bowel incontinence occurs, the goal should be to identify and remove the cause, if possible. Any associated symptoms such as weight loss, fever, rectal bleeding, or steatorrhea should be documented. Environmental changes such as placing a bedside commode near the patient, ensuring a clear path to the bathroom, ensuring proper lighting, and removing any physical restraints should be made (Arthur, 2016). Skin should be properly cleansed after each episode of incontinence and a barrier cream or ointment may be used, if needed.

Ascites

Ascites is the accumulation of fluid in the abdominal cavity due to portal hypertension and hypoalbuminemia. Other causes of ascites include malignancy and heart failure. Regardless of the cause, ascites is an indication of end-stage disease. It causes abdominal discomfort, altered body image, decreased mobility, and dyspnea as the fluid increases pressure on the diaphragm. Ascites may also lead to umbilical herniation, cellulitis, or bacterial peritonitis (Bodtke & Lingon, 2016).

Interventions for ascites include the following:

- Sodium restriction to 2 g/d
- Fluid restriction
- Spironolactone 50 to 400 mg daily
- Furosemide 20 to 150 mg daily
- Paracentesis (if >4 L, add IV albumin)
- Transjugular intrahepatic portosystemic shunt (TIPS) procedure (Medici & Meyers, 2016)

If paracentesis is used frequently to alleviate symptoms, then the patient should consider placement of an indwelling abdominal catheter (Bodtke & Lingon, 2016). When weighing benefits and risks of treatment options, patients and caregivers should be taught that the TIPS procedure may induce hepatic encephalopathy, which compromises cognitive functioning. Treatment choices should always be consistent with the goals of care, and the hospice or palliative care nurse serves as a source of information and support as treatment options are considered.

Hiccups

Hiccups are "sudden, involuntary contractions of one or both sides of the diaphragm and intercostal muscles, terminated by an abrupt closure of the glottis producing the sound of 'hic'" (Dahlin & Cohen, 2015, p. 210). Hiccups are categorized as follows:

- Benign, which last from a few minutes up to 2 days
- Persistent, which last between 2 days and 1 month
- Intractable, which last longer than 1 month

Frequent hiccups can cause indigestion, bloating, pain, abdominal distention, insomnia, and fatigue. The effect on the quality of the patient's life should be determined and interventions should be chosen that are in alignment with the goals of care. Nonpharmacological interventions include the following:

- Holding one's breath
- Rebreathing in a paper bag
- Compressing the diaphragm
- Applying ice in the mouth
- Inducing a cough or sneeze
- Placing pressure on the nose
- Swallowing sugar
- Eating a lemon wedge with bitters
- Eating soft bread

- Touching the palate with a cotton swab
- Ocular compression
- Carotid massage
- Cognitive behavioral therapy
- Repositioning
- Fasting
- Inserting a nasogastric tube
- Acupuncture
- Inducing vomiting
- Disrupting the action of the phrenic nerve (ablation is a last resort because of the risk to pulmonary function)
  (Dahlin & Cohen, 2015; Walker, 2016)

In addition to nonpharmacological interventions, several pharmacological interventions may be used to treat hiccups. Some examples include the following:

- Simethicone 15 to 30 mL PO every 4 hours to decrease gastric distension
- Baclofen 5 to 10 mg PO every 6 to 12 hours up to 15 to 37 mg daily or midazolam 5 to 10 mg PO every 4 hours to reduce muscle spasms
- Gabapentin 300 to 600 mg PO TID for its anticonvulsant effects
- Amitriptyline 10 to 50 mg PO or sertraline 50 to 150 mg PO QID for central nervous system effects
- Haloperidol 2 to 10 mg PO/IV/SQ every 4 to 12 hours to block dopamine and alpha-adrenergic receptors
  (Dahlin & Cohen, 2015; Walker, 2016)

Nausea or Vomiting

In the presence of advanced disease, nausea and vomiting are frequently experienced due to tumors, obstruction, increased ICP, vestibular disturbances, decreased gastric motility, medication side effects (including chemotherapy), or psychological stress. Nausea is a subjective feeling described as the need to vomit and is commonly experienced as pressure in the back of the throat or epigastrium. It is associated with increased salivation, loss of appetite, and diaphoresis. Vomiting is an objective finding that involves uncontrollable expulsion of stomach contents from the mouth. Although nausea and vomiting are often co-occurring, they should always be assessed separately (Chow, Cogan, & Mun, 2015).

Understanding the pathophysiology of nausea and vomiting is crucial for determining the most appropriate interventions. Vomiting can be stimulated when the vomiting center is triggered in the medulla oblongata. The chemoreceptor zone and the cortex are central neural pathways that also can stimulate the vomiting center. Likewise, disturbances in the vestibular apparatus from motion or vertigo also stimulate nausea and vomiting (see Figure 16.5; Chow et al., 2015).

Management of nausea and vomiting requires both pharmacological and nonpharmacological approaches. Nonpharmacological approaches should include withholding routine medications (if possible), offering small meals or full liquid diet, provision of adequate hydration, cognitive behavioral therapy, complementary and alternative approaches (i.e., aromatherapy, relaxation, mediation), repositioning, alleviation of pressure caused by tumor growth through surgery, stenting, decompression, or insertion of a nasogastric tube (Bodtke & Ligon, 2016; Chow et al., 2015).

Pharmacological interventions should be aimed specifically toward alleviating the trigger of the vomiting center. A summary of antiemetic therapy is presented in Table 16.3.

Bowel Obstruction

Malignant bowel obstruction (MBO) is commonly related to intraabdominal cancers. MBO can partially or fully obstruct the large or small intestine, which places the patient at risk for sepsis, perforation, and necrosis. The prognosis is generally poor, only 30 to 90 days after onset. Signs of MBO include nausea and vomiting of undigested food. In the advanced stage, there is a possibility of vomiting fecal matter. Bowel sounds will be hyperactive with borborygmi. Pain and/or abdominal distention is more common with obstruction of the large intestine (Chow & Korateng, 2015).

Management of MBO is primarily palliative and directed at easing nausea, vomiting, pain, and colic. If the patient is not able to tolerate food or fluids, parenteral fluid may be initiated for comfort. A nasogastric tube may be inserted to help decrease abdominal distention. Frequent oral care and ice chips may be offered to ease dry mouth.

Pharmacological interventions such as the use of opioids, anticholinergics, and corticosteroids may be useful palliative options. For nausea associated with MBO, metoclopramide 10 mg every 6 to 8 hours is considered a first-line intervention. Octreotide, 50 to 100 mcg SC or IV every 8 to 12 hours, may also be helpful due to its antisecretory effect. However, its use may be limited due its high cost and side effects such as diarrhea, flatulence, abdominal pain, nausea, and constipation (Arthur, 2016).

Genitourinary Symptoms

At the end of life, genitourinary symptoms may arise for a variety of reasons, including infection, cancer, medical interventions, or as sequelae of other end-stage disease. Common end-of-life genitourinary symptoms include bladder spasms, urinary incontinence, and urinary retention. Each of these are reviewed in the following sections.

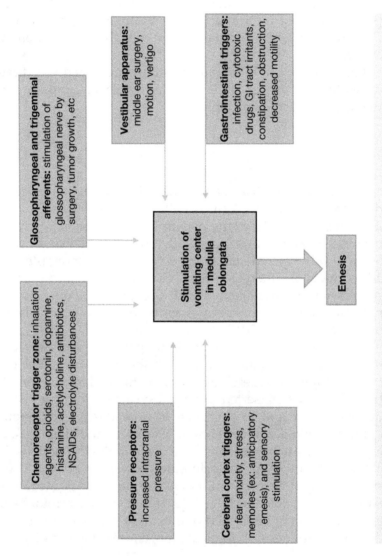

FIGURE 16.5 Pathophysiology of nausea and vomiting.

Table 16.3 Antiemetics

Antiemetic Class	Examples	Key Points
Anticholinergic agents	Hyoscine (scopolamine) 1.5 mg patch, ½–3 patches transdermally every 72 hours or 0.6–1 mg SC/IV every 6–8 hours	Hyoscine is specifically indicated for nausea and vomiting related to motion or obstruction. Use cautiously in older adults due to anticholinergic side effects.
	Atropine eye drops 1%, 1–2 drops sublingually every 8 hours as needed	
	Hyoscyamine 0.4–0.6 mg subcutaneously every 4 hours as needed	
Antihistaminic agents	Diphenhydramine 25–50 mg PO/SC/IV every 6 hours PRN	The antiemetic effects of these drugs is due to their ability to block H1 receptors in the vomiting center, CTZ, and vestibular nuclei.
	Cyclizine 50 mg PO every 4–6 hour PRN to a maximum of 200 mg daily	Use diphenhydramine cautiously in older adults due to risk for extrapyramidal side effects. Cyclizine is recommended for nausea and vomiting related to increased ICP, motion sickness, pharyngeal stimulation, or mechanical bowel obstruction.
Benzodiazepines	Lorazepam 0.5–2 mg PO/SC/IV every 8–12 hours	Synergistic effect with psychological techniques Should be used in combination with another agent unless anxiety is the cause of the nausea/vomiting
Cannabinoids	Dronabinol 5–10 mg PO every 3–6 hours Nabilone 1–2 mg PO BID	Useful for chemotherapy-related nausea and vomiting if other treatments fail
Corticosteroids	Dexamethasone 4 mg PO every 6 hours (with food)	May be used prophylactically during chemotherapy or radiation therapy. May help reduce bowel obstruction

(continued)

Table 16.3 Antiemetics *(continued)*

Antiemetic Class	Examples	Key Points
Dopamine receptor antagonists	Haloperidol 0.5–2 mg PO/SC/IV every 4–6 hours Prochlorperazine 10–20 mg PO/SC/IV every 6 hours or 25 mg rectally (best for opioid-induced nausea)	Blocks dopamine in the chemoreceptor zone. Sedating effect may be beneficial for patients who are near death.
Octreotide	Octreotide 100–400 mcg SC every 8 hours	Used to decrease nausea and vomiting associated with bowel obstruction
Prokinetic agents	Metoclopramide 10–20 mg PO/SC/IV every 4–6 hours up to 40 mg for chemo-induced nausea and vomiting	Indicated for gastric stasis; typically administered prior to meals. Dose reduction is appropriate in renal disease and in older adults Contraindicated in bowel obstruction, perforation, or in the immediate postoperative period
Selective 5-HT3 receptor antagonists	Ondansetron 4–8 mg PO/SC/IV every 8 hours on day 1 of chemotherapy; 16–24 mg PO once, or 8–16 mg IV once (maximum dose of 16 mg)	Specifically indicated for preventing chemotherapy or radiation-induced nausea and vomiting
Substance P antagonists (NKI receptor antagonists)	Aprepitant 125 mg PO once on day 1 of chemotherapy, then 80 mg PO every morning on days 2–3. Start 1 hour prior to chemotherapy on day 1. Give with a corticosteroid and a 5-HT3 antagonist.	May be used in combination with ondansetron to prevent chemotherapy or radiation-induced nausea and vomiting

CTZ, chemoreceptor trigger zones; ICP, increased intracranial pressure.
Sources: Bodtke, S. & Lingon, K. (2016). Hospice and palliative medicine handbook: A clinical guide. Retrieved from www.hpmhandbook.com; Chow, K., Cogan, D., & Mun, S. (2015). Nausea and vomiting. In B. R. Ferrell, N. Coyle, & J. A. Paice (Eds.), *Oxford textbook of palliative nursing* (4th ed., pp. 174–190). New York, NY: Oxford University Press.

Bladder Spasms

Bladder spasms are sudden, painful contractions of the bladder caused by the action of the detrusor muscle against a blocked or partially blocked bladder outlet. Blockage of the bladder outlet may be secondary to tumor, blood clots, or a foreign object such as a urinary catheter or stent. An indwelling urinary catheter that is too large, blocked, or kinked may also block the bladder outlet (Gray & Sims, 2015).

Diagnosis of bladder spasm is primarily based on the patient's report of symptoms such as stabbing, cramping, or colicky pain in the suprapubic area. The pain may be associated with urinary urgency or leakage. Management of bladder spasm involves addressing the underlying etiology, if possible. If a urinary catheter is in place, it should be changed to a smaller size. The balloon should be inflated to the appropriate size. Patients who experience bladder spasm should be taught to drink sufficient fluids and avoid bladder irritants such as caffeine and alcohol. Anticholinergic medications may also be used to inhibit contractions. In severe cases, injection of botulinum toxin A into the detrusor can help to decrease feelings of urinary urgency (Gray & Sims, 2015).

Urinary Incontinence

Urinary incontinence is the uncontrollable loss of urine. It may be transient in patients with delirium, urinary tract infection, immobility, or severe constipation. It can also be a side effect of certain medications. Some physical conditions that diminish the contraction of the detrusor can also cause chronic urinary incontinence (Gray & Sims, 2015).

Assessment of urinary incontinence should begin with a review of medications to identify any drugs that may cause incontinence or sedating medications that can reduce sensitivity to bladder fullness, causing overflow incontinence. Further, the timing of incontinence should be noted along with whether it occurs only at night, with stress (sneezing, coughing), or involves continual leaking. Management of urinary incontinence should be discussed with the patient and caregiver(s). Proper skin care should be provided after each episode of incontinence. If the patient is bedbound, proper technique for changing adult briefs or bed linens should be reviewed with the caregiver(s). An indwelling urinary catheter may be inserted if sphincter insufficiency is severe (Gray & Sims, 2015). However, the insertion of an indwelling urinary catheter may increase the risk for complicated urinary tract infection (Flores-Mireles, Walker, Caparon, & Hultgren, 2015). Inquiring about signs and symptoms of urinary tract infection and obtaining a urine sample for urinalysis are important steps in establishing etiology and treatment.

Urinary Retention

Urinary retention is the inability to pass urine. Causes of urinary obstruction include the following:

- Urinary tract infection
- Mechanical obstruction (most common in patients who have benign prostatic hypertrophy, colon, or pelvic cancer)
- Neurological issues
- Medications such as
  - Anticholinergics

- Antihistamines
- Antidepressants
- Antihypertensives
- Anti-Parkinson agents
- Antipsychotics
- Sympathomimetics
- Opioids (especially when used in combination with anticholinergics)
(Bodtke & Ligon, 2016; Wong & Reddy, 2016)

When urinary retention occurs, a medication review should be completed to identify causative agents. Medications that cause urinary retention should be discontinued, if possible. Insertion of an indwelling urinary catheter may be warranted by bladder firmness on palpation, bladder scan results indicating over 300 mL of urine, or straight catheterization residual of 200 to 300 mL of urine (Bodtke & Ligon, 2016)

Musculoskeletal Symptoms

At the end of life, musculoskeletal symptoms may arise for a variety of reasons, including immobility, metastasis, pain, debility, or as sequelae of other end-stage disease. Common end-of-life musculoskeletal problems include impaired mobility, deconditioning, and pathological fractures. Each of these are reviewed in the following sections.

Impaired Mobility or Complications of Immobility

Immobility can be related to numerous end-stage diseases or conditions, such as pain, edema, ascites, and others. Immobility increases the risk for skin breakdown, physical deconditioning, activity intolerance, and pathological fractures. When a patient becomes immobile temporarily or permanently, frequent assessment of the condition of the skin and of risk factors for ulceration should be conducted regularly using a reliable tool, such as the Braden scale (see Figure 16.6).

Immobility is a key risk factor for pressure ulcers due to the compression of the skin and underlying tissue between the bed or chair surface and the bones. Immobility combined with sensory loss, incontinence, and poor nutrition increases the risk for pressure ulcers exponentially. Further, patients who must rely on others for repositioning in bed or for transfers are at risk for skin shear injuries or friction abrasions (Bates-Jensen & Petch, 2015).

Prevention of pressure ulcers is a priority for patients' ongoing comfort and well-being. Active participation in repositioning should be encouraged through the use of side rails and/or trapeze bars, which

BRADEN SCALE – For Predicting Pressure Sore Risk

SEVERE RISK: Total score ≤9 HIGH RISK: Total score 10–12 MODERATE RISK: Total score 13–14 MILD RISK: Total score 15–18				DATE OF ASSESS →				
RISK FACTOR	**SCORE/DESCRIPTION**				1	2	3	4
SENSORY PERCEPTION Ability to respond meaningfully to pressure-related discomfort	**1. COMPLETELY LIMITED** Unresponsive (does not moan, flinch, or grasp) to painful stimuli due to diminished level of consciousness or sedation OR limited ability to feel pain over most of body surface.	**2. VERY LIMITED** Responds only to painful stimuli. Cannot communicate discomfort except by moaning or restlessness OR has a sensory impairment which limits the ability to feel pain or discomfort over ½ of body.	**3. SLIGHTLY LIMITED** Responds to verbal commands but cannot always communicate discomfort or need to be turned OR has some sensory impairment which limits ability to feel pain or discomfort in 1 or 2 extremities.	**4. NO IMPAIRMENT** Responds to verbal commands. Has no sensory deficit which would limit ability to feel or voice pain or discomfort.				
MOISTURE Degree to which skin is exposed to moisture	**1. CONSTANTLY MOIST** Skin is kept moist almost constantly by perspiration, urine, etc. Dampness is detected every time patient is moved or turned.	**2. OFTEN MOIST** Skin is often but not always moist. Linen must be changed at least once a shift.	**3. OCCASIONALLY MOIST** Skin is occasionally moist, requiring an extra linen change approximately once a day.	**4. RARELY MOIST** Skin is usually dry; linen only requires changing at routine intervals.				
ACTIVITY Degree of physical activity	**1. BEDFAST** Confined to bed.	**2. CHAIRFAST** Ability to walk severely limited or nonexistent. Cannot bear own weight and/or must be assisted into chair or wheelchair.	**3. WALKS OCCASIONALLY** Walks occasionally during day, but for very short distances, with or without assistance. Spends majority of each shift in bed or chair.	**4. WALKS FREQUENTLY** Walks outside the room at least twice a day and inside room at least once every 2 hours during waking hours.				
MOBILITY Ability to change and control body position	**1. COMPLETELY IMMOBILE** Does not make even slight changes in body or extremity position without assistance.	**2. VERY LIMITED** Makes occasional slight changes in body or extremity position but unable to make frequent or significant changes independently.	**3. SLIGHTLY LIMITED** Makes frequent though slight changes in body or extremity position independently.	**4. NO LIMITATIONS** Makes major and frequent changes in position without assistance.				
NUTRITION Usual food intake pattern [1]NPO: Nothing by mouth. [2]IV: Intravenously. [3]TPN: Total parenteral nutrition.	**1. VERY POOR** Never eats a complete meal. Rarely eats more than ⅓ of any food offered. Eats 2 servings or less of protein (meat or daily products) per day. Takes fluids poorly. Does not take a liquid dietary supplement OR is NPO[1] and/or maintained on clear liquids or IV[2] for more than 5 days.	**2. PROBABLY INADEQUATE** Rarely eats a complete meal and generally eats only about ½ of any food offered. Protein intake includes only 3 servings of meats or dairy products per day. Occasionally will take a dietary supplement OR receives less than optimum amount of liquid diet or tube feeding.	**3. ADEQUATE** Eats over half of most meals. Eats a total of 4 servings of protein (meat, dairy products) each day. Occasionally refuses a meal, but will usually take a supplement if offered OR is on a tube feeding or TPN[3] regimen, which probably meets most of nutritional needs.	**4. EXCELLENT** Eats most of every meal. Usually eats a total of 4 or more servings of meat and dairy products. Occasionally eats between meals. Does not require supplementation.				
FRICTION AND SHEAR	**1. PROBLEM** Requires moderate to maximum assistance in moving. Complete lifting without sliding against sheets is impossible. Frequently slides down in bed or chair, requiring frequent repositioning with maximum assistance. Spasticity, contractures, or agitation leads to almost constant friction.	**2. POTENTIAL PROBLEM** Moves feebly or requires minimum assistance. During a move, skin probably slides to some extent against sheets, chair, restraints, or other device. Maintains relatively good position in chair or bed most of the time but occasionally slides down.	**3. NO APPARENT PROBLEM** Moves in bed and in chair independently and has sufficient muscle strength to lift up completely during move. Maintains good position in bed or chair at all times.					
TOTAL SCORE	**Total score of 12 or less represents HIGH RISK**							

ASSESS	DATE	EVALUATOR SIGNATURE/TITLE	ASSESS	DATE	EVALUATOR SIGNATURE/TITLE
1	/ /		3	/ /	
2	/ /		4	/ /	

NAME—Last	First	Middle	Attending physician	Record No.	Room/Bed

FIGURE 16.6 Braden scale.

allow the patient to use upper body strength to assist with repositioning. Immobile patients should be assisted with repositioning frequently to alleviate pressure on bony surfaces. Pillows, cushions, or antipressure devices or mattresses should be used when possible (Bates-Jensen & Petch, 2015).

A nutritional assessment should be conducted to identify any nutritional deficiencies, loss of body weight, or cachexia. There is a direct correlation between pressure ulcer risk and severity and nutritional deficiencies, particularly low protein and albumin. If appropriate, nutritional supplements may be considered (Bates-Jensen & Petch, 2015).

Deconditioning and Activity Intolerance

Prolonged immobility can lead to deconditioning and activity intolerance, generally manifested by fatigue, weakness, and/or decreased stamina. Activity intolerance can severely impact the patient's quality of life, diminish participation in the activities of daily living, and increase the risk of falls when the patient attempts to ambulate. Signs of physical decompensation related to immobility include weakness, dyspnea with exertion, and fatigue with activity.

Any potential medical causes of fatigue or dyspnea, such as medication side effects, anemia, or disease progression, should be identified and addressed. Physical stamina can be at least partially preserved in patients who are nonambulatory through passive or active range of motion exercises, as tolerated. Steps to avoid falls include ensuring proper lighting, providing assistance with transfers and during ambulation, and placing needed objects, such as glasses, a telephone, or call bell, within the patient's reach (Kresevic, 2015).

Pathological Fractures

Pathological fractures result from disease and commonly occur in patients who have osteoporosis (Gordon, 2015). Bone metastasis is also a common cause of pathological fractures in the hospice and palliative care setting. The most common site of pathological fractures is the femur, of which 75% occur in the proximal end (Willeumier, van der Linden, van der Sande, & Dijkstra, 2016). Other common sites of pathological fractures are the tibia, humerus, ribs, and spine.

Symptoms of pathological fractures include localized pain and swelling, and possibly numbness in the affected limb. If the pathological fracture involves the femur, the affected leg generally appears shorter than the unaffected leg and may be externally rotated. Treatment options for pathological fractures depend on the patient's overall condition. Surgical stabilization with or without joint replacement is a common intervention for pathological fractures, but may be contraindicated if bone metastasis is widespread or if the patient's life expectancy is <6 months (Willeumier et al., 2016). Nursing management of pathological fractures centers on determining risks and providing teaching regarding proper positioning and patient safety. If a pathological fracture occurs, pain management and joint stabilization are priorities. The interdisciplinary team should collaborate with the patient and family to develop a plan of care that promotes quality of life and is consistent with the goals of care.

Skin and Mucous Membranes

At the end of life, problems related to skin and mucous membranes arise for a variety of reasons, including medications commonly used in the end-of-life setting, disease progression, or poor hydration and nutrition. Common end-of-life epidermal problems include xerostomia, pruritus, and pressure ulcers. Each of these are reviewed in the following sections.

Xerostomia (Dry Mouth)

Xerostomia is a subjective feeling of dry mouth and hyposalivation. There may be no objective findings, but associated signs such as thrush, oral dryness, poor dentition or dry lips may be noticeable. Xerostomia can affect the patient's ability to eat, talk, and to wear dentures or other dentifrices. It also increases the patient's risk for halitosis, dental caries, thrush, or taste changes (Villa, Connell, & Abati, 2014).

Common causes of xerostomia include medication side effects, radiotherapy of the head and neck, Sjögren's syndrome, depression, anxiety, stress, and malnutrition. Management of xerostomia involves identifying and removing reversible causes, especially related to medication side effects. Other interventions include ensuring proper hydration and alleviating the feeling of dry mouth by frequently offering sips of water, ice chips, or sugar-free gum or candy (Villa et al., 2014).

Pharmacological interventions such as pilocarpine (5 mg TID) or cevimeline (30 mg TID) may be helpful in increasing salivation. However, side effects such as excessive sweating, diarrhea, nausea, and emesis may deter use. Sialagogue, an oral topical agent, can be used to increase salivation and oral comfort without the systemic side effects (Villa et al., 2014).

Pruritus

Pruritus, or itchy skin, is a common symptom in many healthcare settings. The urge to scratch itchy skin can disrupt the patient's ability to carry out activities of daily living and affect sleep patterns. Usually, pruritus is self-limiting, but may be chronic in certain cases, such as in patients who have liver disease, renal disease, hyperthyroidism or hypothyroidism, anemia, malignancies, or HIV. Many medications also contribute to pruritus, such as opioids (Bobb & Fletcher, 2015).

Treatments depend on the cause, so a thorough assessment of the patient's skin is necessary, using a Woods lamp, if available. The skin should be examined for parasites, skin infections (bacterial or fungal), and lesions. If these are identified, treatment should be initiated accordingly. If no treatable cause can be identified, topical ointments, barrier creams, or soaks can be trialed (i.e., calamine, menthol, oatmeal bath, antihistamine cream, steroids, or capsaicin). Systemic therapies such as antihistamines may be helpful, but should be used with caution in older adults due to anticholinergic side effects (Bobb & Fletcher, 2015).

Wounds (e.g., Pressure Ulcers, Tumor Extrusions, Nonhealing Wounds)

Pressure ulcers are lesions that result from anoxia secondary to prolonged pressure against the skin. Most frequently, the pressure is caused by remaining in the same position for an extended period of time. But pressure ulcers can also be caused by medical devices such as casts and traction. The pressure and associated tissue anoxia can cause damage to the skin in as little as 20 to 40 minutes (Kohn & Trofino, 2015).

Initially, a pressure ulcer appears as a nonblanchable erythematous lesion. If the ulcer progresses, more extensive skin damage and discomfort occur. If the integrity of the epidermis is degraded, the patient is exposed to infection due to compromised skin integrity. Assessment of pressure ulcers involves determining wound severity. Wound classification generally indicates the depth and condition of the wound (see Figure 16.7). Other data that should be gathered include the following:

- Length and width of the wound (mm)
- Wound depth (mm)
- Description of wound edges
- Presence of undermining
- Presence and amount of necrotic tissue
- Exudate (if present, describe)
- Condition of surrounding tissue
- Granulation tissue and epithelialization
  (Bates-Jensen & Petch, 2015)

Management of pressure ulcers involves frequent repositioning, ensuring adequate nutrition and hydration, implementing appropriate wound care, and managing odors. Repositioning of bedbound patients should occur every 2 to 4 hours on a pressure-reducing surface and away from the site of the ulcer. If movement causes pain, the patient should be premedicated 20 to 30 minutes prior to repositioning. For patients who are actively dying or are comfortable in only one position,

Pressure Ulcer Staging

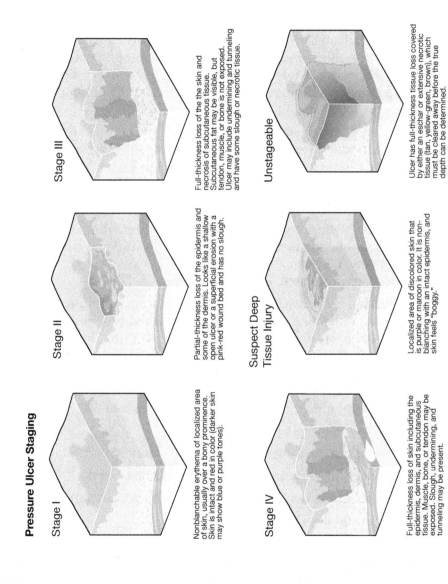

Stage I

Nonblanchable erythema of localized area of skin, usually over a bony prominence. Skin is intact and red in color (darker skin may show blue or purple tones).

Stage II

Partial-thickness loss of the epidermis and some of the dermis. Looks like a shallow open ulcer or a superficial erosion with a pink-red wound bed and has no slough.

Stage III

Full-thickness loss of the the skin and necrosis of subcutaneous tissue. Subcutaneous fat may be visible, but tendon, muscle, or bone is not exposed. Ulcer may include undermining and tunneling and have some slough or necrotic tissue.

Stage IV

Full-thickness loss of skin including the epidermis, dermis, and subcutaneous tissue. Muscle, bone, or tendon may be exposed. Slough, undermining, and tunneling may be present.

Suspect Deep Tissue Injury

Localized area of discolored skin that is purple or maroon in color. It is non-blanching with an intact epidermis, and skin feels "boggy."

Unstageable

Ulcer has full-thickness tissue loss covered by either an eschar or extensive necrotic tissue (tan, yellow-green, brown), which must be cleared away before the true depth can be determined.

FIGURE 16.7 Pressure ulcer staging.

flexibility in the turning schedule is required to promote the patient's comfort.

Wound healing is supported with proper nutrition and hydration. The use of oral, subcutaneous, or intravenous hydration may be an option for some patients. Nutritional supplements may also be considered, if appropriate. However, decisions regarding the use of supplemental nutrition and hydration should always be made in light of the goals of care and the patient's prognosis.

Proper management of a pressure ulcer depends on the stage of the ulcer, the goals of care, and the patient's prognosis. For large wounds, negative pressure wound therapy may be a good choice to remove excess drainage and infectious or necrotic tissue. Necrotic tissue may also be removed through wound debridement. Debridement options include the following:

- Mechanical debridement through wound irrigation or hydrotherapy, enzymatic debridement through the use of topical agents that destroy necrotic tissue (the dressing is changed daily)

- Biosurgical debridement through application of medical maggots (this may not be an acceptable option for all patients)

- Autolytic debridement using a moisture-retaining dressing that causes self-destruction of necrotic tissue (the dressing is changed only once every 3–5 days)
  (Bates-Jensen & Petch, 2015; Kohn & Trofino, 2015)

As with any open wound, partial or full-thickness pressure ulcers incur risk for infection. Wound debridement and proper wound cleansing are often sufficient for preventing infection. But for high-risk wounds, silver-release topical dressings should be considered to prevent infection. Medical-grade honey dressings are also effective in promoting healing and decreasing the risk of infection. Other types of dressings appropriate for pressure ulcers are as follows:

- Thin film dressings to protect skin

- Hydrocolloid dressings for stage 2 or 3 wounds

- Foam dressings for exudative stage 2 pressure ulcers

- Hydrogel dressings for nonexudative or necrotic wounds

- Calcium alginates for absorbing exudate
  (Bates-Jensen & Petch, 2015)

Controlling wound odor is an important quality of life issue for patients. Wound odor is often related to the presence of necrotic tissue and/or bacterial overgrowth. Metronidazole gel (0.77%–1.0%) can be applied daily for 1 week to reduce microbial growth. Dressings that contain activated charcoal are useful for absorbing wound odors. In wounds that are not expected to heal, povidone iodine can be used to reduce wound odor.

Wound pain should be managed with appropriate systemic analgesics. Wound care should be provided gently and slowly to promote comfort. Topical anesthetics such as lidocaine may be used to reduce the pain associated with dressing changes. Low-dose topical morphine may also be useful for reducing wound pain (Bates-Jensen & Petch, 2015).

Psychosocial, Emotional, and Spiritual Issues

At the end of life, psychosocial, emotional, and spiritual issues may arise as patients begin to come to terms with their own mortality. Each patient responds to the news of serious illness differently based on her or his unique coping mechanisms, support systems, and cultural and religious background. The emotional states discussed in the following section may arise in a particular patient or may not. It must also be recognized that some patients are not open to expressing their emotions. Nurses should offer calm reassurance when a patient expresses emotional distress. Validation of the patient's feelings and emotional support should be provided in a nonjudgmental manner using therapeutic communication skills, such as appropriate touch and eye contact, listening attentively, and communicating empathetically. False reassurance and axioms should be avoided. Many patients experience anger, depression, anxiety, denial, fear, grief, hopelessness, and other emotional challenges. These are reviewed in the following sections.

Anger or Hostility

Anger is a common emotion that surfaces from time to time in seriously ill patients. Anger may be related to the illness, the feeling of being out of control in regard to outcomes, family or caregiver reactions to the illness, or dependency. When hostility is directed toward others, it may be arising from family tensions or unresolved altercations. The work of the interdisciplinary team, especially the social worker and chaplain, is to help the patient and loved ones process anger and express it in a safe and nonhurtful manner. If the patient's anger leads to violence, interventions must be immediately directed toward ensuring the safety of the family, caregivers, and the patient. When the patient expresses anger, the nurse should provide reassurance that the feeling is common, but is usually related to another feeling such as fear, depression, or grief. Identifying and coping with underlying emotion may help alleviate the patient's anger.

Depression

Depression is defined as "persistent low mood, or anhedonia (pervasive loss of interest or pleasure) that lasts for more than 2 weeks and is accompanied by at least four of the following symptoms:

- sleep disruption (especially early morning insomnia),
- weight loss or change in appetite
- psychomotor retardation or agitation,
- fatigue or loss of energy,
- feelings of worthlessness or excessive guilt,
- diminished ability to think or concentrate, and
- recurrent thoughts of death or suicidal ideation" (Periyakoil, 2016, p. 247).

Depression can occur at the end of life as patients try to take in the uncertainty of their disease trajectory and the possibility of their own death. Importantly, depression frequently coexists with anxiety, so both should be explored in patients who express depressive symptoms. Therapeutic listening skills should be used to allow the patient to openly express feelings. The interdisciplinary team should collaborate to develop a plan with the patient to use relaxation techniques, meditation, positive self-talk, and cognitive behavioral therapy. Selective serotonin reuptake inhibitors such as citalopram 20 to 60 mg daily, escitalopram 10 to 20 mg daily, paroxetine 20 to 50 mg daily, fluoxetine 20 to 60 mg daily, fluvoxamine 50 to 100 mg twice daily or sertraline 50 to 200 mg daily are useful for decreasing symptoms of depression, but may take several weeks to achieve therapeutic effect. If the patient's life expectancy is thought to be <2 weeks, methylphenidate (Concerta, Ritalin) may be used to treat symptoms of depression (Periyakoil, 2016).

Anxiety

Anxiety is "a state of apprehension and fear resulting from the perception of a current or future threat to oneself" (Periyakoil, 2016, p. 248). In seriously ill patients, anxiety may arise from a fear of death, pain, or distressing symptoms. Anxiety is a very common end-of-life symptom and can be addressed nonpharmacologically by teaching and coaching the patient in deep breathing and relaxation techniques, visualization, meditation, and the use of essential oil (topically or diffused; Buckle, 2015; Martinez-Kratz, 2015). For patients with persistent anxiety with or without depressive features, escitalopram 10 to 20 mg daily may be effective. For patients who have intermittent or situational anxiety, or a life expectancy of <2 weeks, a benzodiazepine such as lorazepam (0.5–1 mg PO/IM/IV/SC BID or TID) is recommended.

Denial

Denial is a state of refusal to believe the truth regarding a present situation. Some patients facing end-of-life situations are not able to accept the reality of their illness. Denial is a protective psychological mechanism that shields patients from the consequences of their illness until they are psychologically ready to cope. Challenging patients to face a situation that they are not ready to handle may cause increased emotional distress. Therapeutic communication skills such as reflection, active listening, and therapeutic silence are useful when working with patients who express denial. Patients should be calmly reassured that the interdisciplinary team is available for emotional support as needed.

Fear

Fear is a psychological response to a real threat to one's safety. Fear may also have physical components such as tachycardia, tachypnea, shaking, insomnia, diaphoresis, a sinking feeling in the pit of the stomach, and/or nightmares. Fear sometimes appears similar to anxiety, but anxiety can occur in response to a perceived threat as well as to a real threat. Fear occurs at the end of life due to many factors, including threats of death, dying alone, being a burden, financial struggles, pain, discomfort, loss of dignity, and loss of loved ones. Interventions to manage fear, such as distraction, deep breathing, meditation, massage, and cognitive behavioral therapy, may be helpful. Focused support should also be provided by the team social worker or chaplain.

Grief

Grief is a feeling of sadness related to an impending or past loss. Grief also entails psychological symptoms such as intrusive thoughts, regret, inability to think clearly, and dulled or heightened emotions. Physical symptoms associated with grief include nausea, fatigue, and myalgias. Grief support should begin with therapeutic listening, empathetic support, and assurance that the experience is normal. The team social worker and chaplain can provide expertise in facilitating life review, teaching cognitive behavioral therapy techniques, and providing spiritual support and guidance.

Loss of Hope or Meaning

Hopelessness occurs in serious or terminal illness as the patient's or family's hope for recovery fails to materialize. The grief and sadness related to the patient's disappointment and loss of hope for recovery must first be recognized and addressed. A goals of care conversation with the interdisciplinary team is warranted to help the patient shift his or her focus of hope from recovery to comfort, preserved function, preserved dignity, or anything that gives the patient comfort.

Hope can often be found in the patient's source of meaning, which may be family, work, or faith. If a source of meaning can be identified, it may also serve as a source of hope. Some patients struggle to identify a source of meaning in their lives. The hospice team can help facilitate life review, which may reveal a source of meaning and hope in the patient's life.

Guilt

Guilt is associated with feelings of regret for actions one has taken or has failed to take. Patients may feel a sense of personal responsibility for their illness or may feel guilty about leaving their family through death. Feelings of guilt are rooted in the individual's moral, social, and cultural beliefs, and so these beliefs must be explored. Nurses must recognize the existential suffering that accompanies guilt and should encourage patients to explore and express such feelings. The nurse should also encourage patients to avail themselves of the skills of the other members of the interdisciplinary team, particularly the social worker and chaplain to address their feelings of guilt.

Nearing Death Awareness

Roughly half of terminally ill patients experience some form of nearing death awareness (NDA). Patient reports of NDA are usually coherent and comforting. In contrast to delirium or hallucinations, NDA usually brings the patient a sense of overall peace and may involve

- Communicating with deceased loved ones
- Preparing for change
- Seeing the afterlife
- Knowing that death is near

NDA is culturally bound and varies from patient to patient. Response to NDA should center on differentiating the experience from delirium or hallucinations and validating the patient's perception of the NDA (Marks & Marchand, 2018).

Sleep Disturbances

Sleep disturbances, including difficulty falling or staying asleep, unusual sleep patterns, or daytime fatigue are common in palliative care. Factors that influence sleep patterns, such as disease progression, socioeconomic factors, pain, medications, and psychological issues, should be reviewed and addressed (Mercadante et al., 2015). Promotion of restful sleep involves good sleep hygiene (i.e., dim lighting, quiet, comfortable temperature), allowing the patient to rest undisturbed, and avoidance of stimulants. Nonpharmacological interventions such as relaxation techniques, massage, aromatherapy, and music may all be used to promote restful sleep and improve the patient's quality of life.

Suicidal Ideation

When patients lose hope or face their own death, they may become fearful or depressed, which can lead to suicidal thoughts or thoughts of self-harm. Some warning signs of suicidal ideation are as follows:

- Changes in behavior
- Giving away prized possessions
- Talking about suicide
- Withdrawing from friends or activities
- Increasing use of alcohol or drugs
  (American Psychological Association, 2018)

The key assessment questions for the nurse to ask are *Are you considering harming yourself?* and *Do you have a plan to harm yourself?* If the answer is *yes* to either of these questions, the patient is considered to be at risk for suicide and steps must be taken urgently to ensure the patient's safety.

Intimacy/Relationship Issues

Serious illness can strain even the closest of relationships. Caregiver stress may cause one to feel angry or disenfranchised, while the patient may feel despondent or angry about being dependent. Sexual intimacy may also be affected by serious illness and this may be a painful loss for some couples. When nurses observe signs of relationship strain, the issue should be raised and discussed openly. As patients and loved ones express their concerns, the nurse should normalize their experience, offer reassurance, and encourage counseling.

Nutritional and Metabolic

At the end of life, nutritional and metabolic issues arise for a variety of reasons, including disease progression, organ failure, or medication side effects. Common end-of-life nutrition and metabolic problems include anorexia, cachexia, dehydration, fatigue, hypercalcemia, and hypo- or hyperglycemia. Each of these are reviewed in the following setions.

Anorexia and Cachexia

Anorexia is loss of appetite that can occur from illness, emotional stress, or medications. Severe or prolonged anorexia can lead to cachexia, but these conditions are actually two separate medical issues that can occur independently of each other. Cachexia is manifested by weight loss, fluid retention, muscle wasting, and metabolic changes. When these two conditions occur together, particularly at the end stage of a disease process, the condition is referred to as anorexia/cachexia syndrome (ACS; Wholihan, 2015).

ACS often occurs in serious illness such as cancer, heart failure, obstructive pulmonary disease, HIV, renal disease, and others. It is a grave sign indicating advanced disease. Typically, ACS is manifested by metabolic changes, systemic inflammation, neurohormonal changes, and catabolism. In addition to serious medical issues, ACS can

> **Key Point**
>
> Mid-arm circumference is a useful measure in assessing malnutrition over time. Progressively decreasing mid-arm circumference is an indicator of both weight loss and muscle wasting. To determine mid-arm circumference, the nurse should measure the arm halfway between the olecranon process and the acromion process of the scapula (in centimeters).

result from medications, treatments, or severe psychological or spiritual distress. The cause of ACS should be identified and removed, if possible. But if ACS is secondary to an end-stage disease process, the patient's prognosis remains poor even with intervention (Wholihan, 2015).

Interventions for ACS may entail oral nutritional supplementation, easing of dietary restrictions, and offering small, frequent meals. Enteral or parenteral nutritional supplementation has not generally been found to be beneficial in end-stage disease. The following criteria should be considered before beginning a trial:

- Potential benefit
- Life expectancy
- Functional status
  - ▩ Karnofsky score should be >50
  - ▩ The patient's medical issues should be manageable
  - ▩ A caregiver should be available
  - ▩ The patient should be able to have follow-up laboratory monitoring
    (Abrahm, 2014)

Pharmacological interventions such as megestrol acetate, glucocorticoids, and cannabinoids have been found to increase appetite and cause weight gain, but their effects on overall quality of life is uncertain (Wholihan, 2015). In cases where depression is thought to be the underlying cause of ACS, mirtazapine (Remeron) 15 mg at bedtime or methylphenidate 2.5 to 10 mg PO at 8 a.m. and noon may be helpful (Abrahm, 2014).

Dehydration

Dehydration at the end of life is commonly related to anorexia, medication side effects, nausea, vomiting, bowel obstruction, dysphagia, or cognitive impairment. Assessment of dehydration involves assessment of the oral cavity for dryness, assessment of skin turgor, and assessment of bowel function (diarrhea is a cause of dehydration; constipation and impaction may be signs of dehydration).

Patients and families may voice concerns about the effects of dehydration on quality of life and distressing symptoms. Delirium, confusion, agitation, and myoclonus may be exacerbated by dehydration, but the symptoms are not usually responsive to fluid replacement. The interdisciplinary team must carefully weigh the potential benefits of artificial hydration against the potential burdens, which include nausea, fluid overload, dyspnea, ascites, edema, and others. Whether the patient is acutely ill and expected to recover or is actively dying are also factors to be considered (Gabriel & Tschanz, 2015).

Fluid replacement can be offered orally or enterally, if tolerated. Parenteral nutrition should be provided via a competent vein or a long-term catheter such as a central venous catheter. If no venous access is available, subcutaneous fluids can be administered, which is called hypodermoclysis. The absorption rate is comparable to intravenous administration. Proctoclysis, administration of fluids to the gastrointestinal tract through a nasogastric catheter inserted into the rectum is possible, but rarely used (Gabriel & Tschanz, 2015).

Fatigue

Fatigue is a generalized feeling of tiredness and lacking energy to carry out daily activities. Reports of fatigue are largely subjective but the effects may be objectively noted. Fatigue is a common symptom related to cancer, heart disease, obstructive pulmonary diseases, renal disease, HIV/AIDS, multiple sclerosis, and others. Fatigue may be secondary to insomnia, the underlying disease process, or distressing symptoms. It may also be secondary to medication side effects, medical treatment, or psychological or spiritual distress (O'Neil, Anderson, & Dean, 2015).

Nonpharmacological interventions for fatigue include exercise as tolerated, proper pain and symptom management, psychological or spiritual counseling, meditation, relaxation, music therapy, proper sleep hygiene, and avoidance of sleep disruption. Pharmacological interventions should be aimed toward enhancing sleep with a benzodiazepine or an antidepressant (Guay & Yennurajalingam, 2016). When fatigue is not related to sleep quantity or quality, psychostimulants such as methylphenidate or modafinil may be used. Corticosteroids also reduce fatigue, and megestrol acetate has been shown to be effective in increasing activity levels as well as appetite in a few studies (Yennurajalingam, 2016).

Hypercalcemia

Hypercalcemia occurs when there is an excess of calcium in circulation. Hypercalcemia can occur in patients with metastatic cancer as bone deteriorates and calcium is released. Hyperparathyroidism, lithium therapy, Addison's disease, Paget's disease, vitamin A, or aluminum toxicity are also causes of hypercalcemia (Bobb, 2015).

Patients who have hypercalcemia may exhibit symptoms such as nausea, vomiting, anorexia, weakness, constipation, thirst, and changes in mentation. Diagnosis of hypercalcemia is confirmed through serum analysis. Patients with a serum calcium level >14 mg/dL require urgent intervention. Even in advanced disease, interventions should be started to reverse hypercalcemia for the patient's comfort. Bisphosphonates such as pamidronate and zoledronate are used most frequently. Intravenous hydration, administration of calcitonin, use of bone reabsorption agents such as gallium nitrate or plicamycin, or dialysis may also be considered (Bobb, 2015; Kuriya & Dev, 2016).

Hypoglycemia and Hyperglycemia

Fluctuations in blood glucose levels may occur at the end of life due to uncontrolled diabetes mellitus, sepsis, organ failure, cortisol imbalance, or altered nutritional intake. In cases of hypoglycemia, patients typically feel symptoms such as diaphoresis, dizziness, pallor, tachycardia, weakness, anxiety, tremors, nausea, and hunger when the blood glucose level is <70 mg/dL. If the blood glucose level continues to drop to <50 mg/dL, patients may experience irritability, blurry vision or double vision, confusion, headache, and slurred speech. Severe reactions such as coma, seizure, and death may occur if blood glucose levels drop below 40 mg/dL (Bodtke & Ligon, 2016; Levesque, 2012). Interventions to manage hypoglycemia may include the following:

- Administering 15 g of a carbohydrate (i.e., a sugary drink, food, or a glucose tablet), waiting 15 minutes, rechecking the blood glucose level, and administering another 15 g of carbohydrates, if necessary. These steps should be repeated until the blood glucose level is over 70 mg/dL

- Administering glucagon 1 mg IV/SC, which can take effect in 5 minutes

- Administering D50W IV/SC, which has an immediate effect

Administration of corticosteroids may also be considered for dual effect for patients who also have symptoms of dyspnea, pain, or inflammation (Bodtke & Ligon, 2016; Levesque, 2012).

Overtreatment of hypoglycemia or noncompliance with a prescribed treatment plan for hypoglycemia can lead to hyperglycemia. Other causes of hyperglycemia include diabetes mellitus, "acute illness, stroke, sepsis, myocardial infarction, pancreatitis, [or medications such as] glucocorticoids, high-dose thiazides, dobutamine, atypical antipsychotics, [and] cocaine" (Bodtke & Ligon, 2016). Hyperglycemia is defined as a fasting blood glucose level above 116 mg/dL or a postprandial blood glucose level above 200 mg/dL. Symptoms of hyperglycemia include polyuria, polydipsia, polyphagia, weight loss, glucosuria, weakness, marked fatigue, blurred vision, increased risk for infection or poor wound healing, and diabetic ketoacidosis (primarily in type 1 diabetes; Levesque, 2012).

Usual medical management of hyperglycemia includes lifestyle modification and medications to improve glycemic control such as

- Metformin (up to 2,250 mg/d)
- Sulfonylureas (such as glipizide, glyburide, or glimepiride)
- Metglitinides (such as matelinide or repaglinide)
- Glucosidase inhibitors (such as acarbose and miglitol)
- Thiazolidinediones (such as pioglitazone and rosiglitazone)
- Dipeptidyl peptidase 4 (DPP-4) inhibitors (such as sitagliptin phosphate)
- Amylin agonists (such as pramlintide)
- Insulin (Levesque, 2012).

For patients who are terminally ill, usual monitoring and management of diabetes may not be feasible due to a patient's inability to take oral medications or to eat. At the end of life, the necessity of finger sticks and strict dietary control should be considered in light of the patient's comfort. Patient and family teaching is crucial if normal routines are modified, and the goals of care should be reviewed in light of the patient's overall condition (Bodtke & Ligon, 2016).

Immune/Lymphatic System

At the end of life, immunological issues arise for a variety of reasons, including disease progression, organ failure, or medication side effects. Common end-of-life immunological and lymphatic problems include infection or fever, myelosuppression, and lymphedema. Each of these are reviewed in the following sections.

Infection or Fever

Fever is typically defined as a single temperature reading of 101.3°F (38.5°C) or three readings of 100.4°F (38°C) or higher 1 hour apart. The body produces pyrogens as it attacks pathogens, which suggests that fever is often, but not always, related to infection (Bobb & Fletcher, 2015). It may also be related to immunological disorders and metabolic imbalances. Fever is experienced in three stages: chills, fever, and then flush. Antipyretics can be administered orally or rectally to treat these symptoms. The use of antibiotics may also be considered to alleviate symptoms and promote comfort (Calton & Ritchie, 2016).

In patients who are very near death, central fever may occur, which manifests as an abnormally high temperature while the patient's skin feels cool to the touch. The patient should be treated with antipyretics for comfort (Berry & Griffie, 2015).

Myelosuppression (i.e., Anemia, Neutropenia, Thrombocytopenia)

Myelosuppression is "a condition in which bone marrow activity is decreased, resulting in fewer red blood cells [anemia], white blood cells [leukopenia/neutropenia], and platelets [thrombocytopenia]. Myelo-suppression is a side effect of some cancer treatments" (National Cancer Institute, 2018). In addition to some cancer treatments, myelo-suppression may also result from a disease process, particularly at the end-stage.

Anemia may occur in many disease states, including heart disease, pulmonary disease, kidney disease, and others. In chronic illness, anemia may be related to inflammatory processes, with older and obese patients at greatest risk (Fraenkel, 2015). Anemia is diagnosed when the patient's hemoglobin (Hb) is <8.0 g/dL (Hui, 2016). Treatment of anemia involves transfusion of packed red blood cells for patients whose hemoglobin is <8.0 g/dL, but for those with advanced disease, the threshold of 9.0 g/dL may be used. Other interventions may include erythropoiesis-stimulating agents such as epoetin-alpha or darbepo-etin. However, these medications should not be used for patients who have advanced cancer as they can accelerate tumor growth and increase mortality (Hui, 2016).

Neutropenia is defined as an absolute neutrophil count (ANC) of <1,000/mm^3 (Hui, 2016). Neutropenia may be related to bone marrow suppression, cancer treatments, infections, medication side effects, or autoimmune disorders (Stöppler, 2017). Neutropenia alone is not considered to be life-threatening. However, patients who have neutropenia are at risk for febrile neutropenia, which is an oncological emergency. Manifestations of febrile neutropenia include a temperature of 100.4°F (38.3°C) for more than 1 hour along with an ANC of less than 500/mm^3 with the expectation that it may decrease even further. Any patient who exhibits a fever while on chemotherapy is presumed to have febrile neutropenia until proven otherwise. Once the diagnosis is confirmed, treatment with broad-spectrum antibiotics should commence. High-risk patients may require hospitalization for intravenous antibiotic therapy if consistent with the goals of care (Hui, 2016).

Thrombocytopenia is diagnosed when a patient's thrombocyte count is <20,000/mm^3 or if a patient exhibits clinically significant active bleeding (Hui, 2016). Thrombocytopenia may result from, among other reasons, cancer, aplastic anemia, chronic alcohol use, side effects of medications, and autoimmune disorders. The first signs of thrombocytopenia are often purpura (purple, brown, or red bruises) and petechiae (small red or purple dots on skin; National Heart, Lung, & Blood Institute, 2018). Severe thrombocytopenia can result in uncontrollable hemorrhage. If hemorrhage occurs, interventions include radiation therapy, palliative TACE, endoscopy, vitamin K, vasopressin, antifibrinolytic agents, octreotide (for bleeding varices), platelet transfusion, or fresh frozen plasma. If bleeding is excessive and visible, dark-colored towels should be available to reduce the visual impact of the bleeding for the patient and caregivers (Kuriya & Dev, 2016).

Lymphedema

Lymphedema is caused by obstruction or removal of the lymph nodes, which is often related to cancer surgeries or other treatments. Lymph accumulation may lead to fibrosis or sclerosis, causing permanent edema. If fibrosis has not yet occurred, elevation and compression of the limb may be helpful. Careful skin care is necessary. Although diuretics are generally not effective for lymphedema, manual lymphatic drainage performed by a trained massage therapist or physical therapist may be helpful in reducing fluid accumulation, promoting mobility, range of motion and quality of life (Bodtke & Ligon, 2016; Walker, 2016).

Mental Status Changes

At the end of life, mental status changes occur for a variety of reasons, including disease progression, organ failure, or medication side effects. Common mental status changes that may occur at the end of life include altered level of consciousness, agitation or terminal restlessness, confusion, delirium, and hallucinations. Each of these are reviewed in the following sections.

Altered Level of Consciousness

According to Boss and Huether (2014), a patient's "level of consciousness is the most critical clinical index of nervous system function or dysfunction" (p. 529). Changes in the patient's level of consciousness at the end of life may be related to central nervous system dysfunction, medication side effects, metabolic imbalances, infection, anxiety, or psychological issues. Confusion, delirium, and hallucinations are manifestations of altered levels of consciousness that are commonly seen in hospice and palliative care settings.

Confusion occurs when a patient is unable to think clearly. When a patient is confused, judgment and decision-making capacity are impaired (Boss & Huether, 2014). Confusion may result from a number of factors, including medical reasons, psychological reasons, or an inability to keep track of time and dates due to illness, hospitalization, or altered sleep cycles. The Confusion Assessment Method (CAM) is used in clinical settings to assess cognitive functioning in older adults on a daily scheduled basis (Heidrich & English, 2015). There are several versions of the CAM, including a short version, a long version, and several translations. The CAM is a valid and reliable tool that is consistently used in clinical settings to detect delirium in confused patients (Institute for Aging Research, 2018).

Delirium is an "an acute disorder of attention and cognition" (Inouye, Westendorp, & Saczynski, 2014, p. 911). It occurs most frequently in older adults, those who are admitted for inpatient care, postoperative patients, and those with advanced illness (Heidrich & English, 2015). Disease states that increase the risk for delirium include infection (such as urinary tract infection), renal failure, hepatic failure, central nervous system disorders, vascular disorders, and pain (Bodtke & Ligon, 2016). Signs and symptoms of delirium include:

- Acute onset
- Fluctuation in symptoms
- Clearly differentiated from dementia
- Perceptual changes
- Sleep–wake cycle alterations
- Delusions
- Hallucinations
- Paranoia
- Hyperactivity or lethargy
  (Bodtke & Ligon, 2016)

Management of delirium involves determining and reversing the cause, if possible. Safety is a nursing priority, so a sitter may be needed, or the presence of a family member. The environment should be kept quiet and restful, with minimal disturbance. Although there are no specific treatments for delirium, medications such as haloperidol (2 mg) or risperidone (1 mg) have been used to treat symptoms (Bodtke & Ligon, 2016).

Terminal delirium, also called terminal agitation, is delirium that occurs during the dying process. In some patients, the symptoms may be reversible, but for more than half of dying patients, they are not.

The following pharmacological treatments for terminal delirium may be helpful:

- Haloperidol 2 to 4 mg PO/SC/IV every 30 minutes up to a total daily dose of 20 mg/24 hr
- Olanzapine 2.5 to 5 mg sublingual at hour of sleep to BID plus PRN every 4 hours
  (Abrahm, 2014)

CONCLUSION

In the course of serious illness, patients experience myriad symptoms that can be secondary to the disease process, medication side effects, or drug interactions. Some symptoms may also be iatrogenic. The hospice and palliative care nurse must be able to identify end-of-life symptoms and possible etiologies as well as treatment options. The nurse must also be prepared to provide emotional support for the patient and family as well as appropriate teaching regarding symptoms, symptom management, and disease progression.

Chapter Summary

- End-of-life symptoms may be iatrogenic or related to the terminal diagnosis, multisystem organ failure, medication interactions, or medication side effects.
- **Neurological symptoms**
  - *Aphasia* is the inability to understand written or spoken words or to express oneself verbally or in writing. Aphasia may be secondary to stroke, tumor growth, or degenerative diseases. Use of phonetic boards or computers may help improve communication.
  - *Dysphagia* is difficulty swallowing that can result from stroke, tumor growth, or nerve damage. Patients may exhibit choking, drooling, or hoarseness. Patients should remain NPO until a swallowing screen is completed and dietary recommendations, including appropriate food texture, are in place.
  - *Altered level of consciousness* may be related to disease progression, metabolic changes, or tumor growth. It may be reversible if it is not related to the underlying disease process.
  - *Myoclonus* is manifested as uncontrollable jerking or muscle twitching. It is often treatable with clonazepam, midazolam agents, benzodiazepines, baclofen, or dantrolene. If myoclonus is a manifestation of opioid-induced neurotoxicity, the dose of the opioid should be lowered or the opioid should be rotated.
  - *Paresthesias and neuropathies* manifest as abnormal sensations such as tingling or burning. Gabapentinoids, tricyclic antidepressants, or serotonin–norepinephrine reuptake inhibitors are first-line treatments.
  - *Seizures* result from abnormal impulses in the brain. Lorazepam, phenytoin, or valproic acid are used to treat seizures.
  - *EPSs* are a type of dyskinesia related to neurological disorders or medications such as antipsychotics. If possible, the cause of the EPS should be removed. Pharmacological interventions include lorazepam, propranolol, benztropine, or diphenhydramine.
  - *Paralysis* is characterized by the extent of the nerve damage. Communication, decreasing risk for injury, and emotional and spiritual support are priorities.

(continued)

Chapter Summary (*continued*)

- ▦ *SCC* occurs when the thecal sac is compressed by the vertebrae. It is a medical emergency and may cause irreparable damage. Treatment with corticosteroids and pain management are priorities. Surgery and/or radiation therapy may be recommended for some patients.

- ▦ *Increased ICP* occurs due to fluid shifts or tumor growth in the brain. Treatment is dependent on the goals of care and the patient's prognosis.

- **Cardiac symptoms**

  - ▦ *Bleeding and hemorrhage* can be secondary to liver disease, tumor invasion, or certain medical treatments or medications. Management depends on the amount of bleeding and the goals of care.

  - ▦ *DVT* is usually diagnosable by venous doppler. Treatment may include heparin, low-molecular weight heparin, unfractionated heparin, or fondaparinux.

  - ▦ *PE* may occur when a DVT migrates to a pulmonary artery. Initial treatment focuses on stabilization of the patient, improving ventilation, and vascular stabilization. Anticoagulant therapy is also necessary.

  - ▦ *DIC* is characterized by excessive clot formation, which strains the platelet supply, leading to hemorrhage. Patients are at high risk for organ damage due to thrombus formation and migration of blood clots to major vessels. Once platelet supplies are exhausted, patients are at risk for severe internal or external bleeding. Anticoagulants are used to inhibit clot formation. Other treatments used include synthetic protease inhibitors and antifibrinolytic therapy.

  - ▦ *Angina* is chest pain caused by increased oxygen demands on the cardiac muscle. Symptoms include radiating chest pain, shortness of breath, fatigue, and sometimes nausea. Nitroglycerin is the first-line treatment.

  - ▦ *Edema* is fluid retention that is often related to end-stage organ failure. Diuretics may or may not be effective.

  - ▦ *Lymphedema* occurs due to removal of the lymph nodes. Manual lymphatic drainage may be undertaken by a trained professional.

  - ▦ *Syncope* is a temporary loss of consciousness related to insufficient blood flow to the brain. Patient safety and decreasing the patient's anxiety are priorities.

  - ▦ *SVCS* is caused by obstruction of the vena cava or nearby vessels or lymph nodes. A hallmark sign is facial swelling, especially after recumbancy. The prognosis is fair to poor. Treatment interventions should align with the goals of care.

- **Respiratory symptoms**

  - ▦ *Cough* is usually self-limiting (acute) but is considered chronic if it lasts more than 8 weeks. Thorough nursing assessment including frequency, character, timing of the cough, and whether it is productive or nonproductive should be carried out and carefully documented. Nonpharmacological and pharmacological interventions should be used to manage cough (see Table 16.1)

  - ▦ *Dyspnea* is defined as increased effort to breathe with associated air hunger. Chronic dyspnea is related to obstructive pulmonary disorders or cardiac disease. Management of dyspnea includes nonpharmacological interventions such as fans and relaxation, or pharmacological interventions such as opioids and anxiolytics.

  - ▦ *PE* is the accumulation of fluid between the pleura. It is characterized by acute-onset pleuritic pain with dyspnea and tachycardia. The least invasive approach to reducing PE is pleuroscopy.

  - ▦ *Pneumothorax* means air is trapped in the pleural space. Symptoms include sudden dyspnea, chest pain, tachycardia, restlessness, and anxiety. The patient's prognosis is poor without intervention. Treatment involves placement of a chest tube or Heimlich valve.

(continued)

Chapter Summary (*continued*)

▦ *Terminal secretions* occur at the end of life due to the patient's inability to clear secretions from the airway. Repositioning may decrease the associated "rattling" sound. Deep suctioning is not recommended. Anticholinergic medications can be used to dry secretions.

- **Gastrointestinal symptoms**

▦ *Constipation* is a very common end-of-life symptom often associated with decreased fluid intake or opioid use. Laxatives should be used for all patients who are taking opioids and the dose should be increased if the opioid dose is increased.

▦ *Diarrhea* results when fecal matter passes through the intestines too quickly for water to be properly absorbed from the stool. Antidiarrheals may be used, but caution is warranted if infection is suspected. The nurse should monitor the patient for signs of dehydration.

▦ *Bowel incontinence* may result from muscle atrophy or weakness, neurological disease, or severe diarrhea. The cause should be removed, if possible. The nurse should provide easy access to the commode and proper skin care after each episode of incontinence.

▦ *Ascites* is the accumulation of fluid in the abdomen due to portal hypertension and hypoalbuminemia. Ascites may also occur due to cancer or heart failure. It is indicative of end-stage disease. Interventions to reduce ascites should be consistent with the patient's goals of care.

▦ *Hiccups* may be benign, persistent, or intractable. Nonpharmacological and pharmacological interventions may be used to treat hiccups and increase the patient's quality of life.

▦ *Nausea and vomiting* are separate but related symptoms. Pharmacological treatments should be congruent with the cause of the vomiting (see Table 16.3).

▦ *Bowel obstruction* is primarily related to tumor growth and has a poor prognosis. Management is primarily palliative.

- **Genitourinary symptoms**

▦ *Bladder spasms* occur due to a blocked or partially blocked bladder outlet. If possible, the cause should be removed and steps should be taken to alleviate the blockage, such as insertion of a urinary catheter.

▦ *Urinary incontinence* may be transient or persistent. It may be related to an underlying disease process, poor muscle or sphincter tone, or infection. The cause should be addressed, if possible. The nurse should provide easy access to a commode and proper skin care after each episode of incontinence.

▦ *Urinary retention* is the inability to pass urine. If urinary retention occurs, a medication review should be undertaken to identify possible pharmacological causes. Placement of a urinary catheter should be considered.

- **Musculoskeletal symptoms**

▦ *Impaired mobility* increases risk for skin breakdown, physical deconditioning, and pathological fractures. The interdisciplinary team should develop a plan of care, together with the patient and family, to reduce risk for injury and to preserve function to the greatest extent possible within the limits of the disease processes.

- **Skin and mucous membranes**

▦ *Xerostomia* is a subjective feeling of dry mouth. Pharmacological treatments and proper oral care should be used to alleviate the patient's symptoms.

▦ *Pruritus* is itchy skin and can occur due to numerous medications, medical interventions, or dermatological issues. Treatment should be consistent with the cause.

▦ *Wounds* at the end of life may be iatrogenic or related to immobility. Some wounds are nonhealing due to the patient's condition. The priority nursing interventions focus on

(*continued*)

Chapter Summary (*continued*)

pain management, promotion of wound healing, prevention of further deterioration, and odor control.

- **Psychosocial, emotional, and spiritual issues**

  ▨ At the end of life, patients may experience fear, denial, anger, depression, grief, and/or hopelessness. Patients may also struggle with the meaning of their life or of their suffering. Manifestations of these emotions are culturally based and should be addressed by the interdisciplinary team in a compassionate and culturally sensitive manner.

  ▨ *NDA* may occur with the patient relating specific information about an afterlife. These experiences are often comforting to the patient and should not be negated by the healthcare provider.

  ▨ *Sleep disturbances* are very common at the end of life. The nurse should promote good sleep hygiene and manage symptoms that interfere with restful sleep.

  ▨ *Suicidal ideation* may occur if patients become fearful or deeply depressed. The nurse should determine whether the patient has a plan to implement self-harm and the means to do so. If so, interventions must be taken urgently to ensure the patient's safety.

  ▨ *Intimacy* may be affected by serious illness. The nurse should encourage patients to express their concerns and normalize their experience.

- **Nutritional and metabolic issues**

  ▨ *Anorexia* is the loss of appetite, and it may lead to cachexia or muscle wasting and weight loss. When anorexia and cachexia occur together, it is referred to as ACS. ACS is manifested in many end-stage diseases and treatment should be consistent with the goals of care and the patient's prognosis. Family support is needed, especially if ACS is related to a terminal illness.

  ▨ *Dehydration* is commonly related to anorexia at the end of life. Fluid replacement may be offered, if tolerated, and if consistent with the goals of care.

  ▨ *Fatigue* is a feeling of tiredness and lack of energy. It is a very common end-of-life symptom that causes distress and decreased quality of life. Interventions should be aimed toward enhancing restful sleep or stimulating alertness when the patient is awake.

  ▨ *Hypercalcemia* may occur at the end of life due to bone deterioration secondary to metastasis. It may also occur due to hyperparathyroidism, lithium treatment, Addison's disease, Paget's disease, vitamin A, or aluminum toxicity. Hypercalcemia should be identified through blood analysis and treated promptly to promote the patient's comfort.

- **Immune and lymphatic issues**

  ▨ *Infection* or fever may occur at the end of life for various reasons. Fever is defined as a single temperature reading of 101.3°F (38.5°C) or three single readings of 100.4°F (38°C) or higher 1 hour apart. Antipyretics should be used and, if appropriate, antibiotics.

  ▨ *Myelosuppression* may result from some cancer treatments and manifest as anemia, neutropenia, or thrombocytopenia. Interventions should be aimed at replenishing the depleted blood components, if consistent with the goals of care and the patient's prognosis.

- **Mental status changes**

  ▨ Altered level of consciousness occurs due to infection, anxiety, or psychological issues. The patient may exhibit confusion, delirium, or hallucinations. The nurse must differentiate among these manifestations, provide proper interventions, and offer family teaching and support.

▨ PRACTICE QUESTIONS

1. A hospice nurse is assisting a patient with a meal and observes that when the patient takes liquids, he coughs and drools. The nurse should

   a. Change the patient's diet to pureed

   b. Conduct a swallowing screen

   c. Suction the patient's oropharynx

   d. Administer an analgesic

2. A hospice patient is not able to accurately state the time, date, or place. The patient is

   a. Confused

   b. Disoriented

   c. Delirious

   d. Lethargic

3. A palliative care patient reports a sensation of pins and needles in her legs after sitting in a wheel chair for an extended period of time. The nurse knows that the symptoms are most likely related to

   a. Diabetes

   b. Impingement

   c. Skin breakdown

   d. Nerve damage

4. For the patient in the previous question, which of the following interventions should be implemented?

   a. Assist the patient with a position change

   b. Administer an analgesic

   c. Request a referral to a wound care specialist

   d. Administer a gabapentenoid

5. A patient in an inpatient hospice unit is experiencing a myoclonic seizure. The nurse should immediately

   a. Remove visitors from the room

   b. Initiate intravenous access

   c. Administer lorazepam

   d. Protect the patient's airway

6. An on-call hospice nurse receives a call from a patient's family member who states that when the patient was transferred from the bed to the wheelchair, he experienced sharp back pain and bladder incontinence. The nurse's best response is

   a. "He most likely has a pathologic fracture."

   b. "Does he have a history of herniated disc?"

    c. "This is an emergency, I will be there soon."

    d. "Administer his pain medication and allow him to rest now."

7. A home care hospice patient fell in the bathroom, hitting her head on the toilet. An hour later, her family found her with slurred speech, blurred vision, nausea, and behavioral changes. The patient's symptoms indicate

    a. Syncope

    b. Brain metastasis

    c. Increased intracranial pressure

    d. A pathological fracture

8. A patient is at risk for internal hemorrhage due to esophageal varices. The nurse should keep which of the following at the bedside?

    a. Dark-colored towels

    b. A hemostat

    c. Petroleum gauze

    d. An obturator

9. The family members of a hospice patient who is actively dying are very concerned that the patient has signs of a deep vein thrombosis (DVT). Which of the following should the nurse do first?

    a. Assess blood flow using a Doppler

    b. Apply compression stockings

    c. Review goals of care with the family

    d. Apply moist heat

10. A palliative care patient calls the nurse to report severe chest pain. The patient has taken three doses of sublingual nitroglycerin and is very anxious. The palliative care nurse should

    a. Recommend an opioid

    b. Advise the patient to take another dose of nitroglycerin

    c. Arrange for supplemental oxygen to be delivered to the home

    d. Determine if the patient wants to seek emergency treatment at this time

11. A homebound palliative care patient who has end-stage cardiac disease has been experiencing increased cough, dyspnea, and syncope for the past 2 weeks. He calls the on-call nurse to report facial swelling and is very concerned and anxious about this new development. The nurse should

    a. Arrange for a home x-ray

    b. Advise the patient to take sublingual nitroglycerin

c. Recommend reduced sodium intake

d. Arrange for transport to the hospital

12. Mrs. Artz is a 63-year-old palliative care patient who has end-stage renal disease. She recently began taking lisinopril and hydrochlorothiazide. Today, she reports a dry and persistent cough. The nurse knows that

a. The cough is related to the hydrochlorothiazide

b. Guaifenesin should be started immediately

c. The patient may require an antibiotic

d. Angiotensin-converting enzyme inhibitors may cause cough

13. An actively dying hospice patient has terminal secretions that are very distressing to the family members. During a home visit, which of the following interventions should the nurse implement first?

a. Administer scopolamine

b. Suction the patient's oropharynx

c. Reposition the patient

d. Auscultate the patient's lungs

14. A palliative care patient who has breast cancer reports abdominal bloating, cramping, and leakage of liquid stool. The nurse should first

a. Administer an enema

b. Check for impaction

c. Recommend a laxative

d. Conduct a nutritional assessment

15. Which of the following is an appropriate intervention for hiccups?

a. Calcium carbonate

b. Simethicone

c. Milk of magnesia

d. Propranolol

16. A palliative care patient experiences severe nausea and vomiting several days each week. The patient has a history of severe anxiety and panic disorder. Which of the following would be most helpful to treat the patient's symptoms?

a. Diphenhydramine

b. Dexamethasone

c. Ondansetron

d. Lorazepam

17. The wife of a home care hospice patient who has end-stage prostate cancer calls the nurse to report that the patient is experiencing severe bladder spasms, suprapubic pain, and urinary retention. The nurse should

   a. Recommend that the patient remain nothing by mouth (NPO) until he voids

   b. Visit the home and insert a urinary catheter

   c. Arrange for a transfer to the inpatient hospice unit

   d. Advise administration of scopolamine now

18. A patient in an inpatient hospice unit who has end-stage lung cancer with widespread metastasis develops joint swelling and severe pain in her left arm after being repositioned in bed. The most likely cause of the patient's symptoms is

   a. Hypercalcemia

   b. Compression fracture

   c. Tumor growth

   d. Pathological fracture

19. The nurse visits a hospice patient who has recently returned home after a respite stay at a long-term care facility. The patient has end-stage colon cancer and has recently begun taking morphine 5 mg orally every 4 hours as needed for pain. During today's visit, the patient reports new-onset pruritus. The nurse's best response is

   a. "The dose of your morphine is probably too high"

   b. "I will need to carefully check your skin to assess for rash, infection, or infestation"

   c. "Morphine allergy is very common and itching is a key sign"

   d. "I will call the long-term care facility to see if anyone else is having this problem"

20. A patient who has end-stage colon cancer has had a nonhealing abdominal wound with foul odor for the past 8 weeks. The patient is in poor condition and was transferred to the hospice inpatient unit for pain management. The best intervention to control the wound odor at this time is

   a. Applying metronidazole gel to the wound

   b. Administering oral antibiotics

   c. Applying a wound vac

   d. Referring the patient for surgical debridement

21. A home care hospice patient who has end-stage brain cancer has recently become violent with her spouse and exhibits spontaneous angry outbursts. The nursing priority for this patient is

a. Decreasing intracranial pressure

b. Sedating the patient

c. Ensuring safety

d. Providing calm reassurance

22. A hospice patient who has end-stage pancreatic cancer tells the nurse that he no longer needs hospice care because he feels fine. This is an example of

    a. Fear

    b. Control

    c. Denial

    d. Disbelief

23. A patient who has advanced cancer of the larynx has become dehydrated. The patient and family are very concerned about this development and request a meeting with the interdisciplinary team to develop a plan. The team should

    a. Recommend intravenous fluids

    b. Review goals of care

    c. Assess the patient for signs of dehydration

    d. Measure intake and output daily

24. A home care hospice patient who has end-stage liver cancer recently reported nausea, vomiting, and changes in mentation. Laboratory testing reveals hypercalcemia. Which treatment is recommended at this time?

    a. Bismuth salicylate

    b. A bisphosphonate

    c. Lactulose

    d. Haloperidol

25. A home care hospice patient who has chronic obstructive pulmonary disease (COPD) is transferred to the hospice inpatient unit for symptom management due to new-onset chest pain and fever. After 2 days in the inpatient unit, the patient becomes disoriented to time and place and begins hallucinating that there are bugs on the wall. Based on these symptoms, the nurse knows that the patient has

    a. Pneumonia

    b. Dementia

    c. Delirium

    d. Terminal agitation

■ REFERENCES

Abrahm, J. L. (2014). *A physician's guide to pain and symptom management in cancer patients* (3rd ed.). Baltimore, MD: Johns Hopkins University Press.

American Heart Association. (2018). *Syncope (fainting)*. Retrieved from http://www.heart.org/HEARTORG/Conditions/Arrhythmia/SymptomsDiagnosisMonitoringofArrhythmia/Syncope-Fainting_UCM_430006_Article.jsp#W136dtVKipo

American Psychological Association. (2018). *Suicide warning signs*. Retrieved from http://www.apa.org/topics/suicide/signs.aspx

American Speech-Language-Hearing Association. (2018). *Adult dysphagia*. Retrieved from https://www.asha.org/PRPSpecificTopic.aspx?folderid=8589942550&section=Signs_and_Symptoms

Armour, B. S., Courtney-Long, E. A., Fox, M. H., Fredine, H., & Cahill, A. (2016). Prevalence and causes of paralysis—United States, 2013. *American Journal of Public Health, 106*(10), 1855–1857. doi:10.2105/AJPH.2016.303270

Arthur, J. A. (2016). Constipation and bowel obstruction. In S. Yennurajalingam & E. Bruera (Eds.), *Oxford American handbook of hospice and palliative medicine and supportive care* (2nd ed., pp. 137–151). New York, NY: Oxford University Press.

Bates-Jensen, B. M., & Petch, S. (2015). Pressure ulcers: Prevention and management. In B. R. Ferrell, N. Coyle, & J. A. Paice (Eds.), *Oxford textbook of palliative nursing* (4th ed., pp. 297–324). New York, NY: Oxford University Press.

Berry, P., & Griffie, J. (2015). Preparing for the actual death. In B. R. Ferrell, N. Coyle, & J. A. Paice (Eds.), *Oxford textbook of palliative nursing* (4th ed., pp. 515–530). New York, NY: Oxford University Press.

Blevins, T. (2015). Nursing care of patients with valvular, inflammatory, and infectious cardiac or venous disorders. In L. S. Williams & P. D. Hopper (Eds.), *Understanding medical-surgical nursing* (5th ed., pp. 432–461). Philadelphia, PA: F.A. Davis Company.

Bobb, B. T. (2015). Urgent symptoms at the end of life. In B. R. Ferrell, N. Coyle, & J. A. Paice (Eds.), *Oxford textbook of palliative nursing* (4th ed., pp. 422–439). New York, NY: Oxford University Press.

Bobb, B. T., & Fletcher, D. (2015). Challenging symptoms: Dry mouth, hiccups, fevers, pruritus, and sleep disorders. In C. Dahlin, P. J. Coyne, & B. R. Ferrell (Eds.), *Advanced practice palliative nursing.* (pp. 270–288). New York, NY: Oxford University Press.

Bodtke, S., & Ligon, K. (2016). *Hospice and palliative medicine handbook: A clinical guide*. Retrieved from www.hpmhandbook.com

Boss, B. J., & Huether, S. E. (2014). Disorders of the central and peripheral nervous systems and the neuromuscular junction. In K. L. McCance & S. E. Huether (Eds.), *Pathophysiology: The biologic basis for disease in adults and children* (7th ed., pp. 581–640). St. Louis, MO: Elsevier.

Buckle, J. (2015). *Clinical aromatherapy: Essential oils in healthcare*. St. Louis, MO: Elsevier.

Calton, B. A., & Ritchie, C. S. (2016). Palliative care in older adults. In S. Yennurajalingam & E. Bruera (Eds.), *Oxford American handbook of hospice and palliative medicine and supportive care* (2nd ed., pp. 69–81). New York, NY: Oxford University Press.

Carney, N., Totten, A. M., O'Reilly, C., Ullman, J. S., Hawryluk, G. W., Bell, M. J., . . . Ghajar, J. (2016). Guidelines for the management of severe traumatic brain injury. *Neurosurgery, 80*(1), 6–15. doi:10.1227/NEU.0000000000001432

Chow, K., Cogan, D., & Mun, S. (2015). Nausea and vomiting. In B. R. Ferrell, N. Coyle, & J. A. Paice (Eds.), *Oxford textbook of palliative nursing* (4th ed., pp. 174–190). New York, NY: Oxford University Press.

Chow, K., & Korateng, L. (2015). Bowel symptoms: Constipation, diarrhea, and obstruction. In B. R. Ferrell, N. Coyle, & J. A. Paice (Eds.), *Oxford textbook of palliative nursing* (4th ed., pp. 243–253). New York, NY: Oxford University Press.

Cichero, J. A., Lam, P., Steele, C. M., Hanson, B., Chen, J., Dantas, R. O., . . . Stanschus, S. (2017). Development of international terminology and definitions for texture-modified foods and thickened fluids used in dysphagia management: The IDDSI framework. *Dysphagia, 32*(2), 293–314. doi:10.1007/s00455-016-9758-y

Cleveland Clinic Foundation. (2018). *Paralysis*. Retrieved from https://my.clevelandclinic.org/health/diseases/15345-paralysis

Dahlin, C. M., & Cohen, A. K. (2015). Dysphagia, xerostomia, and hiccups. In B. R. Ferrell, N. Coyle, & J. A. Paice (Eds.), *Oxford textbook of palliative nursing* (4th ed., pp. 191–216). New York, NY: Oxford University Press.

Dalal, S. (2016). Dehydration. In S. Yennurajalingam & E. Bruera (Eds.), *Oxford American handbook of hospice and palliative medicine and supportive care* (2nd ed., pp. 93–96). New York, NY: Oxford University Press.

Demertzi, A., Jox, R. J., Racine, E., & Laureys, S. (2014). A European survey on attitudes towards pain and end-of-life issues in locked-in syndrome. *Brain Injury, 28*(9), 1209–1215. doi:10.3109/02699052.2014.920526

Dudgeon, D. (2015). Dyspnea, terminal secretions, and cough. In B. R. Ferrell, N. Coyle, & J. A. Paice (Eds.), *Oxford textbook of palliative nursing* (4th ed., pp. 246–261). New York, NY: Oxford University Press.

Dudgeon, D. (2016). Dyspnea, death rattle and cough. In J. A. Paice (pp. (Ed.), *Care of the imminently dying patient* (pp. 23–38). New York, NY: Oxford University Press.

Engleka, J. (2016). Cough. In C. Dahlin, P. J. Coyne, & B. R. Ferrell(pp. (Eds.), *Advanced practice palliative nursing* (pp. 260–269). New York, NY: Oxford University Press.

Fedder, W. N. (2017). Review of evidenced-based nursing protocols for dysphagia assessment. *Stroke, 48*(4), e99–e101. doi:10.1161/STROKEAHA.116.011738

Flevari, P., Leftheriotis, D., Repasos, E., Katsaras, D., Katsimardos, A., & Lekakis, J. (2017). Fluoxetine vs. placebo for the treatment of recurrent vasovagal syncope with anxiety sensitivity. *EP Europace, 19*(1), 127–131. doi:10.1093/europace/euw153

Flores-Mireles, A. L., Walker, J. N., Caparon, M., & Hultgren, S. J. (2015). Urinary tract infections: Epidemiology, mechanisms of infection and treatment options. *Nature Reviews Microbiology, 13*(5), 269. doi:10.1038/nrmicro3432

Fraenkel, P. G. (2015). Understanding anemia of chronic disease. *ASH Education Program Book, 2015*(1), 14–18. Retrieved from http://asheducationbook.hematologylibrary.org/content/2015/1/14.full.pdf?hw-tma-check=true

Gabriel, M. S., & Tschanz, J. A. (2015). Artificial nutrition and hydration. In B. R. Ferrell, N. Coyle, & J. A. Paice (Eds.), *Oxford textbook of palliative nursing* (4th ed., pp. 237–246). New York, NY: Oxford University Press.

Gordon, S. (2015). Nursing care of patients with musculoskeletal and connective tissue disorders. In L. S. Williams & P. D. Hopper (Eds.), *Understanding medical-surgical nursing* (5th ed., pp. 641–683). Philadelphia, PA: F.A. Davis Company.

Gray, M., & Sims, T. (2015). Urinary tract disorders. In B. R. Ferrell, N. Coyle, & J. A. Paice (Eds.), *Oxford textbook of palliative nursing* (4th ed., pp. 262–278). New York, NY: Oxford University Press.

Groninger, H., & Vijayan, J. (2014). Pharmacologic pain management at end of life. *American Family Physician, 90*(1), 26–32. Retrieved from

Guay, M. O. D., & Yennurajalingam, S. (2016). Sleep disturbances. In S. Yennurajalingam & E. Bruera (Eds.), *Oxford American handbook of hospice and palliative medicine and supportive care* (2nd ed., pp. 113–123). New York, NY: Oxford University Press.

Heidrich, D. E., & English, N. K. (2015). Delirium, confusion, agitation, and restlessness. In B. R. Ferrell, N. Coyle, & J. A. Paice (Eds.), *Oxford textbook of palliative nursing* (4th ed., pp. 385–403). New York, NY: Oxford University Press.

Hines, S., Kynoch, K., & Munday, J. (2016). Nursing interventions for identifying and managing acute dysphagia are effective for improving patient outcomes: A systematic review update. *Journal of Neuroscience Nursing, 48*(4), 215–223. doi:10.1097/JNN.0000000000000200

Hopper, P. D. (2015). Nursing care of patients with lower respiratory tract disorders. In L. S. Williams & P. D. Hopper (Eds.), *Understanding medical-surgical nursing* (5th ed., pp. 641–683). Philadelphia, PA: F.A. Davis Company.

Hosker, C. M., & Bennett, M. I. (2016). Delirium and agitation at the end of life. *BMJ, 353*, i3085. doi:10.1136/bmj.i3085

Hui, D., dos Santos, R., Chisholm, G. B., & Bruera, E. (2015). Symptom expression in the last seven days of life among cancer patients admitted to acute palliative care units. *Journal of Pain and Symptom Management, 50*(4), 488–494. doi:https://doi.org/10.1016/j.jpainsymman.2014.09.003

Hui, D. (2016). Management of cancer treatment-related adverse effects. In S. Yennurajalingam & E. Bruera (Eds.), *Oxford American handbook of hospice and palliative medicine and supportive care* (2nd ed., pp. 207–221). New York, NY: Oxford University Press.

Hwang, C. S., Weng, H. H., Wang, L. F., Tsai, C. H., & Chang, H. T. (2014). An eye-tracking assistive device improves the quality of life for ALS patients and reduces caregivers' burden. *Journal of Motor Behavior, 46*(4), 233–238. doi:10.1080/00222895.2014.891970

Inouye, S. K., Westendorp, R. G., & Saczynski, J. S. (2014). Delirium in elderly people. *The Lancet, 383*(9920), 911–922. doi:10.1016/S0140-6736(13)60688-1

Institute for Aging Research. (2018). *Confusion assessment method.* Retrieved from https://www.instituteforagingresearch.org/research/aging-brain-center/confusion-assessment-method

Johns Hopkins Medicine. (2018). *Increased intracranial pressure.* Retrieved from https://www.hopkinsmedicine.org/healthlibrary/conditions/nervous_system_disorders/increased_intracranial_pressure_icp_headache_134,67

Kohn, M., & Trofino, R. B. (2015). Nursing care of the patient with skin disorders. In L. S. Williams & P. D. Hopper (Eds.), *Understanding medical-surgical nursing* (5th ed., pp. 1288–1319). Philadelphia, PA: F.A. Davis Company.

Kojovic, M., Cordivari, C., & Bhatia, K. (2011). Myoclonic disorders: A practical approach for diagnosis and treatment. *Therapeutic Advances in Neurological Disorders, 4*(1), 47–62. doi:10.1177/1756285610395653

Kovach, C. R., & Reynolds, S. (2015). Neurological disorders. In M. Matzo & D. W. Sherman (Eds.), *Palliative care nursing: Quality care to the end of life* (4th ed., pp. 347–371). New York, NY: Springer Publishing Company.

Kresevic, D. M. (2015). Reducing functional decline in hospitalized older adults. *American Nurse Today, 10*(5), 58–67. Retrieved from https://www.americannursetoday.com/reducing-functional-decline-hospitalized-older/

Kuriya, M., & Dev, R. (2016). Emergencies in palliative care. In S. Yennurajalingam & E. Bruera (Eds.), *Oxford American handbook of hospice and palliative medicine and supportive care* (2nd ed., pp. 185–194). New York, NY: Oxford University Press.

Lavorini, F., Di Bello, V., De Rimini, M. L., Lucignani, G., Marconi, L., Palareti, G., . . . Pistolesi, M. (2013). Diagnosis and treatment of pulmonary embolism: A multidisciplinary approach. *Multidisciplinary Respiratory Medicine, 8*(1), 75. Retrieved from https://www.ncbi.nlm.nih.gov/pmc/articles/PMC3878229/pdf/2049-6958-8-75.pdf

Levesque, C. (2012). Endocrine problems. In J. G. W. Foster & S. S. Prevost (Eds.), *Advanced practice nursing of adults in acute care* (pp. 444–524). Philadelphia, PA: F.A. Davis.

Lippincott Nursing Center. (2007). Guide to care for patients: Managing seizures. *The Nurse Practitioner, 32*(5), 19–20. Retrieved from https://www.nursingcenter.com/journalarticle?Article_ID=715092&Journal_ID=54012&Issue_ID=715080

Manthey, D. E., & Ellis, L. R. (2016). Superior vena cava syndrome (SVCS). In K. H. Todd & C. R. Thomas (Eds.), *Oncologic emergency medicine* (pp. 212–218). Switzerland: Springer International Publishing. doi:10.1007/978-3-319-26387-8_18

Marks, A., & Marchand, L. (2018). *Fast facts and concepts #118: Near death awareness.* Retrieved from https://www.mypcnow.org/blank-rnt14

Martinez-Kratz, M. (2015). Nursing care of patients with mental health disorders. In L. S. Williams & P. D. Hopper (Eds.), *Understanding medical-surgical nursing* (5th ed., pp. 432–461). Philadelphia, PA: F.A. Davis Company.

McDonald, M. (2015). Nursing care of patients with occlusive cardiovascular disorders. In L. S. Williams & P. D. Hopper (Eds.), *Understanding medical-surgical nursing* (5th ed., pp. 462–498). Philadelphia, PA: F.A. Davis Company.

Medici, V., & Meyers, F. J. (2016). Palliative care in end stage liver disease. In S. Yennurajalingam & E. Bruera (Eds.), *Oxford American handbook of hospice and palliative medicine and supportive care* (2nd ed., pp. 385–396). New York, NY: Oxford University Press.

Mercadante, S., Aielli, F., Adile, C., Ferrera, P., Valle, A., Cartoni, C., . . . Porzio, G. (2015). Sleep disturbances in patients with advanced cancer in different palliative care settings. *Journal of Pain and Symptom Management, 50*(6), 786–792. doi:10.1016/j.jpainsymman.2015.06.018

Morici, B. (2014). Diagnosis and management of acute pulmonary embolism. *Journal of the American Academy of PAs, 27*(4), 18–22. doi:10.1097/01.JAA.0000444729.09046.09

National Cancer Institute. (2018). *NCI dictionary of cancer terms.* Retrieved from https://www.cancer.gov/publications/dictionaries/cancer-terms/def/myelosuppression

National Heart, Lung, and Blood Institute (2018). *Thrombocytopenia.* Retrieved from https://www.nhlbi.nih.gov/health-topics/thrombocytopenia

National Institute of Diabetes and Digestive and Kidney Diseases. (2018). *Symptoms and causes of constipation.* Retrieved from https://www.niddk.nih.gov/health-information/digestive-diseases/constipation/symptoms-causes

National Institute of Neurological Disorders and Stroke. (2018a). *What is myoclonus?* Retrieved from https://www.ninds.nih.gov/Disorders/Patient-Caregiver-Education/Fact-Sheets/Myoclonus-Fact-Sheet

National Institute of Neurological Disorders and Stroke. (2018b). *Paresthesia information page.* Retrieved from https://www.ninds.nih.gov/Disorders/All-Disorders/Paresthesia-Information-Page

National Institute of Neurological Disorders and Stroke. (2018c). *What is peripheral neuropathy?* Retrieved from https://www.ninds.nih.gov/Disorders/Patient-Caregiver-Education/Fact-Sheets/Peripheral-Neuropathy-Fact-Sheet

National Institute of Neurological Disorders and Stroke. (2018d). *The epilepsies and seizures: Hope through research.* Retrieved from https://www.ninds.nih.gov/Disorders/Patient-Caregiver-Education/Hope-Through-Research/Epilepsies-and-Seizures-Hope-Through#3109_9

Nightingale, F. (1860). *Notes on nursing.* Retrieved from http://digital.library.upenn.edu/women/nightingale/nursing/nursing.html

Nowicki, L. V. (2015). Nursing care of patients with lower gastrointestinal tract disorders. In L. S. Williams & P. D. Hopper (Eds.), *Understanding medical-surgical nursing* (5th ed., pp. 744–778). Philadelphia, PA: F.A. Davis Company.

O'Neil, E., Anderson, P. R., & Dean, G. E. (2015). Fatigue. In B. R. Ferrell, N. Coyle, & J. A. Paice (Eds.), *Oxford textbook of palliative nursing* (4th ed., pp. 154–166). New York, NY: Oxford University Press.

Paice, J.A. (2015). Pain at the end of life. In B. R. Ferrell, N. Coyle, & J. A. Paice (Eds.), *Oxford textbook of palliative nursing* (pp. 135–153). New York, NY: Oxford University Press.

Periyakoil, V. S. (2016). Psychosocial and cultural considerations in palliative care. In S. Yennurajalingam & E. Bruera (Eds.), *Oxford American handbook of hospice and palliative medicine and supportive care* (2nd ed., pp. 93–96). New York, NY: Oxford University Press.

Powers, J., & Jones, D. (2012). Musculoskeletal problems. In J. G. W. Foster & S. S. Prevost (Eds.), *Advanced practice nursing of adults in acute care* (pp. 711–732). Philadelphia, PA: F.A. Davis Company.

Rogers, L. C., Frykberg, R. G., Armstrong, D. G., Boulton, A. J., Edmonds, M., Van, G. H., . . . Uccoli, L. (2011). The Charcot foot in diabetes. *Diabetes Care, 34*(9), 2123–2129. doi:10.2337/dc11-0844

Schimpf, M. M. (2012). Diagnosing increased intracranial pressure. *Journal of Trauma Nursing, 19*(3), 160–167. doi:10.1097/JTN.0b013e318261cfb4

Sharfman, G., & Braun, U. K. (2017). Palliative and end of life issues in patients with advanced respiratory distress. In A. Sharafkhaneh, A. M. Yohannes, N. A. Hanania, & M. E. Kunik (Eds.), *Depression and anxiety in patients with chronic respiratory distress* (pp. 183–194). New York, NY: Springer Science & Business Media, LLC.

Shelton, B. K. (2012). Hematology and oncology problems. In J. G. W. Foster & S. S. Prevost (Eds.), *Advanced practice nursing of adults in acute care* (pp. 591–651). Philadelphia, PA: F.A. Davis Company.

Smith, H. S. (2012). Opioids and neuropathic pain. *Pain Physician, 15*, ES93–ES110. Retrieved from http://painphysicianjournal.com/2012/july/2012;: 15;: ES93-ES110.pdf

Son, D. S., Seong, J. W., Kim, Y., Chee, Y., & Hwang, C. H. (2013). The effects of removable denture on swallowing. *Annals of Rehabilitation Medicine, 37*(2), 247–253. doi:10.5535/arm.2013.37.2.247

Spiess, J. L. (2017). Hospice in heart failure: Why, when, and what then? *Heart Failure Reviews, 22*, 593–604. doi:10.1007/s10741-017-9595-6

Stöppler, M. C. (2017). *Neutropenia causes, symptoms, ranges, levels, and treatment.* Retrieved from https://www.medicinenet.com/neutropenia/article.htm#neutropenia_definition_and_facts

Tradounsky, G. (2013). Seizures in palliative care. *Canadian Family Physician, 29*(9), 951–955. Retrieved from https://www.ncbi.nlm.nih.gov/pmc/articles/PMC3771721/pdf/0590951.pdf

Twomey, S., & Dowling, M. (2013). Management of death rattle at end of life. *British Journal of Nursing, 22*(2), 81–85. doi:10.12968/bjon.2013.22.2.81

Villa, A., Connell, C. L., & Abati, S. (2015). Diagnosis and management of xerostomia and hyposalivation. *Therapeutics and Clinical Risk Management, 11*, 45–51. doi:10.2147/TCRM.S76282

Wada, H., Matsumoto, T., & Yamashita, Y. (2014). Diagnosis and treatment of disseminated intravascular coagulation (DIC) according to four DIC guidelines. *Journal of Intensive Care, 2*(1), 15. doi:10.1186/2052-0492-2-15

Walbert, T. (2016). Palliative care in end stage neurological disease. In S. Yennurajalingam & E. Bruera (Eds.), *Oxford American handbook of hospice and palliative medicine and supportive care* (2nd ed., pp. 419–434). New York, NY: Oxford University Press.

Walker, P. W. (2016). Other symptoms: Xerostomia, hiccups, pruritus, pressure ulcers and wound care, lymphedema and myoclonus. In S. Yennurajalingam & E. Bruera (Eds.), *Oxford American handbook of hospice and palliative medicine and supportive care* (2nd ed., pp. 195–206). New York, NY: Oxford University Press.

Weaver, D. L. (2015). Nursing care of patients with central nervous system disorders. In L. S. Williams & P. D. Hopper (Eds.), *Understanding medical-surgical nursing* (5th ed., pp. 1118–1170). Philadelphia, PA: F.A. Davis.

Wholihan, D. (2015). Anorexia and cachexia. In B. R. Ferrell, N. Coyle, & J. A. Paice (Eds.), *Oxford textbook of palliative nursing* (4th ed., pp. 167–174). New York, NY: Oxford University Press.

Willeumier, J. J., van der Linden, Y. M., van de Sande, M. A., & Dijkstra, P. S. (2016). Treatment of pathological fractures of the long bones. *EFORT Open Reviews, 1*(5), 136–145. doi:10.1302/2058-5241.1.000008

Wong, A., & Reddy, S. K. (2016). Pain assessment and management. In S. Yennurajalingam & E. Bruera (Eds.), *Oxford American handbook of hospice and palliative medicine and supportive care* (2nd ed., pp. 27–67). New York, NY: Oxford University Press.

Yennurajalingam, S. (2016). Fatigue. In S. Yennurajalingam & E. Bruera (Eds.), *Oxford American handbook of hospice and palliative medicine and supportive care* (2nd ed., pp. 69–81). New York, NY: Oxford University Press.

V

Patient and Family Care, Education, and Advocacy

17 Establishing Goals of Care and Managing Resources

The goal of [hospice and] palliative care is achievement of the best quality of life for patients and their families.
—Becker (2009)

LEARNING OBJECTIVES

After completing this section, the nurse will be able to

1. Approach goals of care conversations with terminally ill patients and their families.
2. Establish hospice eligibility
3. Discuss hospice benefits, coverage, and eligibility

ESTABLISHING GOALS OF CARE

Advance care planning is a collaborative effort between healthcare providers, patients, and families through which the patient establishes their preferences for future medical treatments (Moore, 2007). Patients may express their advance directives through the development of a living will or by designating a medical power of attorney (see Table 17.1; Wright, 2017). Advance directives are used to guide care only when patients are unable to speak or make decisions for themselves (see also, Chapter 3, Disease Progression and Imminent Death).

A type of advance directive that is used specifically for patients who have a life expectancy of 1 year or less is a physician (or provider) order for life-sustaining treatment (POLST), also called a medical order for life-sustaining treatment (MOLST). The POLST form specifies which treatments the patient would choose to have in the case of a medical emergency. Unlike an advance directive, the POLST can be followed by emergency care providers because it is a medical order (see Table 17.1).

Table 17.1 POLST Versus Advance Directives

	POLST Paradigm Form	Advance Directive
Type of document	Medical order	Legal document
Who completes the document	Healthcare professional (which healthcare professional can sign varies by state)	Individual
Who should have one	Any seriously ill or frail individual (regardless of age) whose healthcare professional would not be surprised if he or she died in the year	All competent adults
What document communicates	Specific medical orders	General treatment wishes
Can document appoint a surrogate decision-maker?	No	Yes
Surrogate decision-maker role	Can engage in discussion and update or void form if patient lacks capacity	Cannot complete
Can emergency personnel follow this document?	Yes	No
Ease in locating/portability	Patient has original; a copy is in patient's medical record. A copy may be in a state registry (if state has one)	No set location. Individuals must make sure surrogates have most recent version
Periodic review	Healthcare professional responsible for reviewing with patient or surrogate	Patient responsible for periodically reviewing

POLST, physician (or provider) order for life-sustaining treatment.
Source: National POLST Paradigm. (2018). *Advance care planning: Advance directives vs. POLST forms.* Retrieved from https://polst.org/wp-content/uploads/2019/05/2019.04.30-POLST-vs-ADs-chart.pdf. Used with permission.

Patients may change their goals or wishes as a disease process progresses. Thus hospice and palliative care nurses must be prepared to establish and reestablish goals of care with patients and families regularly. Goals of care conversations should first focus on establishing the patient's values, clarifying the issues at hand, and weighing the risks and benefits of various treatment options (You, Fowler, & Heyland, 2014). If possible, family members or surrogate decision-makers should be included in goals of care conversations to ensure that they receive accurate information. Hearing the patient's wishes firsthand may lead to greater congruency between the patient's wishes and the decisions made by surrogates. If possible, the patient's wishes should be documented and signed in the presence of her or his family (Perrin, 2015; You et al., 2014).

Clinicians can open goals of care conversations by asking patients to verbalize their perceptions of their illnesses, what their hopes are, and what they worry about (see Table 17.2). The nurse should provide active listening in a nonjudgmental manner to establish a patient's understanding of his or her illness and perceptions about life-sustaining treatments (Perrin, 2015).

Key Point
When discussing goals of care with families of terminally ill patients who cannot speak for themselves, the nurse should avoid questions such as "Do you want us to do everything?" or "Should we discontinue care now?" These phrases convey the misperception that all care will be discontinued if curative treatments are stopped (Perrin, 2015).

Table 17.2 Suggested Statements for Leading a Goals of Care Discussion

Determining a Patient's Values

- "Have you previously had an experience with serious illness, or has someone close to you had an experience with serious illness or death?" (You et al., 2014)
- "If you were in this situation (again), what would you hope for? What would worry you most?" (You et al., 2014)
- "Did this situation make you think about states of being that would be so unacceptable to you that you would consider them to be worse than death?" (You et al., 2014)

Establishing Leeway in Substitute Decision-Making

- "What if, based on changes in your health, the doctors recommend something different from what you have told your loved one(s)?" (You et al., 2014)
- "Will you give your loved one(s) permission to work with your doctors to make the best decision possible for you, even if it may differ from what you said you wanted in the past?" (You et al., 2014)
- "Are there certain decisions about your health that you would never want your loved one(s) to change under any circumstances?" (You et al., 2014)

Aligning Language With the Patient's Preferred Mode of Decision-Making

- Shared decision-making: "Based on what you've said, it seems to me that the most reasonable course of action is . . . " (i.e., avoid asking "What would you like us to do?" to avoid placing the burden of the decision solely on the patient)
- Active decision-maker: "It is up to you to decide, but many people in your circumstances would consider it acceptable to . . ." (i.e., legitimize the difficult option, but leave the patient as the final decision-maker)
- Passive decision-maker: "I recommend that we do the following . . ." (i.e., declare the plan)

Note: The suggested wording contained here can and should be modified by clinicians to suit their own communication style and to meet the individual's needs and preferences of patients. Statements without references are based on the authors' experiences.

Source: You, J. J., Fowler, R. A., & Heyland, D. K. (2014). Just ask: Discussing goals of care with patients in hospital with serious illness. *Canadian Medical Association Journal*, *186*(6), 425–432. doi:10.1503 /cmaj.12127. Used with permission.

In some cases, patients will want to be well informed about their illness and will want to consider every treatment option before making a medical decisions. On the other end of the spectrum, patients may rely heavily on the healthcare provider to advise them about what they believe is their best option (You et al., 2014). Thus the patient's preference for participation in goal setting is important to establish and honor.

When establishing goals, the nurse should ensure that every goal is measurable so that results can be observed and quantified. A goal may be somewhat broad in its scope and thus may have associated objectives. Objectives are more specific than goals and can be seen as steps that need to be achieved to meet the overall goal. Both goals and objectives should be developed according to the patient's preferences and should be specific to the situation, measurable, and realistic. A commonly used mnemonic used to describe the necessary components of goals and objectives is the SMART model (see Figure 17.1).

If goals and objectives are properly created, evaluation of progress is easily tracked by determining whether the goals were met, partially met, or unmet by the expected date of completion. After determining if the goals were met, the goals should be reviewed to determine if they should be modified, extended, or discontinued. Then the plan of care should be modified to incorporate the revised goals. The process of goal setting, implementation, evaluation, and revision is ongoing and requires the skills of the interdisciplinary team as well as frequent involvement of the patient and family (see Figure 17.2).

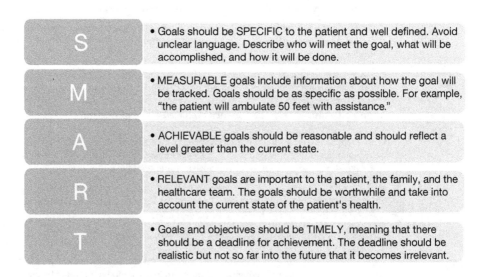

S	• Goals should be SPECIFIC to the patient and well defined. Avoid unclear language. Describe who will meet the goal, what will be accomplished, and how it will be done.
M	• MEASURABLE goals include information about how the goal will be tracked. Goals should be as specific as possible. For example, "the patient will ambulate 50 feet with assistance."
A	• ACHIEVABLE goals should be reasonable and should reflect a level greater than the current state.
R	• RELEVANT goals are important to the patient, the family, and the healthcare team. The goals should be worthwhile and take into account the current state of the patient's health.
T	• Goals and objectives should be TIMELY, meaning that there should be a deadline for achievement. The deadline should be realistic but not so far into the future that it becomes irrelevant.

FIGURE 17.1 SMART goals and objectives.

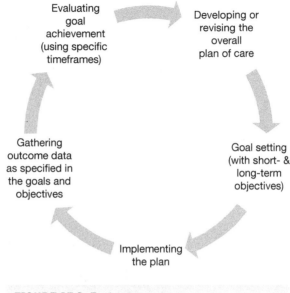

FIGURE 17.2 Evaluation process.

The plan of care is sometimes influenced by availability of services, insurance coverage, and patient preferences. The hospice and palliative care nurse can provide in-depth education regarding hospice and/or palliative care. When patients and families are aware of their care options, they are empowered to make well-informed choices in light of the available community resources.

Resource Management

Palliative Care Coverage

For patients who have serious illnesses and need expert symptom management, a palliative care referral is warranted. Palliative care involves a team of healthcare professionals who approach care in a holistic manner, with the goal of addressing patients' physical, emotional, spiritual, and psychosocial needs. The palliative care team can also help address concerns about cost, co-pays, and insurance coverage. Most private insurances, as well as Medicare and Medicaid, will cover the costs of palliative care that is provided in an inpatient setting, such as a hospital. Medicare Part A may cover the cost of community-based palliative care services and Medicare Part B may cover supplies related to the serious illness. Patients who wish to access palliative care services should talk with a palliative care social worker or to the insurance or Medicare/Medicaid representative regarding coverage and co-payments (Center to Advance Palliative Care, 2018).

Hospice Coverage

For patients who have been diagnosed with a terminal illness and have a life expectancy of approximately 6 months, hospice services may be an option. Patients who are eligible for Medicare Part A may receive services provided that they

> **Key Point**
>
> According to the American Nurses Association, nurses must be prepared to provide holistic palliative and end of life care and to assist patients with end-of-life decision-making (American Nurses Association, 2016).

- Accept hospice care instead of curative treatments

- Sign a statement choosing hospice care and revoking Medicare benefits for curative treatment of the terminal condition

- Receive certification of terminality (life expectancy of 6 months or less) from *both* the primary care physician *and* the hospice medical director
(Centers for Medicare & Medicaid Services, 2015a)

Other criteria used to support terminality and eligibility for services, such as local coverage determinations (LCDs), are also used to determine eligibility for hospice care (see Figure 3.8).

When an eligible patient chooses hospice services, the first benefit period is for 6 months (two 90-day periods). After two 90-day periods, recertification of the terminal illness is required every 60 days for as long as the patient continues to meet the eligibility requirements (see Figure 17.3). The initial certification must be obtained within 2 days after the patient is admitted. Subsequent certifications must be completed 15 days prior to the recertification date or less than 2 days after it (Centers for Medicare & Medicaid Services, 2015a). When documenting a patient's ongoing eligibility for hospice care, the hospice nurse should reference the LCD guidelines and appropriate assessment tools, such as the Palliative Performance Scale, the FAST Scale, and any others that are appropriate to the patient's diagnosis (see also, Chapter 3, Disease Progression and Imminent Death).

Face-to-Face Encounters

As a result of the Affordable Care Act, Medicare now requires that hospice patients be seen by the hospice nurse practitioner (who must be employed by the hospice) or the hospice medical director prior to the

> **Key Point**
>
> The Medicare Benefit Policy Manual for Hospice Services can be accessed at https://www.cms.gov/Regulations-and-Guidance/Guidance/Manuals/downloads/bp102c09.pdf

third benefit period. The purpose of the face-to-face encounter is to verify continued eligibility for hospice services (Centers for Medicare & Medicaid Services, 2015b). The nurse practitioner or medical director should work closely with the hospice nurse to review the patient's status when determining ongoing eligibility.

| Admission eligibility: terminality certified by two physicians (usually the hospice medical director and the patient's primary care provider). Patient receives care for a period of 90 days. | After 90 days of hospice care, terminality and the need for ongoing hospice services are certified by 1 physician and the hospice interdisciplinary team for a second 90-day period. | Every 60 days after the initial two 90-day periods, a face-to-face visit must be made to the patient by the hospice physician or nurse practitioner to verify ongoing eligibility for hospice services. |

FIGURE 17.3 Hospice certification and recertification requirements.

Levels of Care

Hospice care involves four levels of care. The appropriate level of care is determined through conversations between the patient, the patient's family, and the interdisciplinary team. Levels of care in hospice are as follows:

- *Routine home care* is provided in the patient's home, which may be a long-term care facility. Visits from members of the hospice team are scheduled regularly as indicated by the patient's needs.

- *Continuous home care* is provided in the patient's home, predominantly by nurses, but also by hospice nurses' aides. The goal of continuous home care is to provide support for patients and families during a short-term crisis, such as a pain crisis.

- *Inpatient respite care* may be provided in an approved facility for a short period of time to allow respite for the caregiver(s).

- *General inpatient (GIP) care* takes place in an inpatient facility with the goal of addressing acute pain or other symptoms.
  (Centers for Medicare & Medicaid Services, 2015a)

Last 7 Days

In 2016, reimbursement regulations were changed to take into account the intense care that is provided for patients during their final week of life. According to the Centers for Medicare & Medicaid Services (2015b), in order to receive the additional reimbursement, the following criteria must be met:

- The patient's level of care must be "routine home care"

- The billing dates of care occur within the last 7 days of the patient's life

- Direct patient care is provided by a RN or licensed social worker

The care needs of terminally ill patients may change frequently; thus, the nurse must update and coordinate the plan of care regularly. To ensure proper coordination of care and interdisciplinary collaboration, the plan of care must be reviewed and revised by the interdisciplinary team at least every 15 days (National Hospice and Palliative Care Organization, 2009).

Hospice Medicare/Medicaid Benefits

Hospice care necessarily involves the coordination of services and the development of a plan of care by an interdisciplinary team. Core hospice services that are covered by Medicare and Medicaid include the following:

- Physician services
- Nursing services, with 24 h/d, 7 d/w availability
- Medical social services
- Counseling

Noncare services must also be provided according to the patient's unique needs, condition, and living arrangements. These services include the following:

- Physical, occupational, and speech therapy
- Hospice aide services
- Homemaker services
- Volunteers
- Medical supplies and medications related to the terminal illness
- Short-term inpatient care for acute or chronic symptom management in a Medicare/Medicaid participating facility
  (Centers for Medicare & Medicaid Services, 2015a)

Private Insurance Coverage

Although the majority of adult hospice patients are able to access services through Medicare or Medicaid, those who are not eligible may utilize veterans' benefits or private health coverage. The Veterans Health Administration provides hospice care coverage that is very similar to Medicaid and Medicare coverage. Many private insurances also cover hospice services, but some may limit the length of services or require specific co-payments for medications or medical supplies. Patients should contact their insurance provider to verify benefits. Uninsured patients may be able to receive hospice care from a hospice agency gratis or arrange sliding scale payments (American Hospice Foundation, 2018).

Patient Discharge

When a patient is no longer eligible for hospice due to an improvement in health, the patient will be discharged from the service. Patients who choose curative treatment rather than palliative and end-of-life care may also initiate discharge by revoking the hospice benefit. When a patient is discharged, a discharge order must be written by the hospice medical director, and the hospice team must include the patient and family in the discharge planning process (National Hospice and Palliative Care Organization, n.d.).

Patient Death

When a patient dies at home, the hospice nurse must go to the home to complete an assessment and to support the family. Upon arrival to the home, the nurse should (Berry & Griffie, 2015)

- Maintain a calm approach
- Identify the patient
- Assess the patient for breathing, motion, or other signs of life
- Assess for lack of pupillary response, absent carotid pulses, and apical pulses (auscultate for 1 minute in most situations)
- Provide respectful, culturally appropriate postmortem care

Documentation of the patient's death should include the following:

- The patient's name
- Time of the call, who called, who was present at the time of death
- Physical exam findings
- Who made the pronouncement of death, and the time of the pronouncement
- Who was notified of the patient's death
- To whom the patient's body was released

Prior to leaving a patient's home after a death, the nurse must dispose of controlled medications by removing medications from their containers, mixing them with cat litter or used coffee grounds, and placing them in a plastic bag or tub to prevent diversion (Nathan & Deamant, 2015). When disposing of fentanyl patches, each patch should be folded in half with the sticky side inward and flushed down a toilet. Labels on medication bottles should be removed and the bottles should be placed in the trash or recycle container, as appropriate. The nurse should document that medications were properly disposed of, following all agency policies and procedures (Wright, 2017).

■ CONCLUSION

Hospice and palliative care nurses must possess expertise in discussing goals of care with patients and their families. Goals may need to be revised as the patient's condition changes. When goals are developed, they should be measurable and achievable. The types of services available to the patient should also be discussed to help in care planning. Hospice and palliative care services are covered by Medicare and Medicaid and by most private insurances. Patients should be advised to contact the hospice or palliative care social worker or their insurance company with questions about their benefits.

Chapter Summary

- Types of advance directives include living wills, designation of a power of attorney, and development of a POLST (MOLST).
- Nurses should possess expertise in discussing end-of-life care with patients and families.
- Goals should be specific, measureable, achievable, relevant, and timely.
- The interdisciplinary team should meet regularly to determine if the patient's goals of care are met, partially met, or unmet.
- Hospice and palliative care services are typically covered by Medicare and Medicaid.
- Patients must have hospice eligibility certified on admission, after 90 days, and then every 60 days.
- Levels of care in hospice include routine home, continuous home, inpatient respite, and general inpatient.
- Reimbursement for hospice services is increased during the last 7 days of a patient's life.
- Core hospice services include physician services, nursing services, medical social work services, and counseling services.
- Noncore hospice services include physical, occupational, and speech therapy; volunteer services; homemaker services; hospice aide services; medications; and medical supplies.
- Patients are discharged from hospice through death, improvement in condition, or by revoking the hospice benefit.

■ PRACTICE QUESTIONS

1. Advance directives become effective when a patient
   a. Becomes terminally ill
   b. Designates a power of attorney
   c. Completes a physician (or provider) order for life-sustaining treatment (POLST)
   d. Cannot express his or her own wishes

2. A physician (or provider) order for life-sustaining treatment (POLST) is a type of advance directive that can be
   a. Used to designate a surrogate decision-maker
   b. Followed by emergency care providers

    c. Established at any time in the patient's life

    d. Certified by the patient's attorney

3. Goals of care should be

    a. Established by the patient only

    b. Developed within a year of death

    c. Reestablished monthly

    d. Measureable and achievable

4. The family members of a patient on life support tells the palliative care nurse that they are struggling with making medical decisions for their loved one who is not able to express his own wishes and does not have an advance directive. The nurse's best response is

    a. "Do you feel that it's time to discontinue care?"

    b. "Should I call the chaplain for you?"

    c. "Did you ever have a conversation with him about what he might want in this situation?"

    d. "Do you want us to do everything to make him better?"

5. A hospice patient asks the nurse if she can consider an experimental curative treatment. The nurse knows that

    a. Curative treatments are covered by the Medicare hospice benefit

    b. Once the patient chooses hospice care, she cannot receive curative treatments

    c. The patient may receive curative treatments, but must be discharged from hospice first

    d. The patient should be directed to a hospice counselor

6. A patient has been receiving hospice services for almost 6 months. To continue to receive services, the patient must

    a. Obtain certification from the hospice case manager

    b. Have terminality verified by two physicians

    c. Meet with the hospice care team

    d. Receive a face-to-face visit recertification evaluation

7. A nurse practitioner may perform a face-to-face visit with a patient to establish ongoing eligibility for hospice services when

    a. A physician is unavailable

    b. Employed by the hospice

    c. The patient requests a visit

    d. The first 90-day benefit period ends

8. To ensure coordination of care and interdisciplinarity, the hospice interdisciplinary team should meet no less than every

    a. 7 days

    b. 30 days

    c. 15 days

    d. 60 days

9. Which of the following is not a core hospice service?

    a. Physician services

    b. Volunteer services

    c. Counseling services

    d. Nursing services

10. A nurse disposes of a patient's medications upon the patient's death. The nurse mixes liquid morphine with cat litter and places it in the trash. The nurse then folds the fentanyl patches with the sticky sides together and flushes them down the toilet along with the long-acting morphine tablets. What has the nurse done incorrectly?

    a. Coffee grounds should have been used instead of cat litter

    b. The fentanyl patches should have been cut in half and placed in the trash

    c. All of the medications should have been mixed with cat litter

    d. The long-acting morphine tablets should not have been placed in the toilet

■ REFERENCES

American Hospice Foundation. (2018). *FAQ: How is hospice care paid for?* Retrieved from https://americanhospice.org/learning-about-hospice/how-is-hospice-care-paid-for/

American Nurses Association. (2016). *Nurses' roles and responsibilities in providing care and support at the end of life.* Retrieved from https://www.nursingworld.org/~4af078/globalassets/docs/ana/ethics/endoflife-positionstatement.pdf

Becker, R. (2009). Palliative care 1: Principles of a palliative care nursing and end-of-life care. *Nursing Times, 105*(13), 14–16. Retrieved from https://www.nursingtimes.net/

Berry, P., & Griffie, J. (2015). Preparing for the actual death. In B. R. Ferrell, N. Coyle, & J. A. Paice (Eds.), *Oxford textbook of palliative nursing* (pp. 513–530). New York, NY: Oxford University Press.

Center to Advance Palliative Care. (2018). *Palliative care is covered under both public and private insurance plans.* Retrieved from https://getpalliativecare.org/palliative-care-is-covered-under-both-public-and-private-insurance-plans/

Centers for Medicare & Medicaid Services. (2015a). *Local coverage determination (LCD).* Retrieved from https://www.cms.gov/medicare-coverage-database/details/lcd-details

Centers for Medicare & Medicaid Services. (2015b). *Hospice payment system.* Retrieved from https://www.cms.gov/Outreach-and-Education/Medicare-Learning-Network-MLN/MLNProducts/downloads/hospice_pay_sys_fs.pdf

Moore, C. D. (2007). Advance care planning and end of life decision making. In K. K. Kuebler, D. E. Heidrich, & P. Esper (Eds.), *Palliative and end-of-life care: Clinical practice guidelines* (2nd ed., pp. 49–62). St. Louis, MO: Saunders Elsevier.

Nathan, S., & Deamant, C. D. (2015). Medication disposal #286. *Journal of Palliative Medicine, 18*(1), 82–82. doi:10.1089/jpm.2015.0004

National Hospice and Palliative Care Organization. (n.d.). *Discharge from hospice services*. Retrieved from https://dart.nhpco.org/discharge-hospice-services

National Hospice and Palliative Care Organization. (2009). *Hospice admission care map*. Retrieved from http://www.nhpco.org/sites/default/files/public/regulatory/Hospice_admission_map -2009-F_(2).pdf

National POLST Paradigm. (2018). *Advance care planning: Advance directives vs. POLST forms*. Retrieved from https://polst.org/wp-content/uploads/2019/05/2019.04.30-POLST-vs-ADs-chart.pdf

Perrin, K. O. (2015). Legal aspects of end of life decision making. In M. Matzo & D. W. Sherman (Eds.), *Palliative care nursing* (4th ed., pp. 61–87). New York, NY: Springer Publishing Company.

Wright, P. M. (2017). *Fast facts for the hospice nurse*. New York, NY: Springer Publishing Company.

You, J. J., Fowler, R. A., & Heyland, D. K. (2014). Just ask: Discussing goals of care with patients in hospital with serious illness. *Canadian Medical Association Journal, 186*(6), 425–432. doi:10.1503/cmaj.121274

18

Psychosocial, Spiritual, and Cultural Needs

My hope is that my story will resonate with your story, or the story
of someone you love, or someone you are struggling to love.
—Finnegan-Hosey (2018)

◼ LEARNING OBJECTIVES

After completing this section, the nurse will be able to

1. Discuss psychosocial needs of seriously ill patients
2. Identify spiritual beliefs about the end of life
3. Define the influence of culture on end-of-life care

◼ PSYCHOSOCIAL, SPIRITUAL, AND CULTURAL NEEDS

The provision of holistic care for terminally ill patients and their families requires attention to the psychosocial, spiritual, and cultural aspects of the patient's experience. Patients often experience fear, depression, denial, anger, and hopelessness during their final weeks and days. Some patients may find comfort in spiritual beliefs, while others may turn away from their faith. Often rituals surrounding death are religiously and culturally bound. Thus, hospice and palliative care nurses must demonstrate expertise in navigating each patient's unique blend of cultural, spiritual, and psychosocial experiences.

Psychosocial Needs

Psychosocial support addresses the patient's psychological, spiritual, and cultural needs (Legg, 2011). Psychosocial needs underlie the patient's emotional and psychological well-being (Swash, Hulbert-Williams, & Bramwell, 2014). Hospice care is family-based care, and thus the nurse must be aware of the family structure and the influence of the family to develop a therapeutic relationship (Legg, 2011).

The serious illness of one member of the family affects all members of the family and alters normal family processes. The primary caregiver may have multiple domains of their lives affected as they take on the care of the patient and also attempt to balance other responsibilities (Wittenberg, Saada, & Prosser, 2013). The hospice and palliative care nurse must identify the family needs, connect the family with needed resources, and provide support as needed. Further, the nurse should work with the interdisciplinary care team to help manage manifestations of family disputes and/or dysfunction.

Spiritual Needs

Spiritual issues, such as loss of faith or feelings of meaninglessness, may arise at the end of life as patients face the unknown and question what might happen after they take their last breaths. The ability to recognize and address patients' spiritual concerns is central to end-of-life care because "patients learn to cope and understand their suffering through their spiritual beliefs, or the spiritual dimension of their lives" (Pulchalski & Roma, 2000, p. 129). The patient's spiritual needs should be identified by the hospice and palliative care nurse who is responsible for

- Assessing spiritual suffering
- Meeting the patient's immediate needs
- Working with other members of the health team to develop and implement a plan for ongoing support
  (Wright, 2017)

The hospice and palliative care chaplain or social worker is a key member of the interdisciplinary team whose expertise is invaluable in supporting patients through spiritual distress. In collaboration with the other members of the interdisciplinary team, the nurse can take the following steps to provide spiritual support:

> **Key Point**
>
> The FICA tool is commonly used to assess spiritual needs
>
> **F:** Faith or beliefs
>
> **I:** Importance and influence of one's faith in her or his life
>
> **C:** Community of faith (if any)
>
> **A:** Address the patient's spiritual concerns
> (Pulchalski & Roma, 2000)

- Uphold the patient's dignity throughout the course of his or her illness
- Provide a compassionate and caring environment
- Provide active listening, presence, respect, and support
- Be available to listen to the patient's concerns
- Encourage attendance at religious services or a visit from the patient's faith leader
- Facilitate the use of meditation, prayer, or other religious practices

- Encourage life review
- Help patients clarify their beliefs and values, as appropriate
- Provide spiritual music, literature, radio, or television programs for the patient
- Pray with the patient, as appropriate
  (Kisvetrová, Klugar, & Kabelka, 2013)

In providing support for patients from various religious backgrounds, the nurse should be aware of how death is viewed in different faith traditions. For example,

- Most branches of Abrahamic faith traditions, such as Christianity, Islam, and Judaism, teach that there is some form of an afterlife. Some believe that the soul continues on, some believe that there will be a resurrection of the body, and others believe that the afterlife is a new life in the presence of God (Sherman & Free, 2015). Followers of these faith traditions will often be comforted by readings from their religious texts, praying with faith leaders, or listening to music associated with their religious services (Cheraghi, Payne, & Salsali, 2005; Soskice, 2012).

- Eastern faith traditions, such as Hinduism and Buddhism, teach that when the current life ends a new life may begin through reincarnation. The circumstances of death may influence the next reincarnation, so the nurse must take steps to ensure that a calm and peaceful environment is maintained. Religious symbols, threads, or beads may be placed on or near the patient and should not be removed without the family's permission.

Cultural Needs

Hospice and palliative nurses must develop cultural awareness, which is the ability to identify and appreciate cultural differences between themselves and their patients. In healthcare settings, cultural preferences influence medical decisions, family decision-making, and the types of nonmedical interventions the patient might choose. Thus, the delivery of excellent healthcare is contingent on the nurse's ability to understand cultural influences on care and end-of-life preferences. For example, in the allopathic medical model, illness is viewed as a "disruption in physical or biochemical processes that can be manipulated by health care" (Sherman & Free, 2015, p. 93). In holistic or naturopathic health models,

> **Key Point**
>
> The Bible is the primary religious text for Christians.
>
> The Qur'an is the Holy Book of Islam and contains the teachings that God revealed to Muhammad.
>
> The sacred text of Judaism is called the Tanakh, which is composed of the Torah, Nevi'im, and Ketuvim.

illness is viewed as an imbalance in energy, or in yin and yang, the vital life forces. Moreover, some cultures associate illness with evil, sin, or curses (Sherman & Free, 2015).

In addition to the influence of culture on health decisions and beliefs regarding etiology of illness, culture influences each patient's

- Food preferences
- Family roles
- Privacy needs
- Rituals
- Time orientation
- Relationship with healthcare professionals
- Dietary practices
- Perceptions of personal space and appropriate touch (Agency for Healthcare Research and Quality, 2015 ; Ritter & Graham, 2017)

Nondominant cultural groups are at risk for poor access to healthcare services, provider bias, gender inequity, and language barriers. In addition to cultural groups, nurses must be aware that healthcare disparities also affect several other disenfranchised groups such as older adults, patients who have disabilities, veterans, those who have low English proficiency, and those of lower socioeconomic status. Specifically, vulnerable populations may have poor access to transportation, steady healthcare providers, insurance coverage, or needed medications (Ritter & Graham, 2017; Wright & Hanson, 2016).

■ CONCLUSION

Hospice and palliative care are comprehensive, family-centered approaches to the care of seriously ill or terminally ill patients. The provision of holistic care necessitates an understanding of the patient's family structure and the influence of family. Each patient's spiritual or religious beliefs as well as cultural background play an important role in the patient's comfort throughout the disease process.

Chapter Summary

- End-of-life care is family centered. Family processes may be altered or may break down as a result of the patient's illness.
- Spiritual and religious beliefs influence patients' views of death and their beliefs in an afterlife.
- Spiritual needs should be promptly identified and addressed.
- The FICA tool can be used to assess spiritual beliefs and needs.
- Cultural norms influence the patient's approach to illness and health as well as healthcare decisions.

■ PRACTICE QUESTIONS

1. A hospice nurse visits the home of a patient and overhears the primary caregiver telling another family member that she "just can't take it anymore" and that no one else is helping with the care of the patient. The nurse should

   a. Gently approach the caregiver and open a discussion regarding respite care

   b. Offer to provide 24-hour aide services in the home

   c. Determine if other family members are available to help with the patient's care

   d. Discuss home physical therapy services to improve the patient's function

2. The family of a hospice patient in an inpatient unit asks if a hospice volunteer can read to the patient from the Qur'an because the patient finds great comfort in this. The nurse knows that the Qur'an is the religious text of

   a. Judaism

   b. Hinduism

   c. Islam

   d. Zoroastrianism

3. A palliative care patient tells the nurse that he feels hopeless and does not understand why God has abandoned him. The nurse's best response is

   a. "God hasn't abandoned you, have faith."

   b. "Would you like me to pray with you?"

   c. "You feel that God has abandoned you?"

   d. "I will call the chaplain for you."

4. The nurse's primary role in meeting the spiritual needs of seriously ill patients is

   a. Praying with them

   b. Identifying patient's needs and providing support

   c. Performing in-depth spiritual evaluations

   d. Assisting with rituals that bring spiritual comfort

5. A hospice nurse conducts a home visit to discuss hospice admission with a patient. The patient tells the nurse that she cannot make a decision about her care without her husband present. The nurse should

   a. Tell the patient that she is capable of making her own decisions

   b. Ask the social worker to speak with the patient

   c. Ask if another family member is available now

   d. Arrange another visit when the patient's husband can be present

REFERENCES

Agency for Healthcare Research & Quality. (2015). *Health literacy universal precautions toolkit* (2nd ed.). Retrieved from https://psnet.ahrq.gov/resources/resource/18204/health-literacy-universal-precautions-toolkit-second-edition

Cheraghi, M. A., Payne, S., & Salsali, M. (2005). Spiritual aspects of end-of-life care for Muslim patients: Experiences from Iran. *International Journal of Palliative Nursing, 11,* 468–474. Retrieved from http://www.magonlinelibrary.com/toc/ijpn/current

Finnegan-Hosey, D. (2018). *Christ on the psych ward.* New York, NY: Church Publishing.

Kisvetrová, H., Klugar, M., & Kabelka, L. (2013). Spiritual support interventions in nursing care for patients suffering death anxiety in the final phase of life. *International Journal of Palliative Nursing, 19*(12), 599–605. doi:10.12968/ijpn.2013.19.12.599

Legg, M. J. (2011). What is psychosocial care and how can nurses better provide it to adult oncology patients. *The Australian Journal of Advanced Nursing, 28*(3), 62–67. Retrieved from http://www.ajan.com.au/Vol28/28-3.pdf#page=62

Pulchalski, C., & Romer, A. (2000). Taking a spiritual history allows clinicians to understand patients more fully. *Journal of Palliative Medicine, 3*(1), 129–137. doi:10.1089/jpm.2000.3.129

Ritter, L. A., & Graham, D. H. (2017). *Multicultural health* (2nd ed.). Burlington, MA: Jones & Bartlett.

Sherman, D. W., & Free, D. (2015). Culture and spirituality as domains of quality palliative care. In M. Matzo & D. W. Sherman (Eds.), *Palliative care nursing: Quality care to the end of life* (4th ed., pp. 91–127). New York, NY: Springer Publishing Company.

Soskice, J. (2012). "Dying well in Christianity." Religious understandings of a good death: Hinduism. In H. Coward, K. I. Stajduhar, & D. Maguire (Eds.), *Religious understandings of a good death in hospice and palliative care* (pp. 29–50). Albany: State University of New York Press.

Swash, B., Hulbert-Williams, N., & Bramwell, R. (2014). Unmet psychosocial needs in haematological cancer: A systematic review. *Supportive Care in Cancer, 22*(4), 1131–1141. Retrieved from https://chesterrep.openrepository.com/bitstream/handle/10034/344398/swash%2c%20hulbert-williams%2cbramwell2014.pdf?sequence=7&isAllowed=y

Wittenberg, E., Saada, A., & Prosser, L. A. (2013). How illness affects family members: A qualitative interview survey. *The Patient-Patient-Centered Outcomes Research, 6*(4), 257–268. doi:10.1007/s40271-013-0030-3

Wright, P. M. (2017). *Fast facts for the hospice nurse.* New York, NY: Springer Publishing Company.

Wright, P. M., & Hanson, M. J. (2016). Interprofessional graduate students' perspectives on caring for vulnerable populations. *Nursing Education Perspectives, 37*(5), 281–282. doi:10.1097/01.NEP.0000000000000036

19

Grief and Loss

The expectation that we can be immersed in suffering and loss daily and not be touched by it is as unrealistic as expecting to be able to walk through water without getting wet.
—Remen (2006, p. 51)

LEARNING OBJECTIVES

After completing this section, the nurse will be able to

1. Identify typical and atypical grief reactions
2. Assess grief responses in families
3. Provide age-appropriate grief and bereavement support

GRIEF AND LOSS

Hospice and palliative care nurses work at the nexus of life and death on a daily basis. A thorough understanding of the features of grief and grief theories fosters therapeutic communication and the implementation of effective grief support (Wright & Hogan, 2008). This chapter discusses the grief and bereavement experienced by patients and their families, along with appropriate support interventions.

Grief Related to Dying

Patients who are facing their own death must struggle with how to let go of all they hold dear in their lives. Throughout their illness, they may have sustained multiple losses, possibly including the loss of mobility, speech, comfort, and continence. As patients near death, they may experience myriad emotions that can change over time and as symptoms ebb and flow.

Kübler-Ross's (1969) work on reactions to one's own impending death indicates that dying patients experience denial that death may actually be near as well anger about their own circumstances. Patients may engage in bargaining with their higher power or with themselves through "if-then" statements such as "if I recover from this illness, then I will never smoke again." Depression may set in as patients take in the inevitability of their death and may feel hopeless at times. Ultimately, the patient accepts that death is near and may take time to resolve past grievances or mend damaged relationships, if possible.

Family Grief

Family members, close friends, and caregivers can also be deeply affected by the illness and death of the patient. The grief they experience is influenced by their relationship with the patient, their age, their involvement in patient care and medical decision-making, previous experiences with death, culture, spiritual beliefs, and their individual coping mechanisms.

Grief is the manifestation of physical and emotional responses to an impending or actual loss. Grief involves deep sorrow and emotions such as sadness, guilt, anger, despair, and shame (Potter & Wynne, 2015). Typically, the intensity of grief symptoms slowly lessens over time. As the intensity of grief decreases, the person is more and more able to reengage in usual activities.

Complicated grief is a form of grief that involves dysfunctional or maladaptive responses that are prolonged and debilitating and interfere with the person's ability to engage in usual activities on an ongoing basis (Prigerson et al., 1995; Stroebe, Schut, & van den Bout, 2013). The following symptoms are associated with complicated grief:

- Longing
- Yearning
- Hallucinations
- Preoccupation with thoughts of the deceased
- Intrusive thoughts about the deceased
- Avoidance of people and places that can trigger grief
- Altered sleep patterns
- Failure to adapt to the loss over time
  (Horowitz et al., 2003; Prigerson et al., 1996; Shear, 2015; Worden, 1991).

Complicated grief responses are more common among those who have a history of mental illness or those who have experienced disenfranchised grief. Disenfranchised grief results when a significant loss is not openly or publicly recognized, such as in the case of suicide, pregnancy loss, or loss at war (Doka, 2008). The social recognition of loss and grief are critical to garnering support and sharing grief with others.

Families who share the same loss may grieve together, but the reactions of individual family members may vary according to their relationship with the decreased, family dynamics, and age. For example, children may not fully understand the permanence of death. Hospice and palliative care nurses must be prepared to teach family members how children understand death at various ages and how to best support children according to their developmental level (see Table 19.1).

Peri-Death and Bereavement Support

Around the time of the patient's death, family members may draw near to spend last days or hours with the patient. Often, this time is referred to as the "death vigil." Hospice and palliative care nurses can provide support for families by teaching them about the process of dying

Table 19.1 Children's Grief Responses and Appropriate Interventions		
Age Group	Common Reactions to Loss	Grief Interventions
Babies and toddlers (up to 18 months)	Searching for deceased Irritability and/or hyperactivity and wakefulnes Increased crying Need to be held and comforted Decreased appetite	Maintain routines Pick up and comfort when crying Speak softly and calmly Provide comfort items such as favorite blanket or toy
Preschool-aged children (18 months to 4 years)	Searching for deceased Dreaming of the deceased Feeling fearful and anxious Wanting to be close with loved ones or social withdrawal Changes in appetite Disturbed sleeping patterns Regression	Maintain routine Spend as much time as possible together Speak calmly and softly Encourage the children to express themselves through play Explain death as a change Offer snacks and small meals Explain that the deceased will not come back (children of this age do not understand finality so they may ask over and over when the decreased will return)

(continued)

Table 19.1 Children's Grief Responses and Appropriate Interventions *(continued)*

Age Group	Common Reactions to Loss	Grief Interventions
Primary school children (age 5–9 years)	Searching for deceased Dreaming of the deceased "Magical thinking"— believing that they may have caused the death Fearfulness, irritability, defiance Wanting to be near loved ones more frequently or withdrawing Regression	Maintain routine Offer reassurance of safety of the child and others Explain death as a change—avoid terms like "passed on" or "gone to sleep" Allow the child to participate in the funeral or other services, if desired Encourage expression of feelings through art or play
Tweens (age 10–12 years)	Anxiety about safety of self and friends Wanting to please parents Strong emotional responses but may hide them May ask questions about the loss and may want to talk about it with friends or others Understand that death is permanent—ability to think abstractly	Encourage child to express feelings verbally or through art or writing Offer assurance of safety Answer questions openly and honestly Do not expect the child to respond to the loss like an adult
Teenagers (age 13+)	May be overwhelmed by emotions—may engage in risky behaviors May exhibit attention deficit, anxiety, and distraction Feelings of isolation Withdrawal from family but draw nearer to friends	Be honest and available Maintain routine Encourage involvement in services Locate teen support groups, if available

Sources: KidsHealth. (2018). Bereavement reactions by age group. Retrieved from https://www .kidshealth.org.nz/bereavement-reactions-age-group; McNiel, A., & Schuurman, D. L. (2016). Supporting grieving children. In B. P. Black, P. M. Wright, & R. Limbo (Eds.), *Perinatal and pediatric bereavement in nursing and other health professions* (pp. 327–344). New York, NY: Springer Publishing Company.

(see Chapter 3, Disease Progression and Imminent Death). The nurse should also encourage the family and caregivers to say their goodbyes and to seek closure, as appropriate.

After the patient's death, the hospice or palliative care nurse should help the family break the news to loved ones, as necessary, and remain with the family to offer support. Initial assessment of the family's bereavement reactions should be documented and reassessed as needed. The hospice bereavement coordinator or social worker should develop a bereavement plan of care with the input from the interdisciplinary care team. Bereavement care may include visits, cards, invitations to memorial services, and/or support group attendance. Bereavement care should continue to at least 12 months after the patient's death, as required by Medicare.

Key Point
Bereavement is the condition of being separated from someone, usually through death. It is often seen as a period of mourning.

CONCLUSION

Patients nearing the end of life may experience profound grief and myriad emotions such as anger, deep sorrow, and denial. Family members and other loved ones of the patient may also experience sadness and grief during the patient's illness and after the patient's death. Patients and family members need excellent support throughout their grief. Grieving children require age-appropriate support from the entire interdisciplinary team. The hospice nurse must be aware of usual grief experiences as well as complicated grief reactions.

Chapter Summary
• Hospice and palliative care nurses must be adept at identifying grief and providing support along with the interdisciplinary team.
• Patients facing death often experience denial, anger, bargaining, depression, and acceptance.
• Family grief is influenced by the relationship between the patient and each of the family members.
• Grief in children is manifested according to age and developmental level (see Table 19.1).
• After the patient's death, bereavement care should be offered for at least 12 months.

PRACTICE QUESTIONS

1. A 4-year-old child asks when her recently deceased grandmother will return. Her mother explains that she cannot come back. The child nods but asks the same question later. This is an example of

   a. Congruence with developmental level

   b. Denial regarding the permanence of the death

   c. Regression to earlier stage of development

   d. A sign of advanced developmental level

2. A 59-year-old hospice patient with end-stage liver disease is nearing death and tells the nurse that if God will let him live, he will never drink alcohol again. This is an example of

   a. Anger

   b. Denial

   c. Bargaining

   d. Acceptance

3. During a bereavement follow-up call, a widow tells the nurse that she has not been able to stop thinking about her husband since he died 8 months ago and is not able to leave the house due to her sadness. The nurse knows that

   a. This is a typical grief reaction

   b. Recovery from grief can take 12 months

   c. The woman is experiencing complicated grief

   d. This is a sign of spiritual distress

4. Following the death of a patient, bereavement support for the family should continue for

   a. 6 months

   b. 18 months

   c. 12 months

   d. 3 months

5. After the death of a loved one, teenagers are at risk for

   a. Regression

   b. Risky behaviors

   c. Social isolation

   d. Magical thinking

▪ REFERENCES

Doka, K. J. (2008). Disenfranchised grief in historical and cultural perspective. In M. S. Stroebe, R. O. Hansson, H. Schut, & W. Stroebe (Eds.), *Handbook of bereavement research and practice: Advances in theory and intervention* (pp. 223–240). Washington, DC: American Psychological Association.

Horowitz, M. J., Siegel, B., Holen, A., Bonanno, G. A., Milbrath, C., & Stinson, C. H. (2003). Diagnostic criteria for complicated grief disorders. *PsychiatryOnline, 1*, 290–298. doi:10.1176/foc.1.3.290

KidsHealth. (2018). *Bereavement reactions by age group*. Retrieved from https://www.kidshealth.org.nz/bereavement-reactions-age-group

Kübler-Ross, E. (1969). *On death and dying*. New York, NY: Scribner.

McNiel, A., & Schuurman, D. L. (2016). Supporting grieving children. In B. P. Black, P. M. Wright, & R. Limbo (Eds.), *Perinatal and pediatric bereavement in nursing and other health professions* (pp. 327–344). New York, NY: Springer Publishing Company.

Potter, M. L., & Wynne, B. P. (2015). Loss, suffering, bereavement, and grief. In M. Matzo & D. W. Sherman (Eds.), *Palliative care nursing: Quality to the end of life* (4th ed., pp. 205–234). New York, NY: Springer Publishing Company.

Prigerson, H. G., Bierhals, A. J., Kasl, S. V., Reynolds, C. F., 3rd., Shear, M. K., Newsom, J. T., . . . Jacobs, S. (1996). Complicated grief as a disorder distinct from bereavement-related depression and anxiety: A replication study. *American Journal of Psychiatry, 153,* 1484–1486. doi:10.1176/ajp.153.11.1484

Prigerson, H. G., Frank, E., Kasl, S. V., Reynolds, C. F., 3rd., Anderson, B., Zubenko, G. S., . . . Kupfer, D. J. (1995). Complicated grief and bereavement-related depression as distinct disorders: Preliminary empirical validation in elderly bereaved spouses. *American Journal of Psychiatry, 152,* 22–30. doi:10.1176/ajp.152.1.22

Remen, R. N. (2006). *Kitchen table wisdom.* New York, NY: Riverhead Books.

Shear, M. K. (2015). Complicated grief. *New England Journal of Medicine, 372,* 153–160. doi:10.1056/NEJMcp1315618

Stroebe, M., Schut, H., & van den Bout, J. (2013). Introduction. In In M. Stroebe, H. Schut, & J. van den Bout (Eds.), *Complicated grief: Scientific foundations for health care professionals* (pp. 1–10). New York, NY: Routledge.

Worden, J. W. (1991). *Grief counselling and grief therapy: A handbook for the mental health practitioner* (2nd ed.). New York, NY: Routledge.

Wright, P. M., & Hogan, N. S. (2008). Grief theories and models: Applications to hospice nursing practice. *Journal of Hospice & Palliative Care, 10*(6), 350–356. doi:10.1097/01.NJH. 0000319194.16778.e5

20

Caregiver Education, Support, and Advocacy

Nurses possess necessary technical knowledge and are viewed as being in the best position to advocate for the interests and well-being of patients and their families.
—Choi (2015, p. 53)

LEARNING OBJECTIVES

After completing this section, the nurse will be able to

1. Identify caregiver stress
2. Assess family support needs
3. Advocate for the patient through education and collaboration

CAREGIVER SUPPORT

A family caregiver is a relative, partner, friend, or other significant person in the life of the patient. The caregiver takes responsibility for meeting the daily needs of the patient. Taking on the role of a family caregiver can impact the health and well-being of the caregiver in terms of time, physical and mental strain, and the need to balance other responsibilities (Sherman & Cheon, 2015).

When a family caregiver is unable to fulfill his or her usual roles, the entire family system is strained, which can lead to disharmony. The nurse must assess the strength and resilience of the family unit in terms of

- Affection and appreciation shown for each other
- Spiritual well-being
- Commitment to each other
- Spending time with each other and sharing positive experiences

- Demonstrating the ability to cope with stressors and deal with crises (Sherman & Cheon, 2015)

Although everyone in the family is affected by the illness of a single member, the primary caregiver bears the heaviest burden. The caregiver must possess the necessary technical skills to provide care and be able to withstand the financial and social effects of caring for a loved one (Sherman & Cheon, 2015). The hospice and palliative nurse should frequently assess the well-being of the caregiver for signs of role strain such as

- Feeling tired and overwhelmed
- Insomnia or increased somnolence
- Unplanned weight changes
- Irritability
- Loss of interest in previously enjoyable activities
- Somatic complaints
- Overuse or reliance on drugs (prescription or nonprescription) or alcohol
  (Mayo Clinic, 2018)

Interventions to help alleviate caregiver burden include the following:

- Offering respite care
- Encouraging the caregiver to accept help from others
- Setting realistic goals
- Connecting with others through classes, support groups, or community services
- Maintaining healthy living patterns
  (Mayo Clinic, 2018; Sherman & Cheon, 2015)

Education

In order to provide proper care for the patient, the family must be well informed regarding the illness, disease progression, medication use, and use of equipment. The nurse must identify barriers to family education such as low English proficiency, low literacy, caregiver confidence, family dynamics, and cultural beliefs regarding care during illness. Verbal instructions should be supplemented with written instructions. The nurse can use the teach-back method to ensure the caregiver's ability to complete skills. The nurse must also consider the learning style of the caregiver. Some common learning styles include the following:

- *Narrative learners:* Retain knowledge better through spoken or written language
- *Numerical learners:* Access information best through numbers or patterns

- *Foundational learners:* Access material best through myths or the arts
- *Aesthetic learners:* Retain information better when it is presented in a balanced and harmonious way
- *Hands-on learners:* Comprehend material best when they can manipulate materials or carry out experiments
- *Social learners:* Learn best in groups where they can assume different roles and take in other points of view
  (Gardner, 2009)

Patient Advocacy

When patients are cared for at home, caregiver stress, lack of support, resentment, or other issues can sometimes lead to aggressive behavior toward the patient. Thus, the nurse and other members of the interdisciplinary team must monitor for signs of abuse such as

- Bruising in unusual places
- Burns
- Preventable decubiti
- Dehydration
- Evidence of sexual abuse
- Malnutrition
- Withheld medications
- Unexplained fractures
- Urine burns
- Inattention to hygiene
  (Hoover & Polson, 2014)

Dependency and the declining condition of the patient may prevent the patient from voicing his or her own wishes at the end of life. Thus, to effectively advocate for the patient, the nurse must rely on written documents, conversations with the patient, and the documentation in the medical record to ascertain the patient's stated wishes. Family disagreements can occur regarding the plan of care, especially when the patient's condition is deteriorating. The nurse must collaborate with the interdisciplinary team to plan family discussions and to mediate conflict. Family meetings are structured by

- Setting an agenda
- Inviting family members to share their feelings about the current circumstances
- Discussing the patient's daily care needs
- Determining who is the primary decision-maker

- Discussing how other members of the family can offer input and feel heard
- Problem-solving regarding how to honor the patient's wishes, ensure comfort, and promote dignity
  (Family Caregiver Alliance, 2018)

▪ CONCLUSION

As a patient's condition deteriorates, the need for advocacy and family education increase. The hospice and palliative care nurse is in an excellent position to determine the needs of the patient, caregiver, and family and to implement interventions, along with the other members of the interdisciplinary team, to safeguard the patient's dignity and safety, and to ensure that end-of-life wishes are honored.

Chapter Summary

- When a family caregiver provides care in a patient's home, the nurse must assess the needs of the caregiver and monitor for caregiver stress.
- If caregiver stress is noted, the nurse must take steps to alleviate the caregiver's burden by offering respite care and connecting the caregiver with needed resources.
- Patient and family education is needed when a patient is being cared for at home. The nurse must assess the family members' learning styles and tailor educational resources to their needs.
- As the patient's condition changes, the nurse must determine the patient's safety in the home and advocate for the implementation of the patient's end-of-life wishes.

▪ PRACTICE QUESTIONS

1. A family caregiver informs the hospice nurse that he quit his job to care for his wife at home and now is unable to pay their bills. The nurse should
   a. Discharge the patient from hospice because the family cannot afford care
   b. Offer to connect the family with different insurance options
   c. Contact community agencies to identify helpful programs
   d. Collaborate with the interdisciplinary team to identify appropriate resources

2. A home hospice patient is actively dying and his son asks if emergency services should be called. The best response is
   a. "What would you want them to do for your father?"
   b. "They will only provide life-sustaining care."

c. "Keeping him home and comfortable is consistent with his wishes."

d. "Have you changed your mind about hospice care?"

3. A nurse must teach a family caregiver how to administer medications subcutaneously for a patient at home. The best approach is to

a. Demonstrate the skill and then ask the caregiver to demonstrate it

b. Leave literature in the home for the caregiver about the procedure

c. Tell the caregiver to call the on-call nurse when the patient needs medication

d. Develop a mnemonic to help the caregiver remember the steps of the process

4. A dependent patient is admitted to the palliative care unit from home. The palliative care nurse notes bruising on the patient's back and forearms and a perineal rash. The nurse should first

a. Carefully document the findings

b. Ask the patient how the bruising happened

c. Remove the patient's caregiver from the room

d. Inform the members of the interdisciplinary team

5. A hospice patient informed the nurse that he does "not feel emotionally strong enough to deal with bad news anymore" and asks that all communication about his condition take place with his family. The nurse should

a. Tell the patient that he is in charge of his own decisions

b. Ask the patient if his family members are aware of his wishes

c. Determine if the patient has assigned a power of attorney

d. Arrange a family meeting with the hospice team

■ REFERENCES

Choi, P. P. (2015). Patient advocacy: The role of the nurse. *Nursing Standard, 29*(41), 52. doi:10.7748/ns.29.41.52.e9772

Family Caregiver Alliance. (2018). *Holding a family meeting.* Retrieved from https://www.caregiver.org/holding-family-meeting

Gardner, H. (2009). Multiple approaches to learning. In K. Illerus (Ed.), *Contemporary theories of learning: Learning theorists in their own words.* New York, NY: Routledge.

Hoover, R. M., & Polson, M. (2014). Detecting elder abuse and neglect: Assessment and intervention. *American Family Physician, 89*(6), 453–460. Retrieved from www.aafp.org

Mayo Clinic. (2018). *Caregiver stress: Tips for taking care of yourself.* Retrieved from https://www.mayoclinic.org/healthy-lifestyle/stress-management/in-depth/caregiver-stress/art-20044784

Sherman, D. W., & Cheon, J. (2015). Family caregivers. In M. Matzo & D. W. Sherman (Eds.), *Palliative care nursing: Quality care to the end of life* (pp. 147–167). New York, NY: Springer Publishing Company.

VI

Practice Issues

21 Care Coordination and Collaboration

Coming together is a beginning. Keeping together is progress.
Working together is success.
—Henry Ford

LEARNING OBJECTIVES

After completing this section, the nurse will be able to

1. Discuss coordination of care in hospice and palliative care
2. Determine the roles of each member of the hospice and palliative care team
3. Appropriately delegate tasks to other members of the team

CARE COORDINATION AND COLLABORATION

Interdisciplinary teams have shared goals and work collaboratively to plan the best care for the patient. The Centers for Medicare & Medicaid Services (2015) outline the services covered by members of the hospice team, including:

- *Nursing care:* These services "require the skills of a registered nurse (RN), or a licensed practical nurse (LPN) or a licensed vocational nurse (LVN), under the supervision of a Registered Nurse, and must be reasonable and necessary for the palliation and management of the patient's terminal illness and related conditions" (p. 19).

- *Medical social services:* Include assessments of social, emotional, and financial factors that have bearing on the patient's terminal condition. The hospice social worker assesses the patient's medical and nursing needs, home situation, financial resources, and community resources, and also provides counseling services as needed. The hospice social worker aims to remove impediments to the provision of effective end-of-life care.

- *Physician services:* The hospice medical director must be prepared as either a Doctor of Osteopathic Medicine (DO) or a Medical Doctor (MD) in order to verify the patient's terminality and oversee medical care. The hospice medical director may complete the required face-to-face visits to verify continued eligibility for hospice, and may also serve as the attending physician for hospice patients. The attending physician has "the most significant role in the determination and delivery of the individual's medical care" (p. 21). A nurse practitioner may serve as the attending physician if employed by the hospice and provided that the patient has the option to receive care from a physician. (*Note:* Nurse practitioners cannot certify or recertify terminality or prognosis, but may complete the required face-to-face visits to verify continued eligibility for hospice services.)

- *Hospice aide and homemaker services:* Hospice aides provide personal care services as well as household services as needed to maintain a safe and clean environment for the patient. The hospice aide is assigned and supervised by the RN.

- *Physical therapy, occupational therapy, and speech therapy:* These services are provided for the purpose of symptom control or to enable the individual to maintain activities of daily living and basic functional skills.

Together, the hospice interdisciplinary team addresses the biomedical, psychosocial, and spiritual care of the patient (Moore, Bastian, & Apenteng, 2015). The team gathers assessment information such as

- Terminality and prognosis
- The patient's ability to perform activities of daily living
- Availability of a caregiver
- Safety hazards in the home such as throw rugs, fire hazards, accessibility, cords, and tubing in paths where the patient walks
- Use of community resources (adult day care, meal delivery services, grocery delivery)
- Financial ability to pay for caregivers in the home
- Qualification for financial assistance or access to programs

With the appropriate information gathered, the hospice team can determine the appropriate level of care for the patient (see Chapter 17, Establishing Goals of Care and Managing Resources). The levels of care are as follows:

- Routine
- Continuous
- Inpatient respite
- General inpatient

The level of care is determined through collaboration of the hospice team and the patient and family. In addition to the provision of care in the home or a hospice inpatient unit, routine hospice care can be provided in a long-term care facility (LTCF). If hospice care is provided to a patient who resides in a LTCF, care will be provided according to a written agreement that specifies

- What services the hospice will provide
- The hospice team's role in developing the patient's plan of care
- How information will be communicated between the hospice team and the staff of the LTCF
- How the staff at the LTCF will immediately notify the hospice team regarding
  - Significant changes in the patient's condition
  - Any changes that may warrant modification of the plan of care
  - The need to transfer the patient from the LTCF
  - The patient's death
- That the hospice assumes responsibility for determining an appropriate end-of-life plan of care, including the level of care
- The LTCF's responsibility in providing room and board and meeting the patient's personal care and nursing needs and for coordinating care with the hospice team
- The hospice team's responsibility for providing
  - Medical direction and medical management for the patient
  - Nursing care
  - Counseling services
  - Social work
  - Supplies, medical equipment, and medicines related to the terminal illness
  - All other hospice services that are warranted by the patient's life-limiting condition and related issues
- That the staff of the LTCF may assist in the provision of necessary treatments and therapies as allowed by state law and facility policies
- That the staff of the LTCF will immediately report any alleged violations, including mistreatment, neglect, abuse, or misappropriation of the patient's belongings by hospice staff to the hospice administrator
- Designate the responsibilities of the hospice and the LTCF staff to provide bereavement services
(National Hospice & Palliative Care Organization, 2013)

Coordination of Care

Because hospice care is holistic and family centered, it is critical that the patient and/or family be invited to participate in interdisciplinary team meetings. During team meetings, the nurse offers input regarding nursing assessments, changes in the patient's condition, responses to medication or treatment changes, and the types of supportive care needed. The nurse should also take part in

- Encouraging patient and caregiver participation in team meetings
- Reducing any role conflicts or interprofessional tensions that may arise
- Ensuring that everyone's contributions are taken seriously and that everyone is included in the decision-making process
- Being open to sharing negative patient experiences while ensuring that this sharing results in unburdening for team members and allows for mutual support
  (Moore et al., 2015)

All members of the hospice team share in the responsibility for ensuring that the appropriate care is provided. Communication with the patient's specialists, caretakers, patient educators, therapists, or others involved in the patient's care is paramount to delivering excellent hospice care without overlapping services with other providers. Communication must be especially clear and transparent during times of transition.

Communicating During Patient Transitions

During patient transitions, such as transfer to an inpatient setting from home, or at the time of a patient's death, the use of a standard communication tool, such as the SBAR (Pope, Rodzen, & Spross, 2008), has been recommended to facilitate smooth transitions (The Joint Commission, 2012). SBAR is used in healthcare settings to convey the

- *Situation:* Identify yourself, identify the patient, and succinctly explain what the issue is. In hospice settings this may also entail information about the patient's home situation and family dynamics.
- *Background:* Provide information that helps to situate the current problem, such as pertinent medical history, lab results, and any recent changes in condition.
- *Assessment:* Describe what you think the problem is and the severity of the problem.
- *Recommendation:* Provide a recommendation for what should happen next. This recommendation may be the need to prescribe a different prescription drug or change the dosage of currently used

medications. Other recommendations may include a change in the level of care, such as a transfer from home to the inpatient unit for symptom management.

As the nurse works with the hospice team and others who take part in the care of the hospice patient, effective communication skills are essential. The nurse must also possess the skills and knowledge to determine ongoing patient care needs, to develop appropriate interventions, and to delegate tasks to other team members as necessary.

Delegation

A RN may delegate certain tasks to licensed practical nurses/licensed vocational nurses (LPNs/LVNs) and to unlicensed assistive personnel (UAP). "Delegation is the act of empowering another person to act. Delegation occurs in a downward manner" (Williams, Block, & Shannon, 2015, p. 24). The nurse who chooses to delegate tasks must be aware of the state laws and regulations related to delegation, because the delegator remains responsible for the outcomes of the delegate's tasks (National Council of State Boards of Nursing, 2018). Prior to delegating a task, the RN should determine whether the

- Task can be delegated according to the state practice act
- Delegate has the appropriate knowledge and training to perform the task
- Patient would benefit from delegation of the task
  (Williams et al., 2015)

The RN can use the delegation decision tree offered jointly by the American Nurses Association and the National Council of State Boards of Nursing (2005; see https://www.ncsbn.org/Delegation_joint_statement_NCSBN-ANA.pdf) as the first step in the delegation process. Delegation involves excellent communication between the delegator and the delegate. Proper communication between the delegator and the delegate is crucial. The process of communication is explicated in steps 2 through 4 of the delegation process below. Before the delegate carries out delegated tasks, the RN should check the five rights of delegation

1. The right task
2. Under the right circumstances
3. To the right person
4. With the right directions and communication
5. Under the right supervision and evaluation
   (American Nurses Association/National Council of State Boards of Nursing, 2005)

Step One—Use delegation decision tree
(See: https://www.ncsbn.org/Delegation_joint_statement_NCSBN-ANA.pdf)

Step Two—Communication
Communication must be a two-way process.

The nurse	The nursing assistive personnel	Documentation:
• Assesses the assistant's understanding ▪ How the task is to be accomplished ▪ When and what information is to be reported, including – Expected observations to report and record – Specific client concerns that would require prompt reporting • Individualizes for the nursing assistive personnel and client situation • Addresses any unique client requirements and characteristics, and clear expectations of • Assesses the assistant's understanding of expectations, providing clarification if needed • Communicates his or her willingness and availability to guide and support assistant • Assures appropriate accountability by verifying that the receiving person accepts the delegation and accompanying responsibility	• Ask questions regarding the delegation and seek clarification of expectations if needed • Inform the nurse if the assistant has not done a task/function/activity before, or has only done it infrequently • Ask for additional training or supervision • Affirm understanding of expectations • Determine the communication method between the nurse and the assistive personnel • Determine the communication and plan of action in emergency situations	Timely, complete, and accurate documentation of provided care • Facilitates communication with other members of the healthcare team • Records the nursing care provided

Step Three—Surveillance and Supervision

The purpose of surveillance and monitoring is related to the nurse's responsibility for client care within the context of a client population. The nurse supervises the delegation by monitoring the performance of the task or function and assures compliance with standards of practice, policies, and procedures. Frequency, level, and nature of monitoring vary with needs of client and experience of assistant.

The nurse considers the	The nurse determines	The nurse is responsible for
• Client's healthcare status and stability of condition	• The frequency of onsite supervision and assessment based on	• Timely intervening and follow-up on problems and concerns. Examples of the need for intervening include
• Predictability of responses and risks	▪ Needs of the client	
• Setting where care occurs	▪ Complexity of the delegated function/task/activity	• Alertness to subtle signs and symptoms (which allows nurse and assistant to be proactive before a client's condition deteriorates significantly)
• Availability of resources and support infrastructure	▪ Proximity of nurse's location	
• Complexity of the task being performed		• Awareness of assistant's difficulties in completing delegated activities
		• Providing adequate follow-up to problems and/or changing situations is a critical aspect of delegation

Step Four—Evaluation and Feedback

Evaluation is often the forgotten step in delegation.

In considering the effectiveness of delegation, the nurse addresses the following questions:
• Was the delegation successful?
  ▪ Was the task/function/activity performed correctly?
  ▪ Was the client's desired and/or expected outcome achieved?
  ▪ Was the outcome optimal, satisfactory, or unsatisfactory?
  ▪ Was communication timely and effective?
  ▪ What went well; what was challenging?
  ▪ Were there any problems or concerns; if so, how were they addressed?

(continued)

(continued)

- Is there a better way to meet the client need?

- Is there a need to adjust the overall plan of care, or should this approach be continued?

- Were there any "learning moments" for the assistant and/or the nurse?

- Was appropriate feedback provided to the assistant regarding the performance of the delegation?

- Was the assistant acknowledged for accomplishing the task/activity/function?

Source: American Nurses Association and National Council of State Boards of Nursing. (2005). *Joint statement on delegation.* Retrieved from https://www.ncsbn.org/Delegation_joint _statement_NCSBN-ANA.pdf. Used with permission.

CONCLUSION

Excellent communication is the key to excellent patient care. Members of the interdisciplinary team must work in unity to assure that the patient's needs are met and that the right level of hospice and/or palliative care is delivered. RNs may delegate tasks as needed to other members of the team, such as LVN/LPNs or UAPs, provided that the delegate is able to legally perform the task and is competent to do so. The RN retains accountability for delegated tasks.

Chapter Summary

- Interdisciplinary teams have shared goals and work together to deliver the best quality care for the patient.

- Services covered by the Medicare Hospice Benefit include nursing, social work, medical, hospice aide or homemaker services, and needed therapies such as physical therapy or occupational therapy.

- The levels of hospice care are routine, continuous, inpatient respite, and general inpatient care. The level of care is determined through collaboration with the interdisciplinary team and the patient and family needs.

- Hospice care may be delivered in LTCFs, but the terms agreed upon by the LTCF and the hospice must be documented in writing.

- Effective intrateam communication is paramount to excellent patient care, especially during times of transition. A commonly used tool to guide communication is the SBAR.

PRACTICE QUESTIONS

1. Which of the following services is not covered by the Hospice Medicare Benefit?

   a. Personal care

   b. Medication management

   c. Light housekeeping

   d. Pet therapy

2. In order to conduct the required face-to-face visits for patient recertification, a nurse practitioner must be

   a. An employee of the hospice

   b. Working on an as-needed basis

   c. Certified in hospice and palliative care

   d. In attendance at all interdisciplinary team meetings

3. An RN is considering delegating personal care tasks to a hospice aide. Before doing so, the nurse must determine whether

   a. The patient is willing to allow the aide to complete the tasks

   b. The aide is employed by the hospice on a full-time basis

   c. A licensed practical nurse/licensed vocational nurse (LPN/LVN) would be willing to complete the tasks

   d. The aide is competent in performing the needed tasks

4. A hospice patient tells the nurse that he cannot get to the team meetings but would like to participate in the discussions regarding his care. The nurse should

   a. Arrange transportation for the patient

   b. Ask the patient if he can participate by phone

   c. Ask the patient to send a family member

   d. Tell the patient he must attend in person to participate

5. A palliative care patient is diagnosed with end-stage cardiac disease. She is hospitalized and tells the palliative care nurse that she does not want any further curative treatments. The palliative care nurse should

   a. Arrange a hospice consult

   b. Explain that palliative care is strictly curative

   c. Discuss care options such as hospice and palliative care

   d. Encourage the patient to remain hopeful

■ REFERENCES

American Nurses Association and National Council of State Boards of Nursing. (2005). *Joint statement on delegation.* Retrieved from https://www.ncsbn.org/Delegation_joint_statement_NCSBN-ANA.pdf

Centers for Medicare and Medicaid Services. (2015). *Local coverage determination (LCD): Hospice—Determining terminal status (L33393).* Retrieved from https://www.cms.gov/medicare-coverage-database/details/lcd-details.aspx?LCDId=33393&ver=2&kc=59c12399-6&bc=AAAA AAQAAAAAAA%3d%3d&#0

The Joint Commission. (2012). *Transitions of care: The need for a more effective approach to continuing patient care.* Retrieved from http://www.jointcommission.org/assets/1/18/hot_topics_transitions_of_care.pdf

Moore, A. R., Bastian, R. G., & Apenteng, B. A. (2015). Communication within hospice interdisciplinary teams: A narrative review. *American Journal of Hospice & Palliative Medicine, 33*(10), 996–1012. doi:10.1177/1049909115613315

National Council of State Boards of Nursing. (2018). *Delegation*. Retrieved from https://www .ncsbn.org/1625.htm

National Hospice & Palliative Care Organization. (2013). *NHPCO regulatory alert: Long term care facility final rule on hospice care in nursing homes.* Retrieved from https://www.nhpco.org/ sites/default/files/public/regulatory/NH_Comp-Final-Rule_July-2013.pdf

Pope, B. B., Rodzen, L., & Spross, G. (2008). Raising the SBAR: How better communication improves patient outcomes. *Nursing, 38*(3), 41–43. doi:10.1097/01.NURSE.0000312625.74434.e8

Williams, L. S., Block, M., & Shannon, J. (2015). Issues in nursing practice. In L. S. Williams & P. D. Hopper (Eds.), *Understanding medical-surgical nursing* (5th ed., pp. 19–38). Philadelphia, PA: F.A. Davis.

22

Scope and Standards of Practice

Mediocrity will never do. You are capable of something better.
—Hinckley (2003)

LEARNING OBJECTIVES

After completing this section, the nurse will be able to

1. Discuss the scope and standards of hospice and palliative nursing practice
2. Define key ethical principles
3. Identify self-care methods

SCOPE AND STANDARDS OF PRACTICE

Nursing practice is governed by the board of nursing in each state or territory. Every nurse is responsible for adhering to the rules and regulations set forth by the board of nursing. Hospice and palliative nursing is a speciality practice that entails "evaluation, treatment, and management within the eight domains of palliative care outlined in the National Consensus Project" (American Nurses Association, 2014, p. 4).

In 2001, the National Consensus Project (NCP) was undertaken by a group of palliative care experts from multiple disciplines who were dedicated to defining the domains of hospice and palliative care, as well as establishing guidelines for this specialty area. In 2018, this group released the 4th edition of the landmark document *Clinical Practice Guidelines for Quality Palliative Care*. The eight domains of palliative care identified in the Clinical Practice Guidelines (NCP, 2018) are as follows:

1. *Structure and processes of care:* Refers to the composition and qualifications of the interdisciplinary team and defines how the team should collaborate with patients and families.

2. *Physical aspects of care:* Emphasizes management of physical symptoms such as pain, fatigue, anxiety, and others.

3. *Psychological and psychiatric aspects of care:* Defines assessment of the psychosocial needs of patients and families. The requirement for bereavement support is included in this domain.

4. *Social aspects of care:* Focuses on leveraging family strengths and social support mechanisms to alleviate family stress.

5. *Spiritual, religious, and existential aspects of care:* Emphasizes the roles of the members of the interdisciplinary team, especially the chaplain, in recognizing and addressing spiritual and existential distress. Specifically, the competency of all team members in understanding and supporting religious practice preferences of patients and families is stressed.

6. *Cultural aspects of care:* Describes cultural competence and defines processes for the provision of culturally sensitive care.

7. *Care of the patient at the end of life:* Highlights the importance of providing multidimensional interdisciplinary end-of-life care for patients and their families, which includes educating them and guiding them through the dying process.

8. *Ethical and legal aspects of care:* Addresses advance care planning, ethics, and legal aspects of care. The role of the interdisciplinary team in broaching end-of-life conversations and documenting patients' preferences is stressed. Consultation with ethics committees and legal counsel is also emphasized.

The report from the NCP provided the first coherent account of what quality end-of-life care entailed. The Clinical Practice Guidelines were endorsed by the National Quality Forum

> **Key Point**
>
> The Nurse Practice Act Toolkit and links to each state's nurse practice act are available at https://www.ncsbn.org/npa-toolkit.htm

(NQF) in 2006, lending further credence to this excellent work. The Clinical Practice Guidelines underpinned the provision of high-quality, uniform, end-of-life care across multiple practice settings and served as the foundation for many other hospice and palliative care initiatives and guidelines (Dahlin, 2015).

Hospice and palliative nurses should be familiar with the Clinical Practice Guidelines because they serve as a foundational framework for excellence in end-of-life care and during serious illness. Further, the hospice and palliative care nurse must "demonstrate knowledge, attitudes, behaviors, and skills that are consistent with palliative nursing professional standards, codes of ethics, and scope of practice" (American Nurses Association, 2014, p. 23).

Code of Ethics

Every nurse is expected to adhere to an unwavering ethical framework when providing care for patients. The American Nurses Association (2015) set forth provisions of the Code of Ethics for Nurses (see https://www.nursingworld.org/coe-view-only).

In addition to upholding the provisions of the code of ethics set forth by the American Nurses Association, nurses are also expected to provide care in accordance with widely accepted ethical principles such as

Autonomy: The right to make decisions for oneself. Autonomy is the principle that underpins the practice of informed consent

Beneficence: The principle of doing the most good; acting kindly and charitably

Confidentiality: The expectation that the patient's private information will not be disclosed to anyone without the patient's consent

Justice: The promotion of good for all

Nonmaleficence: Doing no harm

Paternalism: Restricting the liberty or rights of another, seemingly for the person's own good

Truthfulness: Providing information with honesty and integrity

Ethical dilemmas occur in clinical practice when treatment options or other aspects of the patient's care, including the patient's treatment preferences, conflict with one or more ethical principles. Lo (2012) recommends the following process for approaching ethical dilemmas:

1. Determine the medical facts of the case

2. Identify the values, concerns, and recommendations of the clinician(s)

3. Identify the values, concerns, and preferences of the patient (or designated surrogate)

4. Identify the ethical issues at hand

5. Consider any practical issues that may have bearing on the case

If the clinician finds that the ethical issues cannot be readily resolved, then a second medical opinion should be sought and the expertise of the interdisciplinary team and possibly a clinical ethicist should be utilized. Frequently facing ethical dilemmas can cause moral distress in healthcare professionals. Moral distress is defined as a negative

> **Key Point**
>
> Hospice and palliative care nurses are expected to develop trusting and therapeutic relationships with their patients while maintaining professional boundaries by avoiding communication with patients outside of work hours, providing only services that are included in one's job description, and openly sharing information about the patient with all members of the team (Perry, 2011).

feeling that emerges when an individual knows the morally correct action to take but feels unable to take that action due to hierarchical or institutional barriers (Jameton, 1984). Repeated exposure to moral distress may contribute to nurse burnout (Wagner, 2015).

Self-Care

Moral distress, grieving, frequent exposure to death and dying, workload pressure, lack of support, existential issues, and intrateam conflicts can lead to occupational stress for hospice nurses. Other factors that can contribute to occupational stress include workplace bullying, generational differences, personality types, and work values. Serious consequences of workplace stress include disengagement, increased absenteeism, decreased job satisfaction, decreased productivity, low morale, and compassion fatigue (Wright, 2017).

Self-care involves taking steps to minimize the effects of occupational stress and/or to address the root causes of the stressors. If workplace conflict is identified as a stressor, then steps should be taken to address the conflict, such as

- *Avoidance*, which is appropriate when the issue is not significant

- *Accommodation*, which occurs when the person accepts the position of the other

- *Competition*, which is a conflict resolution style that entails one person vehemently defending her or his position. Although this approach may end the conflict, it does not support team building

- *Collaboration*, which involves working with the other person until a resolution can be reached. This is usually considered the best approach to conflict resolution
(Saltman, O'dea, & Kidd, 2006)

Engaging in earnest conflict resolution improves the working conditions for nurses. Yet, in light of the various stressors faced by hospice nurses, other self-care strategies should be used to reduce the effects of occupational stress. The World Health Organization (2009) defines self-care as "a deliberate action that individuals, family members and the community should engage in to maintain good health" (p. 2). Self-care activities include the following:

- Eating well
- Exercising
- Pursuing outside interests
- Journaling
- Praying
- Meditating
- Using vacation time

- Massage
- Requesting a change of assignment, if needed

Consistent engagement in self-care activities can help nurses avoid burnout, build resilience, and reduce stress. Self-care is important because "clinicians meeting the criteria for burnout deliver poorer quality of care, make more medial errors, and display low empathy" (Back, Steinhauser, Kamal, & Jackson, 2016, p. 285). Thus, nurses must engage in self-care as part of their professional responsibilities.

Professional Development

Professional development (PD) involves voluntary learning and continuing development with the purpose of remaining abreast of the skills, trends, and knowledge development in one's field. Examples of PD include the following:

- Teaching and mentoring
- Ongoing construction and reconstruction of one's professional identity
- Participating in informal learning opportunities
- Maintaining professional competencies and developing new competencies
- Embracing and engaging in innovative practice changes (Collin, Van der Heijden, & Lewis, 2012).

All nurses must recognize PD as a professional responsibility to themselves, to their patients, and to their profession. Additionally, hospice and palliative care nurses are expected to be aware of emerging trends, policies, legislative efforts, or reimbursement changes that potentially impact the delivery of hospice and palliative care. Nurses can easily remain up to date on the practice issues by joining professional organizations (i.e., Hospice and Palliative Nurses Association), reading professional journals, attending and/or presenting at professional conferences, and serving professional organizations by volunteering to assist with committee work, outreach, or peer review.

▪ CONCLUSION

Hospice and palliative nurses are expected to maintain a high degree of professionalism in the care of their patients and in the workplace. Occupational stress and workplace conflicts also contribute to employee stress and to burnout. Thus, hospice and palliative care nurses have a responsibility to actively resolve conflicts in the clinical arena and in the workplace, to act ethically in all clinical situations, to engage in self-care, and to participate in PD in an ongoing way.

> **Chapter Summary**
>
> - Hospice and palliative care nurses must be familiar with the eight domains of care outlined in the National Consensus Project.
> - Occupational stress is caused by lateral violence, generational differences, differences in work ethic, and moral distress. Nurses must be adept at utilizing conflict resolution strategies to reduce stress and decrease the incidence of burnout.
> - Self-care is an essential part of reducing occupational stress and promoting quality clinical care.
> - PD involves formal and informal learning, teaching and mentoring, participation in professional organizations, and remaining abreast of legal and political trends, policies, and reimbursement changes that can affect hospice and palliative care.

■ PRACTICE QUESTIONS

1. The family of a seriously ill patient asks the palliative care nurse to avoid telling the patient that her illness is incurable. The two ethical principles that are in conflict in this situation are

   a. Truthfulness and justice

   b. Autonomy and paternalism

   c. Confidentiality and beneficence

   d. Nonmaleficence and beneficence

2. A hospice nurse manager implements a policy limiting the number of "on-call" days hospice nurses can be required to work each month. This is an example of

   a. Justice

   b. Paternalism

   c. Autonomy

   d. Beneficence

3. Which of the following is an example of violating professional boundaries?

   a. Assisting a patient with light housekeeping

   b. Offering to contact a patient's doctor for them

   c. Telling the patient to use the on-call service if needed

   d. Checking on the patient when not working

4. The most appropriate way of resolving minor conflict is through

   a. Competition

   b. Collaboration

   c. Accommodation

   d. Avoidance

5. A hospice and palliative care nurse volunteers to lead group meditation for his coworkers. This is an example of

   a. Collaboration

   b. Professional development

   c. Self-care

   d. Teamwork

■ REFERENCES

American Nurses Association. (2014). *Palliative nursing: An essential resource for hospice and palliative nurses.* Silver Spring, MD.

American Nurses Association. (2015). *Code of ethics with interpretive statements.* Silver Spring, MD: Retrieved from https://www.nursingworld.org/practice-policy/nursing-excellence/ethics/code-of-ethics-for-nurses/

Back, A. L., Steinhauser, K. E., Kamal, A. H., & Jackson, V. A. (2016). Building resilience for palliative care clinicians: An approach to burnout prevention based on individual skills and workplace factors. *Journal of Pain and Symptom Management, 52*(2), 284–291. doi:10.1016/j.jpainsymman.2016.02.002

Collin, K., Van der Heijden, B., & Lewis, P. (2012). Continuing professional development. *International Journal of Training and Development, 16*(3), 155–163. doi:10.1111/j.1468-2419.2012.00410.x

Dahlin, C. M. (2015). National consensus project for quality palliative care: Promoting excellence in palliative nursing. In B. R. Ferrell, N. Coyle, & J. A. Paice (Eds.), *Oxford textbook of palliative nursing* (pp. 11–19). New York, NY: Oxford University Press.

Hinckley, G. B. (2003). *Remarks at the inauguration of President Cecil O. Samuelson.* Retrieved from https://speeches.byu.edu/talks/gordon-b-hinckley_remarks-inauguration-president-cecil-o-samuelson/

Jameton, A. (1984). *Nursing practice: The ethical issues.* New York, NY: Prentice Hall.

Lo, B. (2012). *Resolving ethical dilemmas: A guide for clinicians.* Philadelphia, PA: Lippincott Williams & Wilkins.

National Consensus Project for Quality Palliative Care. (2013). *Clinical practice guidelines for quality palliative care* (3rd ed.). Retrieved from http://www.nationalconsensusproject.org/

National Consensus Project for Quality Palliative Care. (2018). *Clinical practice guidelines for quality palliative care* (4th ed.). Richmond, VA. Retrieved from https://www.nationalcoalitiionhpc.org/ncp

Perry, A. (2011). *Real stories of boundary violations and what we can learn from them.* Retrieved from https://www.nhpco.org/sites/default/files/public/newsline/2011/Oct11_NL.pdf

Saltman, D. C., O'Dea, N. A., & Kidd, M. R. (2006). Conflict management: A primer for doctors in training. *Postgraduate Medical Journal, 82*(963), 9–12. doi:10.1136/pgmj.2005.034306

Wagner, C. (2015). Moral distress as a contributor to nurse burnout. *American Journal of Nursing, 115*(4), 11. doi:10.1097/01.NAJ.0000463005.73775.9e

World Health Organization. (2009). *Self-care in the context of primary health care.* Retrieved from http://www.searo.who.int/entity/primary_health_care/documents/sea_hsd_320.pdf

Wright, P. M. (2017). *Fast facts for the hospice nurse.* New York, NY: Springer Publishing Company.

VII

Practice Test

Practice Test

1. Routine hospice care can be provided in any of the following facilities except
   a. The patient's home
   b. A long-term care facility
   c. An acute care facility
   d. An assisted living facility

2. A first-line treatment for dyspnea in the end-of-life setting is
   a. Guaifenesin
   b. Budesonide/formoterol
   c. Morphine
   d. Scopolamine

3. A palliative care patient who has stage 5 renal disease tells the nurse that she is tired of going for hemodialysis and wants to talk about discontinuing it. The nurse's best response is
   a. "Tell me about how dialysis is affecting your quality of life."
   b. "You need to continue dialysis for as long as possible."
   c. "Have you considered peritoneal dialysis?"
   d. "Do you have an advance directive in place?"

4. A palliative care patient tells the nurse that he experiences constipation from time to time. After reviewing the patient's medication list, the nurse determines that medications are not the cause. Thus, the nurse should
   a. Refer the patient to a gastroenterologist
   b. Recommend a high-fiber diet
   c. Teach the patient to restrict sodium intake
   d. Administer a senna laxative when constipation occurs

5. When caring for patients in long-term care facilities, the hospice nurse must

   a. Coordinate end-of-life care

   b. Provide personal care

   c. Provide all personal supplies

   d. Pay for room and board

6. A palliative care patient with a diagnosis of lung cancer reports increased pain in her back, which is sharp and persistent, 8/10. Her previous pain level was 3–4/10. The patient's physician states that the pain medication does not need to be adjusted because she feels "the patient is becoming too dependent on opioids." The nurse should

   a. Provide nonpharmacological pain interventions

   b. Ask the physician if an adjuvant might help

   c. Administer the opioid on the clock and not wait for the patient to ask

   d. Advocate for proper pain management for the patient immediately

7. The cause of death for most patients who have amyotrophic lateral sclerosis is

   a. Respiratory failure

   b. Cardiac arrest

   c. Sepsis

   d. Metabolic imbalances

8. A hospice nurse is called to the home of an 89-year-old patient with end-stage cardiac and renal disease. The patient is experiencing chest pain that she describes as 7/10 along with shortness of breath and does not want to leave her home. The hospice nurse recommends that an opioid pain medication be initiated. The family states that they are very fearful of addiction and ask if a nonopioid can be used. The nurse's best response is

   a. "Is there a history of addiction in the family?"

   b. "Addiction doesn't occur in hospice patients."

   c. "Addiction is not likely when opioids are used appropriately to treat pain."

   d. "Opioids are first line treatment for dyspnea."

9. When administering a patient's medications, the hospice nurse observes the patient coughing and choking when attempting to swallow liquids. The nurse should

   a. Ensure proper positioning to alleviate choking

   b. Suction the patient's airway to prevent aspiration pneumonia

c. Thicken the patient's liquids and offer a puree diet

d. Conduct a swallowing screen to determine the patient's risk level

10. The family caregiver is defined as the person who

    a. Is designated by the patient to make medical decisions

    b. Assumes responsibility for daily care of the patient

    c. Makes arrangements for the patient's needs to be met

    d. Coordinates needed services for the patient in the home

11. When teaching a patient the differences between hospice care and palliative care, the nurse explains that

    a. Palliative care takes place in the home only; hospice care is delivered in many settings

    b. Palliative care can be delivered in conjunction with curative care but hospice cannot

    c. Palliative care is never covered by Medicare; hospice is always covered by Medicare

    d. Hospice and palliative care are provided for terminally ill patients only

12. A 60-year-old hospice patient with a terminal diagnosis of end-stage liver disease experiences a nosebleed. The most appropriate nursing action is

    a. Pack the nostril and remain with the patient until the bleeding stops

    b. Assist the patient to a side-lying position on the opposite side of the bleeding

    c. Instruct the patient to pinch the bridge of the nose and tilt the head back

    d. Obtain red towel to minimize the visual effect of the bleeding

13. A hospice nurse is visiting a home care hospice patient who has end-stage renal disease. Besides evaluating renal status, the most important assessment for the nurse to conduct is

    a. Cardiac status because cardiac failure is the leading cause of death in renal patients

    b. Respiratory status because fluid overload causes dyspnea

    c. Mentation because delirium results from uremia

    d. Skin integrity because the buildup of bile salts causes pruritus

14. A hospice nurse is conducting an inservice on grief and applies Dr. Kübler-Ross's work to a case study involving

    a. The loss of a spouse

    b. A patient who is in remission

    c. The loss of a child

    d. A patient facing his own death

15. Which of the following tools should be used frequently when assessing a patient with immobility?

    a. Glascow scale

    b. Braden scale

    c. Karnofsky scale

    d. Functional Assessment Staging (FAST) scale

16. During a home visit with a 75-year-old hospice patient who has a terminal diagnosis of chronic obstructive pulmonary disease, the nurse notes ankle edema that was not present at the last home visit 3 days ago. The nurse should

    a. Advise the patient to elevate his feet when possible

    b. Reduce fluid intake to 500 mL daily

    c. Assess for additional signs of cor pulmonale

    d. Measure the patient for thromboembolic stockings

17. A hospice patient is admitted to the inpatient unit with intractable nausea and vomiting. The patient is given haloperidol and within a few hours begins to experience hallucinations, paranoia, and insomnia. The most likely explanation for the patient's symptoms is

    a. Delirium

    b. Dementia

    c. Drug reaction

    d. Hypovolemia

18. The best nonpharmacologic pain intervention for a patient who is actively dying is

    a. Yoga

    b. Guided meditation

    c. Deep tissue massage

    d. Reiki

19. The nurse documents that a hospice patient is comatose. This means that

    a. The patient is disoriented to person, place, and time

    b. The patient does not respond to verbal or tactile stimuli

    c. The patient is unable to make decisions, but is responsive

    d. The patient has a delayed response when her name is called

20. A 74-year-old patient who has breast cancer with metastasis to the ribs and spine reports new-onset pain which she describes as

radiating from her upper back to her arms. The priority assessment question is

    a. "Is the pain sharp or stabbing?"

    b. "When did the pain begin?"

    c. "Have you tried applying heat or cold?"

    d. "How have you been treated for diabetic neuropathy in the past?"

21. The most appropriate level of care for a hospice patient who is ambulatory and stable is

    a. General inpatient care

    b. Respite care

    c. Continuous care

    d. Routine care

22. A 77-year-old hospice patient who has liver disease reports severe pruritis. Which of the following would not be recommended to treat the patient's symptoms?

    a. Barrier cream

    b. Prednisone

    c. Diphenhydramine

    d. Calamine lotion

23. Which member of the hospice team is responsible for supervising licensed practical/licensed vocational nurses?

    a. RN

    b. Nurse practitioner

    c. Nurse manager

    d. Medical director

24. When tumor growth or metastasis blocks the bladder outlet, the patient will experience

    a. Hematuria

    b. Bladder spasm

    c. Urinary tract infection

    d. Urethral insufficiency

25. A hospice patient who is approaching death has acute-onset edema in her left lower extremity and the area is warm and tender to touch. The most appropriate intervention at this time is

    a. Make arrangements for a venogram

    b. Discuss goals of care with the patient and family

    c. Use a Doppler to check blood flow in the affected leg

    d. Compare pulses on both lower extremities

26. Assessing family resilience involves

    a. Determining the family's commitment to each other

    b. Using the Family Resilience Tool

    c. Asking the primary caregiver about family coping

    d. Monitoring the level of stress in the household

27. A palliative care patient has a history of substance abuse disorder and reports severe pain (9/10) 1 hour after her pain medication was administered. The nurse should

    a. Provide therapeutic presence until the medication is effective

    b. Contact the prescriber to discuss increasing the dose of the pain medication

    c. Administer an adjuvant to decrease the patient's pain

    d. Contact the chaplain to address the patient's spiritual pain

28. The family of a patient who has advanced breast cancer calls the on-call hospice nurse to report sudden-onset back pain that occurred when transferring the patient from the bed to a chair. The patient was also incontinent of urine. The nurse should first

    a. Recommend administration of an analgesic

    b. Arrange a transfer to the inpatient hospice unit

    c. Advise the family member to transfer the patient back to bed

    d. Obtain an order for corticosteroids

29. A 74-year-old palliative care patient experiences new-onset urinary incontinence that wakes her from sleep. After reviewing the patient's medications, the nurse concludes that the most likely cause is

    a. 25 mcg fentanyl patch changed every 72 hours (began 6 months ago)

    b. Escitalopram (Lexapro) 10 mg by mouth daily (began 2 years ago)

    c. Temazepam (Restoril) 15 mg (began 6 days ago)

    d. Morphine IR 10 mg orally every 4 hours as needed (began 6 months ago)

30. The primary caregiver for an 88-year-old hospice patient admits to overusing prescription drugs to deal with the stress of caregiving. Which intervention is most appropriate?

    a. Arrange a visit from the team social worker

    b. Contact the Area Agency on Aging

    c. Provide a list of local detoxification centers

    d. Transfer the patient to the hospice inpatient center

31. The priority nursing diagnosis for a patient who is immobile is
    a. Risk for aspiration
    b. Risk for impaired skin integrity
    c. Impaired social interaction
    d. Compromised family coping

32. A patient is admitted to an inpatient hospice setting with acute, refractory pain. The patient states, "Why is God doing this to me?" What should the nurse do first?
    a. Contact the chaplain
    b. Arrange a visit from the patient's spiritual leader
    c. Ask the patient why they feel their pain is a punishment
    d. Conduct a FICA screening

33. An advance directive is used to guide care when the patient
    a. Designates a proxy
    b. Is terminally ill
    c. Is unable to make medical decisions
    d. Has a life expectancy of less than 6 months

34. A hospitalized patient who has lung cancer with metastasis meets hospice admission criteria. The family agrees that hospice care would provide the best level of care for the patient. When discussing hospice care with the patient, he exhibits periods of confusion and is disoriented to place and time. The nurse knows that
    a. The patient cannot consent to hospice services
    b. The patient has end-stage delirium
    c. Hypocalcemia is the likely cause of the confusion
    d. The patient must remain hospitalized until he is no longer confused

35. The "classic triad" of symptoms associated with Parkinson's disease is
    a. Bradykinesia, resting tremor, and mask-like expression
    b. Tremor, rigidity, and movement disorder
    c. Bradykinesia, dysphagia, and muscle rigidity
    d. Foot drop, tremor, and rigidity

36. Which is the first step of the World Health Organization's cancer pain management ladder?
    a. Apply heat or cold to the affected area
    b. Administer a nonopioid medication

    c. Advise use of an adjuvant medication

    d. Recommend a low-dose opioid

37. Patient care goals should be

    a. Open-ended and relevant

    b. Specific and measurable

    c. Flexible and achievable

    d. Pertinent and timely

38. A hospice nurse notes thrush in the mouth of a patient who uses inhaled corticosteroids to help manage chronic obstructive pulmonary disease (COPD). The nurse should

    a. Recommend that the patient use oral corticosteroids instead

    b. Encourage proper oral care after using inhaler

    c. Arrange for suction equipment to be delivered to the home

    d. Obtain an order for nebulized morphine

39. During a hospice admission assessment for a patient who has advanced cancer, the patient's wife states that her spouse has been experiencing weight loss, gradual decreased ability to engage in activities of daily living, and a progressive decline in overall condition. The nurse should

    a. Advise that the patient be admitted to inpatient care for symptom management

    b. Teach the patient and family that this is the expected course of the illness

    c. Conduct a "get up and go" test

    d. Review the patient's medication to determine if the symptoms are drug side effects

40. The palliative care nurse is teaching a patient's primary caregiver how to measure oral medication using a dropper. The caregiver has limited education and low English proficiency. What is the best way to ensure that the caregiver understands the instructions?

    a. Provide written instructions after verbal instructions

    b. Provide hands-on learning with a dropper using water to practice

    c. Ask the caregiver to teach back the skill

    d. Arrange for a nurse's aide to administer the medication

41. The medication regimen for a 40-year-old palliative care patient includes oxycodone controlled-release, 40 mg by mouth every 12 hours; immediate-release oxycodone, 20 mg by mouth every 3 hours as needed; senna/docusate sodium, two tablets in the

morning and two tablets in the evening; and polyethylene glycol, 1 capful daily as needed. The patient's last bowel movement was 4 days ago and she reports abdominal pain, cramping, and constipation. Which of the following interventions most effectively meets the patient's needs at this time?

a. Advise the patient to take two extra doses of the senna/docusate today

b. Contact the patient's prescriber to discuss the possible use of methylnaltrexone

c. Auscultate the abdomen

d. Check for impaction

42. A hospice patient who has colon cancer has been experiencing a slow decline in functional status and is now approaching death. The patient expresses feelings of worthlessness and tells the nurse that he never did anything right in his life. The best pharmacological intervention for the patient's depression is

a. Paroxetine (Paxil)

b. Methylphenidate (Ritalin)

c. Lorazepam (Ativan)

d. Escitalopram (Lexapro)

43. A 56-year-old hospice patient who has a terminal diagnosis of AIDS has a full-thickness pressure ulcer in the sacral area. The patient is at greatest risk for

a. Sepsis

b. Hemorrhage

c. Kennedy ulcer

d. Nephropathy

44. The hospice nurse knows that a patient is ineligible for hospice services if he

a. Is eligible for Medicare Part A

b. Chooses to continue curative care

c. Has a life expectancy of 6 months or less

d. Meets local coverage determinations

45. The family of a terminally ill patient who has colon cancer is very concerned about the patient's lack of appetite and requests artificial nutrition. With the patient's permission, a nasogastric tube is placed and enteral feedings are initiated at 15 mL/hr. Within 24 hours of these interventions, the patient reports nausea, vomiting, and abdominal pain. What should the nurse do first?

a. Check residual volume

b. Stop the infusion

    c. Administer an antiemetic

    d. Auscultate bowel sounds

46. A 63-year-old hospice patient who has a terminal diagnosis of chronic obstructive pulmonary disease and a history of heart failure and renal dysfunction reports vague chest pain. On examination, the nurse notes tachycardia, diaphoresis, and a clear S2 heart sound. The nurse should take steps to alleviate the patient's impending

    a. Nausea

    b. Dyspnea

    c. Facial edema

    d. Confusion

47. A nurse is admitting a patient to hospice services with a diagnosis of lung cancer. The patient also has a history of cardiac disease, hypertension, and dementia. The best way to assess the patient's pain is using the

    a. 0 to 10 scale

    b. Wong–Baker FACES Scale

    c. Pain Assessment in Advanced Dementia (PAINAD) Scale

    d. Face, Legs, Activity, Cry, Consolability (FLACC) Scale

48. Which of the following is not generally considered to be a sign of caregiver role strain?

    a. Somatic complaints

    b. Irritability

    c. Unplanned weight changes

    d. Increased reliance on faith

49. A palliative care patient has a shallow open ulcer on his left heel with exudate. Which of the following dressings is most appropriate for this wound?

    a. Foam dressing

    b. Hydrogel dressing

    c. Thin film

    d. Hydrocolloid dressing

50. Which of the following is a sign of patient abuse?

    a. Stained clothing after a meal

    b. Lack of medical equipment

    c. Bruising in unusual places

    d. Stage 1 decubiti on the heels

51. All of the following should be invited to hospice interdisciplinary meetings except
    a. The hospice social worker
    b. The primary caregiver
    c. The patient's spiritual advisor
    d. The bereavement coordinator

52. A hospice patient expresses a loss of faith due to her illness. The patient is experiencing
    a. Spiritual distress
    b. Spiritual doubt
    c. Faith crisis
    d. Faith aversion

53. Grief is expected to
    a. Enhance coping mechanisms
    b. Manifest as anger or blame
    c. Involve persistent sorrow
    d. Slowly lessen over time

54. Visceral pain is described as
    a. Gnawing
    b. Shooting
    c. Sharp
    d. Allodynic

55. An on-call hospice nurse makes a home visit to an 80-year-old female patient who is experiencing bladder spasms. The patient has an indwelling urinary catheter, size 14 Fr with an output of 100 mL in the past 10 hours. The patient reports suprapubic pain and urethral discomfort. The most appropriate intervention is
    a. Change the catheter to a 16 Fr
    b. Administer a pain medication
    c. Discontinue the catheter
    d. Insert a larger catheter

56. The palliative care nurse assesses a patient's spiritual preferences and needs using the
    a. Spiritual Assessment Scale
    b. The FICA tool
    c. The Faith and Religion Checklist
    d. The Religiosity Scale

57. A hospice patient tells the nurse that his pain is sharp, 8/10. The patient appears comfortable at rest and is talking with his family. Objective data are blood pressure (BP): 140/90, temperature: 99.0, pulse: 88, regular rhythm, respirations: 28 per minutes. The patient's skin is moist and warm. In developing interventions for the patient, the most important datum is:

a. BP of 140/90

b. Temperature of 99.0

c. The patient appears comfortable at rest

d. The patient rates his pain as 9/10

58. The hospice patient who is most at risk for development of a pressure ulcer is the

a. 65-year-old patient with limited ambulatory ability and diabetes

b. 76-year-old obese patient who transfers to a chair with assistance

c. 80-year-old patient who is bedbound and has albuminemia

d. 57-year-old frail patient who is able to reposition himself in bed

59. When rotating an opioid, the equianalgesic dose of the newly introduced opioid should be decreased by

a. 10%

b. 20%

c. 40%

d. 50%

60. Which of the following patients is at greatest risk for a complicated grief reaction?

a. A 28-year-old veteran who was recently discharged from services

b. A 53-year-old widow who had a miscarriage 30 years ago

c. A 37-year-old with a history of severe mental illness

d. A 19-year-old whose beloved father has died

61. A home care hospice patient reports that she has been experiencing severe pruritus since she began taking sustained-release morphine for pain 2 weeks ago. The nurse should

a. Administer diphenhydramine for this allergic response

b. Discuss opioid rotation with the patient's prescriber

c. Apply lotion to the patient's skin to alleviate dryness

d. Recommend that the patient take only half of a tablet

62. An 88-year-old palliative care patient is experiencing nausea, vomiting, and diarrhea. The patient has poor skin turgor, incontinence, and the following vital signs: blood pressure (BP): 100/60, temperature: 102.3, pulse: 58 bpm, and respirations: 22. Which of the following should the nurse administer now?

    a. 325 mg of acetaminophen

    b. Loperamide

    c. Electrolyte replacement drink

    d. An antibiotic

63. Symptoms of complicated grief include preoccupation with thoughts of the deceased, avoidance of grief triggers, and

    a. Guilt and regret

    b. Anger and blame

    c. Deep sorrow

    d. Hallucinations

64. A 70-year-old patient who has brain cancer is experiencing diminished level of consciousness, bradycardia, and irregular respirations. The patient is in the hospital and has been given mannitol, 125 mg intravenously, prior to being transferred to the hospice inpatient unit. During the admission assessment, the hospice nurse would expect which of the following findings?

    a. Hypertension

    b. Dyspnea

    c. Severe headache

    d. Diarrhea

65. When caring for patients who have end-stage neurological disease, the hospice nurse's priority nursing diagnosis is

    a. Risk for infection

    b. Altered skin integrity

    c. Risk for falls

    d. Altered family processes

66. When a home care hospice nurse is conveying information to an inpatient hospice nurse about changes in a patient's status, the nurse should first

    a. Explain what the issue is

    b. Give the background of the patient's situation

    c. Describe the severity of the problem

    d. Make recommendations about the patient's care

67. A 54-year-old patient who has metastatic pain has been taking 5 mg of morphine orally every 4 to 6 hours PRN for increased and persistent pain. Following the World Health Organization's cancer pain ladder, which of the following should be done?

a. Add an adjuvant

b. Add another opioid medication

c. Rotate the opioid

d. Use a long-acting opioid

68. A hospice nurse in an inpatient setting finds a patient crying while doing rounds. The patient states, "I am so afraid to die. What if there is nothing after this?" The nurse sits at the bedside and states, "Would you like to talk more about this?" This is an example of

a. Upholding patient dignity

b. Providing active listening and presence

c. Encouraging life review

d. Facilitating prayer and meditation

69. The nurse documents that a hospice patient has cachexia. This means that the patient has

a. Temporal wasting

b. Loss of appetite

c. Metabolic changes

d. Dehydration

70. A palliative care patient is considering accepting hospice care. Her three daughters are in her room arguing over what the best course of action should be. The first step the nurse should take is

a. Ask the daughters to step out of the room

b. Determine who the primary decision-maker is

c. Contact the patient advocate

d. Assess the patient's safety in her home

71. While ambulating at home, a patient with end-stage heart failure experiences chest pain and chest tightness. The nurse should instruct the patient to

a. Rest

b. Develop an exercise routine to increase stamina

c. Lie down and raise feet above the level of the heart

d. Take 81 mg of aspirin now

72. A hospice nurse is making a home visit to a 52-year-old patient whose condition is steadily declining. The patient's 15-year-old daughter appears to be withdrawn and remains in her room

when she is not at school. The nurse should teach the patient that the daughter

a. Does not understand the permanence of death

b. Is feeling angry about being different from peers

c. Is exhibiting age-appropriate grief responses

d. May experience regression to an earlier stage of development

73. A 50-year-old hospice patient who has brain cancer has been taking 325 mg of acetaminophen orally for mild pain every 4 to 6 hours as needed. The patient has taken two doses daily for the past several weeks but is no longer able to swallow and appears uncomfortable. The nurse should

a. Insert a saline lock

b. Administer the acetaminophen rectally

c. Request an order for an opioid medication

d. Offer nonpharmacological pain interventions

74. A 77-year-old palliative care patient with liver disease has ascites. The palliative care nurse knows that ascites is a sign of

a. Sodium overload

b. Hyperalbumemia

c. Portal hypotension

d. End-stage disease

75. Which faith tradition teaches that death may lead to reincarnation?

a. Hinduism

b. Christianity

c. Judaism

d. Islam

76. A palliative care patient who has liver cancer with widespread metastasis exhibits changes in mentation, anorexia, nausea, vomiting, weakness, and constipation. The patient's serum calcium level is 16 mg/dL, blood glucose is 150 mg/dL, and pulse oximetry is 90% on room air. The most likely cause of the patient's symptoms is

a. Infection due to compromised immunity

b. Hypercalcemia due to metastasis

c. Hyperglycemia due to diabetes

d. Hypoxia due to metastasis

77. Hospice nursing practice is governed by the

a. American Nurses Association

b. Hospice and Palliative Nurses Association

c. National League for Nurses

d. State Board of Nursing

78. During a palliative care team meeting a patient states that she cannot make final decisions about her healthcare until her husband approves her choices. To demonstrate cultural awareness, the nurse should

a. Arrange a meeting when the patient's husband can be present

b. Recognize when the nurse's cultural views differ from the patient's

c. Teach the patient that she can make autonomous decisions

d. Ask if the patient's husband is available by phone

79. During an admission visit with a patient who has terminal cancer, the patient states that her illness was caused by an imbalance in her energy. The nurse's best response is

a. "Do you feel you have done something to deserve your illness?"

b. "What do you think caused the imbalance?"

c. "How can we help you to feel more balanced now?"

d. "We can help manage any symptoms with the right medications."

80. Which combination of medications, if prescribed for a palliative care patient, would be most likely to cause urinary retention?

a. Acetaminophen and hydrocodone

b. Atropine and hydromorphone

c. Scopolamine and calcium carbonate

d. Losartan and diphenhydramine

81. A 37-year-old palliative care patient who has type 2 diabetes, cardiac disease, and rheumatoid arthritis reports increased symptoms of acid reflux and gastric distress. When asked about diet and medications, the patient reveals that his arthritic pain has increased and he is now taking 800 mg of ibuprofen approximately every 4 hours daily. Patient teaching should be initiated regarding

a. The effect of ibuprofen on diabetes

b. The use of an H2 agonist

c. The maximum daily dose of ibuprofen

d. The cardiac side effects of nonsteroidal anti-inflammatory drugs (NSAIDs)

82. The husband of an 82-year-old patient who was admitted to the ED with signs of renal disease is very distraught upon learning

that his wife will need dialysis. He asks the palliative care nurse "how could she be so sick and seem fine before this?" The nurse's response is based on the knowledge that

a. Symptoms of renal failure mimic urinary tract infections

b. Patients often do not experience symptoms of renal disease until the glomerular filtration rate (GFR) is <29

c. The symptoms patients experience in stage 1 of renal disease are very subtle

d. Symptoms of renal disease do not usually manifest until 50% of function is lost

83. The National Consensus Project outlined domains of palliative care for the purpose of

a. Establishing the scope of hospice nursing practice

b. Providing a reference guide for hospice nurses

c. Setting standards of practice for hospice professionals

d. Developing uniformity in end-of-life care

84. A hospice nurse is working with a patient who is a recent immigrant and does not speak English. The priority nursing intervention is

a. Improving access to healthcare services

b. Overcoming provider bias

c. Accessing translation services

d. Verifying insurance coverage

85. Which of the following patients is at greatest risk for respiratory depression following the oral administration of an opioid medication?

a. A 67-year-old opioid-naïve patient

b. A 45-year-old patient going through opioid rotation

c. A 27-year-old patient who has cirrhosis and a history of drug and alcohol abuse

d. A 32-year-old patient who has received subcutaneous opioid medications in the past

86. A patient recently diagnosed with HIV is seen in a palliative care setting. He states that he has been feeling well and has stopped taking the prescribed antiretroviral medications because he does not feel he needs them. The most important nursing intervention at this time is

a. Teaching the patient about disease transmission

b. Encouraging proper nutrition

    c. Arranging for a palliative care team meeting

    d. Discussing the effects of drug noncompliance

87. The primary caregiver of an 82-year-old hospice patient who has a primary terminal diagnosis of Alzheimer's-type dementia tells the nurse that she is overwhelmed with caregiving and feels that her "whole family is just falling apart." The nurse should first

    a. Identify the family's needs

    b. Recommend needed resources

    c. Offer inpatient respite care

    d. Arrange for a social work visit

88. An 82-year-old patient who resides in a long-term care facility has a history of stage 4 chronic obstructive pulmonary disease (COPD) with Modified British Medical Council (mMRC) grade 3 dyspnea, dementia (Functional Assessment Staging [FAST] scale score 7C), and colon cancer. When the patient is admitted to hospice, the terminal diagnosis should be

    a. Failure to thrive

    b. Cancer

    c. COPD

    d. End-stage dementia

89. A 55-year-old patient who has breast cancer has a large tumor in her breast with metastasis to nearby lymph nodes but no evidence of any distant metastasis. Her cancer would be described as

    a. T0, N1, MX

    b. T1, N0, M2

    c. T2, N1, M0

    d. TX, N0, M0

90. A hospice RN may delegate tasks to the hospice

    a. Aide

    b. Chaplain

    c. Social worker

    d. Pharmacist

91. A nurse is caring for a 90-year-old patient with end-stage dementia and observes the patient clenching her teeth, grimacing, and calling out from time to time. The nurse immediately takes action to reduce the patient's

    a. Jaw stiffness

    b. Vocalizing

    c. Pain

    d. Confusion

92. A 63-year-old hospice patient was recently admitted to the inpatient setting for pain management. A subcutaneous morphine infusion was started 2 days ago and the patient reported sedation, nausea, dry mouth, and constipation. The nurse knows that all of these initial side effects will dissipate except

   a. Sedation

   b. Nausea

   c. Dry mouth

   d. Constipation

93. A hospice RN delegates medication administration to a licensed practical nurse/licensed vocational nurse. The RN is responsible for

   a. Ensuring that the medications are correct

   b. Providing appropriate supervision

   c. Asking the patient his name and birthdate

   d. Witnessing the medication administration

94. A 47-year-old palliative care patient who has breast cancer tells the nurse that she is very worried about whether she will achieve remission. She is also very worried that she will have uncontrollable pain. She is fearful of infection and no longer goes out of her house. She reports that meditation and visualization exercises have not been helpful. The most appropriate intervention for this patient is

   a. Escitalopram (Lexapro)

   b. Deep breathing exercises

   c. Lorazepam (Ativan)

   d. Alprazolam (Xanax)

95. The condition of being separated from someone through death is

   a. Mourning

   b. Detachment

   c. Complicated grief

   d. Bereavement

96. The daughter of a 92-year-old hospice patient who is actively dying asks the nurse to read the Bible to her mother. The nurse should

   a. Use the FICA tool to assess spiritual needs

   b. Play spiritual music in the patient's room

   c. Ask the daughter if there are particular verses the patient likes

   d. Arrange a visit from the chaplain to read scripture to the patient

97. A palliative care nurse is arranging a family meeting with the palliative care team. The team hopes to resolve family conflict regarding the best course of care for the patient. At the beginning of the meeting, the team should

    a. Lay out all treatment options

    b. Set the agenda for the meeting

    c. Designate a family spokesperson

    d. Review the patient's living will

98. A palliative care patient is exhibiting signs of dementia such as forgetfulness, poor attention span, and frequent falls. In addition to monitoring the effects of pharmacological interventions, the nurse should

    a. Evaluate laboratory findings that indicate dementia

    b. Measure mid-arm circumference

    c. Arrange for home physical and occupational therapy

    d. Conduct a mini mental status exam weekly

99. When a hospice RN delegates a task to a nurse's aide, who is responsible for the outcome of the task?

    a. The hospice manager

    b. The hospice aide

    c. The RN

    d. The licensed practical nurse/licensed vocational nurse

100. During a home care visit to a hospice patient, a neighbor arrives and asks the nurse for an update on the patient's condition. The nurse directs the neighbor to discuss their concerns with the patient or family. The nurse is upholding which ethical principle?

    a. Autonomy

    b. Confidentiality

    c. Justice

    d. Beneficence

101. A palliative care patient is unable to express her own healthcare wishes. In advocating for the patient, the nurse should rely on

    a. Documentation of the patient's wishes

    b. The patient's caregiver

    c. The decisions of the medical director

    d. Hospice team decisions

102. A palliative care patient who has a history of hypertension, glaucoma, type 2 diabetes mellitus, and hypercholesterolemia is

experiencing painful neuropathies. Which condition is the primary contributor to this symptom?

a. Hypertension

b. Hypercholesterolemia

c. Glaucoma

d. Diabetes

103. A 67-year-old palliative care patient who has a history of cardiac disease reports lower abdominal pain that is dull and crampy. The nurse should first

a. Auscultate the patient's bowel sounds

b. Palpate the abdomen

c. Administer pain medication

d. Determine last bowel movement

104. When opioids are initiated, which of the following should be added to the patient's drug regimen?

a. An antidepressant

b. A laxative

c. An antiemetic

d. A stimulant

105. The greatest risk of cancer is

a. Poor diet

b. Lack of exercise

c. Genetic predisposition

d. Advancing age

106. A hospice patient with advanced disease states that he has decided to revoke the hospice benefit and attempt an experimental treatment. The nurse believes that the treatment will cause the patient suffering and will not prolong his life. The nurse is facing a(n)

a. Moral stressor

b. Ethical dilemma

c. Internal conflict

d. Value mismatch

107. A 70-year-old patient who has prostate cancer reports increasing pain. The patient has an allergy to morphine. Which of the following can be used with this patient?

a. Fentanyl

b. Buprenorphine

c. Oxycodone

d. Codeine

108. The leading cause of death for American men and women is

    a. Cancer

    b. Heart disease

    c. Pulmonary disease

    d. Accidents

109. During a death vigil, the most appropriate nursing intervention is

    a. Encouraging family members to remain with the patient

    b. Determining cultural needs at the time of death

    c. Teaching the family about the dying process

    d. Arranging a team meeting to prepare for the loss

110. A hospice nurse confides to a coworker that she is feeling disengaged from her work and is "tired of working with patients who are dying." The nurse is experiencing

    a. Emotional fatigue

    b. Moral distress

    c. Lateral violence

    d. Occupational stress

111. A definitive diagnosis of chronic obstructive pulmonary disease is made by

    a. Analyzing spirometry results

    b. Frequent symptoms assessment

    c. Monitoring blood gases

    d. Determining the effectiveness of interventions

112. When a patient is discharged from hospice due to improvement in their condition, the discharge order must be signed by the

    a. Patient's physician

    b. Hospice team

    c. Patient

    d. Hospice medical director

113. The family member of a patient in an inpatient hospice unit does not visit because another family member died there a few months ago and she says it "brings back bad memories." This reaction to loss is called

    a. Avoidance

    b. Denial

    c. Adaptation

    d. Transferrence

114. A 77-year-old hospice patient has a pathological fracture. Nursing care priorities are

    a. Determining cause and assessing surgical risk

    b. Applying steady pressure and ice to the site

    c. Managing pain and stabilizing the joint

    d. Managing edema and elevating the limb

115. On assessment of a patient with a history of cardiac disease, the nurse notes fatigue with minimal exertion, edema, tachycardia, cyanosis in the extremities, and wheezing at rest. Based on the assessment findings, the patient is at risk for

    a. Congestive heart failure

    b. Left-sided heart failure

    c. Right-sided heart failure

    d. Asthma

116. A 47-year-old patient who has breast cancer with metastasis experiences facial swelling, jugular vein distention, and a ruddy complexion. The cause of these signs of superior vena cava syndrome is most likely

    a. Heart failure

    b. Overexertion

    c. Tracheal deviation

    d. Metastasis

117. The bereavement plan of care is developed by the bereavement coordinator or the

    a. RN

    b. Medical director

    c. Chaplain

    d. Social worker

118. Pain described as shooting, burning, stabbing, tingling, or as pins and needles is

    a. Nociceptive pain

    b. Neuropathic pain

    c. Visceral pain

    d. Radicular pain

119. A patient has received hospice services for 90 days. The patient's next benefit period is for a

    a. 90-day period

    b. 30-day period

    c. 60-day period

    d. 180-day period

120. A 65-year-old patient with an extensive history of cardiac disease exhibits significant cardiac symptoms at rest as well as the inability to carry out minimal activities without dyspnea or angina. The patient tells the palliative care nurse that he is interested in finding out if he is eligible for a left-ventricular assist device (LVAD). The nurse's best response is

    a. "You have stage 4 heart disease so you are not a candidate for an LVAD."

    b. "You will need to talk with your cardiologist about that."

    c. "I will arrange a team meeting to answer all of your questions."

    d. "Do you have an advance directive in place?"

121. When reviewing a hospice patient's chart, the nurse finds that the Face, Legs, Activity, Cry, Consolability (FLACC) scale score was 2 on a previous shift, which means that the

    a. Patient was in severe pain

    b. Patient cannot rate his pain

    c. Dose of analgesia should be increased

    d. Pain should be reassessed hourly

122. A face-to-face visit must be made to hospice patients by the hospice physician or nurse practitioner in order to

    a. Complete a comprehensive examination

    b. Verify ongoing eligibility for hospice care

    c. Reconcile the patient's medications

    d. Determine the appropriate level of care

123. In order for a hospice agency to receive additional reimbursement from Medicare during a patient's last 7 days of life, the patient's level of care must be

    a. Routine home care

    b. Continuous home care

    c. Inpatient respite care

    d. General inpatient care

124. The daughter of a 70-year-old nonverbal home care hospice patient who has end-stage Parkinson's disease with dementia contacts the on-call nurse to report that her father is in severe pain. The nurse's best response is

    a. "Have you given him any medication?"

    b. "What makes you think your father is in pain?"

c. "What medications do you have on hand?"

d. "Can you tell me the location of the pain and the signs of pain that you see?"

125. A hospice nurse is admitting a patient who has a primary terminal diagnosis of pancreatic cancer. The patient has a long-standing history of type 2 diabetes mellitus. Which of the following is most likely related to the patient's diabetes and not to the pancreatic cancer?

a. Weight loss

b. Poor appetite

c. Insulinomas

d. Retinopathy

126. A 60-year-old patient who has throat cancer was found at home unresponsive, with pinpoint pupils and shallow respirations. The patient's caregiver contacts the hospice nurse for direction. The nurse should

a. Reassure the caregiver that the findings are part of the normal dying process

b. Arrange for emergency transport to the hospice inpatient unit

c. Offer to make a home visit now

d. Instruct the caregiver to administer naloxone immediately

127. During a bereavement visit, the nurse learns that a former patient's widow has been experiencing grief, nausea, and nightmares since her husband died 6 weeks ago. The nurse teaches her that

a. Physical symptoms are often part of the grief process

b. Her physical grief symptoms should be resolved by now

c. Bereavement care will continue for 2 more years

d. She is experiencing signs of depression

128. A palliative care patient who has greater trochanteric pain syndrome states, "My pain goal is 5/10, that way, the pain will force me to walk more carefully." The nurse should

a. Recommend in-home physical therapy

b. Teach the patient that chronic pain serves no useful purpose

c. Assess the home for fall risks, such as cords and throw rugs

d. Advise the patient to elevate her legs above the level of the heart when sitting

129. Opioid rotation may become necessary due to

a. Addiction

b. Tolerance

    c. Metabolite accumulation

    d. Cost of the opioid

130. Which of the following patients is at greatest risk for suicide?

    a. A palliative care patient who has a plan and access to weapons

    b. A hospice patient who gave her engagement ring to her grand-daughter

    c. The wife of a hospice patient who states, "I can't live without my husband!"

    d. The hospice patient who states, "If I weren't afraid of hell, I'd kill myself."

131. A palliative care nurse administers 5 mg of immediate-release morphine to a patient as prescribed. After approximately 1 hour of administration, the nurse should assess

    a. Respiratory rate

    b. Level of consciousness

    c. Bowel sounds

    d. Pain level

132. A nurse enters the room of a Jewish patient who is talking with her faith leader. The nurse correctly addresses the faith leader as

    a. Rabbi

    b. Imam

    c. Reverend

    d. Father

133. A 45-year-old unemployed male patient who has chronic back pain, hypertension, obesity, and depression is seen today for pain management. The patient is recently divorced and tells the palliative care nurse that he is worried about getting another job because he did not attend college. He states that he is experiencing anxiety due to his current situation and is overusing alcohol and cigarettes. Also, he recently noticed shortness of breath with minimal exercise. In addition to performing a thorough pain assessment, the palliative care nurse should teach the patient how to decrease his risk for

    a. Chronic obstructive pulmonary disease

    b. Panic disorder

    c. Immobility

    d. Cirrhosis

134. A hospice patient who is experiencing uncontrolled pain should receive which level of care?

    a. Routine home care

    b. Continuous home care

c. Inpatient respite care

d. General inpatient care

135. The conversion guideline for converting an opioid from the oral route to the parenteral route is

a. 1:1

b. 2:1

c. 3:1

d. 5:1

136. A 75-year-old patient who has end-stage cardiac disease is actively dying. The hospice nurse has placed a medical magnet over the patient's automated implantable cardioverter defibrillator (AICD). The next step is to

a. Administer morphine to prevent dyspnea

b. Make arrangements for permanent deactivation of the AICD

c. Advise the patient to limit physical activity

d. Monitor the patient for irregular heart rhythm

137. The nurse knows that a Kennedy ulcer is a sign of

a. Patient neglect

b. Incontinence

c. Approaching death

d. Poor perfusion to the extremities

138. Which of the following is not covered by the Medicare hospice benefit?

a. Hospice aide services

b. Speech therapy

c. Homemaker services

d. Long-term inpatient care

139. A hospice patient has been taking 5 mg of oxycodone immediate release for pain related to colon cancer. The patient reported she was taking only one to two doses daily in previous months, but now the pain has become severe and over the past several days, 10–12 doses were needed daily for comfort. The correct dose of long-acting oxycodone is

a. 30 mg every 12 hours

b. 10 mg every 8 hours

c. 10 mg every 12 hours

d. 30 mg every 8 hours

140. A 70-year-old hospice patient who has end-stage renal disease experiences dyspnea, fatigue, edema, and pain. The nurse should

  a. Explain that after this exacerbation, the patient will return to a lower level of function

  b. Advise the patient to use energy conservation techniques when active

  c. Take steps to prepare for the patient's approaching death

  d. Advise the patient to elevate feet above the level of the heart and limit fluid intake

141. A 63-year-old home care hospice patient has a primary terminal diagnosis of metastatic breast cancer and concomitant diagnoses of osteoarthritis, hyperthyroidism, atrial fibrillation, and gastric esophageal reflux disease. The patient has reported poor appetite and dysphagia for the past 2 weeks. During a home care visit today, the patient is confused, profusely sweating, and has had diarrhea for the past 24 hours. Her vital signs are as follows: temperature: 101.9 F, heart rate (HR) = 124, respiration: 26, blood pressure (BP) = 186/110 mmHg. The most important assessment question for the nurse to ask the patient and/or family is

  a. Has she been taking her medications?

  b. Do you have any nitroglycerin in the house?

  c. Have you taken any antidiarrheal medication?

  d. Do you have a physician (or provider) order for life-sustaining treatment (POLST) in the home?

142. A patient with advanced dementia and throat cancer with metastasis to the lung and bone has developed a pleural effusion. The nurse should develop interventions to address which of the following goals?

  a. Reduction of friction rub

  b. Palliation of symptoms

  c. Chest tube placement

  d. Confirmation of the pleural effusion

143. The most common site of metastasis for lung cancer is

  a. Bone

  b. Lymph nodes

  c. Spine

  d. The opposite lung

144. A palliative care patient in a long-term care facility whose pain in managed via continuous subcutaneous morphine infusion

exhibits jerking movements in her arms and legs. The appropriate action for the nurse to take is

a. Prepare a crash cart

b. Administer naloxone

c. Arrange transport to a hospital

d. Administer lorazepam

145. A palliative care patient has a history of focal seizures. The nurse should prepare for this possibility by

a. Padding the side rails on the bed

b. Teaching the patient to ambulate only with assistance

c. Placing an airway at the bedside

d. Obtaining an order for lorazepam

146. Self-care is especially important for hospice nurses because it

a. Decreases risk for burnout

b. Balances emotional strength

c. Decreases work stress

d. Improves work performance

147. Opioid use stimulates the chemoreceptor trigger zones, resulting in

a. Constipation

b. Nausea and vomiting

c. Respiratory depression

d. Centralized pain relief

148. Which statement by a patient who smokes who has supplemental oxygen in the home should be corrected by the nurse?

a. "I should not smoke near my oxygen concentrator."

b. "It is not too late to consider quitting smoking."

c. "I can smoke while I wear my oxygen."

d. "I need to be careful when walking around the tubing."

149. A palliative care patient is experiencing nausea and vomiting related to chemotherapy treatment. The most appropriate pharmacologic intervention is

a. Octreotide

b. Scopolamine

c. Ondansetron

d. Dronabinol

150. The primary cause of liver disease is
    a. Alcohol abuse
    b. Opioid addiction
    c. Hepatitis C
    d. Gall bladder disease

24

Answers With Rationales

■ **CHAPTER 3**

1. **A:** For patients who have cancer, the trajectory of the disease involves a period of relative wellness followed by a predictable and irreversible decline. During the period of decline, the patient may experience symptoms of weight loss, gradual decreased ability to engage in activities of daily living, and a progressive decline in overall condition.

2. **A:** The trajectory associated with dementia involves a gradual functional decline over a period of 6 to 8 years without acute exacerbation. However, patients may fall subject to acute illnesses, such as pneumonia or cardiac events, that unexpectedly lead to their death.

3. **C:** The FAST scale (Reisberg, 1987) is used for patients who have dementia (see Figure 3.2). The FAST scale accounts for signs of dementia such as the patient's ability to perform activities of daily living, ambulate, manage tasks, and in the later stages identifies incontinence and muscular problems associated with the progression of dementia.

4. **D:** A physician (or provider) orders for life-sustaining treatment (POLST) form, called a medical orders for life-sustaining treatment (MOLST) form in some states, is created during a conversation with a medical provider and lays out the patient's end-of-life wishes (see Figure 3.6). It is considered a medical order and is most useful in times of emergency. Typically, POLST or MOLST forms are intended for patients who have a life expectancy of 1 year or less (Bomba et al., 2012). The forms are often printed on brightly colored paper and the order remains in place regardless of the care setting (e.g., hospital, long-term care facility).

5. **B:** A living will is a type of advance directive in which patients specify which treatments they would want if they could no longer express their own wishes (see Figure 3.7).

6. **B:** Palliative care is a holistic approach to promoting patient comfort within the limits of the disease process. It is a specialty practice centered on the management of symptoms that can be incorporated into the plan of care at any stage of the disease process. Within the palliative care model, an interdisciplinary team plans interventions to meet the patient's physical, emotional, spiritual, and psychological needs. Palliative care should be introduced to the patient and family at the time of diagnosis of a serious or potentially terminal condition. Since palliative care often bears the connotation of end-of-life care, education is needed so that the patient and family understand that palliative care is a type of supportive care that can be utilized in every care setting. If a patient's condition deteriorates to the point that palliative and end-of-life care will be the sole focus, then hospice care should be considered if it is consistent with the patient's goals (see Table 3.1).

7. **C:** The disease trajectory for dementia involves a gradual functional decline over a period of 6 to 8 years without acute exacerbation. A score of 7 or above on the FAST scale indicates advanced disease. Other signs of decline such as weight loss, infection, or aspiration should also be documented to support the patient's need for hospice services.

8. **B.** To be eligible for hospice services with a diagnosis of cancer, clinical signs of malignancy and or metastatic disease should be demonstrable. The patient's Palliative Performance Scale score should be ≤70%, and the patient should not be undergoing curative treatment for the disease. Further, declines in condition, such as weight loss, cachexia, and complications of the disease, should be documented to support eligibility for hospice services (see Figure 3.9).

9. **D:** The patient in the scenario is asking about curative measures, which is not consistent with hospice philosophy. Therefore, the nurse should arrange a meeting with the patient and key members of the interdisciplinary team to clarify the patient's goals of care and treatment wishes. Although the hospice nurse is skilled at leading conversations regarding goals of care, it is always desirable for the interdisciplinary team to collaborate when clarifying patients' end-of-life wishes.

10. **A:** Palliative care is aimed at symptom management in any care setting. Unlike hospice care, the patient may or may not be terminally ill at the time of referral. In the scenario presented in the question, the nurse should arrange for a palliative care consult so that the patient's symptoms can be expertly managed and family support can be provided by the interdisciplinary team.

11. **B:** Usually signs of imminent death occur in clusters rather than as individual symptoms. However, individual symptoms may appear one by one over time in some patients. End-of-life symptoms depend on the terminal diagnosis, other concomitant illnesses, and the patient's overall condition. Common signs of approaching death include (Berry & Griffie, 2015; Kehl & Kowalski, 2012; Kerr et al., 2014) confusion and sometimes visions of loved ones who have passed away, terminal agitation followed by increased somnolence, often leading to unresponsiveness, changes in respirations including apnea, Cheyne–Stokes respirations, agonal breathing, and terminal secretions, temporal wasting, dehydration, pain, cyanosis of extremities or lips, cooling of extremities, hypertension leading to hypotension, peripheral edema, mottling, and incontinence, oliguria, and eventually anuria. As death approaches, patients begin to withdraw from their loved ones and lose the ability to communicate verbally. Despite this, hearing is thought to remain intact. In the final hours, the patient will likely exhibit profound weakness and fatigue, gaunt and pale appearance, withdrawal from others, reduced awareness of surroundings, glassy or cloudy eyes, inability to swallow food, liquids, or medications, little to no urine output, agonal respirations and/or apnea, unresponsiveness, and tachycardia (Berry & Griffie, 2015; Bodtke & Ligon, 2016).

12. **B:** The nurse should be taught that oropharyngeal suctioning may help to remove secretions that cause the sound of the "death rattle." But deep suctioning is not a recommended intervention for terminal secretions. Rather, repositioning the patient as needed and suctioning the oropharynx may help to decrease the sound of secretions moving with respirations. If the secretions are causing dyspnea or distress to the patient, anticholinergic medications such as hyoscyamine (sq), atropine (sl), glycopyrrolate (SL), or scopolamine (topically or sq) can be used to dry excess secretions.

13. **D:** The patient described in the question stem is exhibiting signs of approaching death. The family should be prepared for the symptoms that may follow. Specifically, caregivers should be taught to assess nonverbal indications of pain and discomfort. Pain in the patient's final days is often related to tumor pressure, gastrointestinal distress, frailty, joint stiffness, immobility, or bladder distention.

14. **C:** The patient in the question stem is experiencing increased respiratory section, thus the family should be taught to reposition the patient to reduce dyspnea and to move secretions. If the secretions are causing dyspnea or distress to the patient, anticholinergic medications such as hyoscyamine (sq), atropine (sl), glycopyrrolate (SL), or scopolamine (topically or sq) can be used to dry excess secretions. The nurse should make arrangements to have one of these

medications on hand in the home to quickly treat discomfort related to respiratory secretions.

15. **B:** The patient in the question stem is experiencing labored breathing and should be repositioned to promote comfort. Supplemental oxygen is not effective for decreasing respiratory effort at the end of life. There is no indication of increased respiratory secretions; therefore the administration of an anticholinergic medication or suction is not necessary.

16. **A:** In hospice patients, oral fluid intake should be encouraged for as long as possible. When the patient is no longer able to tolerate fluids, the hospice team should work closely with the family to determine if supplemental hydration is warranted. Most often, in the terminal phase, additional fluids are not necessary. However, there is some evidence that hypodermoclysis, the provision of subcutaneous fluids, may ease some end-of-life symptoms such as delirium, opioid toxicity, agitation, and dehydration when used judiciously. The patient in the question stem is stated to appear to be comfortable and therefore no intervention is necessary to ease symptoms. Ice chips should not be offered since the patient is experiencing dysphagia. If the family's wishes for supplemental hydration are related to cultural or religious beliefs or because the systoms are causing them distress, hypodermoclysis or proctoclysis can be used to provide supplemental fluids. IV fluid replacement in hospice patients is not recommended. There is no indication that the patient is experiencing symptoms that cannot be managed in the home; the patient does not need to be transferred to an inpatient hospice setting.

17. **D:** In a patient who is actively dying, oral extended-release morphine should be changed to either parenteral form or immediate-release liquid. Oral calcium supplementation is not considered to be necessary during the dying process. Lactulose is used as a laxative and to treat hepatic encephalopathy. But, administration of Latulose is not necessary during the dying process and the patient is no longer able to swallow the liquid. The scopolamine should be continued because increased respiratory secretions are common during the dying process and the medication can be delivered topically or subcutaneously.

18. **C:** The patient in the question stem has skin breakdown consistent with the initial onset of a Kennedy ulcer. A Kennedy ulcer, also called a Kennedy terminal ulcer, is a form of decubiti that develops suddenly in patients who are near death. The ulcer may begin as a discoloration or a blister and then quickly deteriorate to a full-thickness ulcer. The ulcer usually appears on the sacral area and is often pear or butterfly shaped. The family members should be taught that, despite intervention, the skin may begin to breakdown

very quickly. The nurse should recommend frequent repositioning and interventions that promote comfort.

19. **A:** The patient in the question stem is experiencing terminal secretions, a condition which is generally not thought to be painful or disturbing to the patient. Repositioning the patient as needed and suctioning the oropharynx may help to decrease the sound of secretions moving with respirations. If the secretions are causing dyspnea or distress to the patient, anticholinergic medications such as hyoscyamine (sq), atropine (sl), glycopyrrolate (SL), or scopolamine (topically or sq) can be used to dry excess secretions. The nurse must first determine if the secretions seem to be causing the patient distress before implementing interventions.

20. **D:** In the case of esophageal varices or tumors, the nurse must take steps to prepare for the possibility of terminal hemorrhage. This event is not usually painful for the patient, but the visual imagery is very distressing for families and caregivers. Hemostatic dressings may be used in cases of chronic bleeding. For acute bleeding, dark-colored towels and blankets should be available to minimize the visual impact. Sedation may be necessary if the patient is awake and alert. The family will need focused attention and emotional support throughout the hemorrhagic event.

▪ CHAPTER 4

1. **D:** The staging of tumors commonly follows the tumor, node, and metastasis (TNM) system. The presence, absence, or extent of the primary tumor (T) is noted. Lymph node involvement, if present, is denoted by the letter N. If metastasis is present, its extent is denoted by the letter M (see Table 4.2). T1, T2, T3, and T4 refer to the size and/or extent of the main tumor. The higher the number after the T, the larger the tumor or the more it has grown into nearby tissues. T's may be further divided to provide more detail, such as T3a and T3b. N0 means that there is no evidence of cancer in nearby lymph nodes. M0 indicates that there is no evidence that cancer has spread to other parts of the body. Therefore, a patient whose cancer is staged as T2, N0, M0 has no evidence of metastasis, no evidence of lymph node involvement, but the primary tumor has been identified and is measurable.

2. **B:** The staging of tumors commonly follows the tumor, node, and metastasis (TNM) system. The presence, absence, or extent of the primary tumor (T) is noted. Lymph node involvement, if present, is denoted by the letter N. If metastasis is present, its extent is denoted by the letter M (see Table 4.2). T1, T2, T3, and T4 refer to the size and/or extent of the main tumor. The higher the number after the T, the larger the tumor or the more it has grown into nearby tissues.

T's may be further divided to provide more detail, such as T3a and T3b. N0 means that there is no evidence of cancer in nearby lymph nodes. M1 indicates that there is evidence that the cancer has spread to other parts of the body. Therefore a patient whose cancer is staged as T1, N0, M1 has evidence of metastasis, no evidence of lymph node involvement, but the primary tumor has been identified and is measurable.

3. **D:** The staging of tumors commonly follows the tumor, node, and metastasis (TNM) system. The presence, absence, or extent of the primary tumor (T) is noted. Lymph node involvement, if present, is denoted by the letter N. If metastasis is present, its extent is denoted by the letter M (see Table 4.2). T0 indicates that there is no evidence of tumor. N0 means that there is no evidence of cancer in nearby lymph nodes. M0 indicates that there is no evidence that cancer has spread to other parts of the body. So a patient whose report indicates T0, N0, M0 has no sign of tumor, lymph node involvement, or metastasis.

4. **A:** The term localized means that cancer cells are present but have not spread to other parts of the body.

5. **C:** The patient in the question scenario has multiple comorbidities and is advanced in age. Although the patient is most likely eligible for hospice, due to having end-stage pulmonary disease and cancer, the patient's goals of care must be clarified before the appropriate type of care can be determined. The nurse should not offer false assurance of curative treatments or ask the patient to determine her own eligibility for surgical procedures. Therefore the most appropriate response is the one that helps the nurse to understand the patient's goals of care.

6. **D:** Chemotherapy can decrease the functioning of bone marrow. Blood cells formed in the bone marrow are affected, leading to anemia, which increases risk for fatigue, lethargy, tachycardia, dizziness, and/or chest pain. The patient in the question scenario has numerous chronic diseases and therefore is at risk for anemia of chronic disease. Chemotherapy can further exacerbate this issue. The other options are less serious.

7. **C:** The patient in the question is experiencing symptoms of brain metastasis, which include morning headache; headache that resolves with vomiting; seizures; changes in vision, hearing, or speech; decreased appetite; nausea/vomiting; changes in mood, personality, behavior, or ability to focus on tasks; balance changes; muscle weakness; and changes in sleep patterns (see Table 4.3).

8. **B:** The two main risk factors for thyroid cancer are exposure to radiation to the head or neck during childhood and genetic predisposition (see Table 4.3).

9. **D:** In metastatic spinal cord compression, the spread of bony metastasis into the spine causes displacement of the spinal nerves and/or vertebral collapse. Acute-onset back pain, paraplegia or tetraplegia, and cauda equine syndrome (neurological deficits in the lower extremities, bowel or bladder incontinence, lower back or leg pain, saddle anesthesia) are common symptoms. Facial swelling would not be an expected finding.

10. **A:** The most common sites of metastasis for lung cancer are the opposite lung, adrenal gland, bone, brain, and liver. Thus, when a patient experiences new-onset symptoms of lung cancer, such as cough/hemoptysis, chest pain, malaise, weight loss, dyspnea, or hoarseness, the symptoms are most likely related to metastasis to the opposite lung.

■ CHAPTER 5

1. **A:** Stimulation of the sympathetic nervous system causes mental alertness, increased heart rate and increased cardiac contractility, bronchodilation, decreased digestion, and peripheral vasodilation.

2. **D:** As amyotrophic lateral sclerosis (ALS) progresses, the patient's speech becomes increasingly impaired, dyspnea becomes more pronounced, and movement impossible. Cognitive impairment is present in some but not all patients (Beeldman et al., 2016). Senses such as touch, hearing, taste, smell, and vision remain largely intact, as does cardiac function (The ALS Association, 2018; Boss & Huether, 2014a). Most patients who have ALS eventually succumb to respiratory failure, which can ensue quickly and unexpectedly. Therefore respiratory distress is most predictive of the terminal stage of the disease.

3. **D:** Although there is no cure for amyotrophic lateral sclerosis (ALS), multiple strategies have been used to both promote comfort and extend the patient's life. The only pharmacological intervention that has been found to extend survival and time to tracheostomy is riluzole. Interventional medical options depend on the patient's goals of care. For example, decisions regarding the use of artificial nutrition, mechanical ventilation, and diaphragm pacing must be considered. Oxygen supplementation does not reduce dyspnea, nor does repositioning. Incentive spirometry may help in the short-term; diaphragm pacing is most effective in overcoming the muscle failure associated with ALS.

4. **B:** Hallmark motor symptoms of Parkinson's disease (PD) are bradykinesia, muscle rigidity, postural instability or unbalance, and resting tremor. Tremor, rigidity, and movement disorder are the three components of the "classic triad" of PD symptoms.

5. **C:** Management of Parkinson's disease usually involves medications such as levodopa, dopamine receptor agonists, catechol-O-methyltransferase inhibitors, selective MAO-B inhibitors, muscarinic receptor agonists, and amantadine (Robertson, 2018), as well as diligent management of symptoms as they arise. Additionally, safety planning is a priority as the patient's ability to ambulate independently becomes compromised.

6. **C:** the cause of death for patients who have muscular dystrophy is most often related to cardiac failure or respiratory failure. Respiratory management involves monitoring respiratory function, assisted coughing, routine assessment of pulse oximetry, determination of candidacy for tracheostomy, if needed, pulmonary function testing, and sleep studies. Extensive discussions regarding advance directives, airway management options (i.e., tracheostomy, ventilator support), goals of care, and preferred place of death must be discussed. As the patient's condition worsens, the family should be prepared for the likelihood that the patient's death will be related to pulmonary arrest or cardiac arrest secondary to pulmonary complications.

7. **A:** Cardiac health is often compromised in patients who have muscular dystrophy. The nurse must frequently assess for signs of heart failure such as marked dyspnea, dependent edema, hypoxia, orthopnea, jugular vein distention, activity intolerance, and marked fatigue. Thus, the nurse is aware that cardiomegaly is an expected finding in patients who have muscular dystrophy.

8. **D:** The nurse should document all goals of care conversations with patients and families in the patients' medical records. In the question stem, the patient's family has stated a desire to forego mechanical ventilation. This critical information should be formalized in writing and may necessitate a meeting with the interdisciplinary team for the development of an advance directive. There is no evidence that the patient should be referred to hospice or that signs of abuse are evident.

9. **B:** Myasthenic crisis requires immediate intervention if the symptoms are to be suppressed. During exacerbations of myasthenia gravis, apheresis and intravenous immunoglobulin therapy are used. Roughly 90% of patients who experience myasthenic crisis require intubation and mechanical ventilation. Therefore, an advance directive should be in place for every patient who has myasthenia gravis so that invasive interventions that are contrary to the patient's stated goals of care are not initiated.

10. **C:** The impairment to nerve signal transmission causes symptomatology related to the affected nerves. Initial symptoms vary depending on the location of the lesions (Brownlee et al., 2017), but often include visual and motor deficits because the optic nerve and motor centers in the brainstem are commonly affected. Other symptoms

include overwhelming fatigue, functional impairment, bowel and bladder incontinence, visual disturbances, dizziness and vertigo, pain, cognitive changes, depression, spasticity, and sexual dysfunction (Kovach & Reynolds, 2015; Schwartz, 2015). Symptoms often occur in clusters. Symptom onset can be categorized as relapsing or progressive. Relapsing MS is generally characterized by an acute episode of "unilateral optic neuritis, a partial myelitis, or a brainstem syndrome" (Brownlee et al., 2017, p. 1337) that occurs over hours or days with peak symptomatology within 4 weeks of onset. Remission is usually spontaneous. Progressive onset of MS symptoms is insidious, occurring over the course of months or even years. Most often, initial presentation involves asymmetric paraparesis, progressive hemiparesis, and cerebellar ataxia. Rarely, blindness or dementia can occur (Brownlee et al., 2017).

■ CHAPTER 6

1. **B:** Patients who have end-stage heart failure are debilitated and experience myriad symptoms such as dyspnea, rales, angina, murmurs, edema, ascites, constipation, orthopnea, nocturia, and paroxysmal nocturnal dyspnea and nocturnal cough. Often the symptoms will be refractory despite traditional interventions. Oliguria is not associated with heart failure.

2. **C:** Heart failure is a "condition in which the heart is unable to generate adequate cardiac output" (Brashers, 2014, p. 1175). This underperformance of the cardiac muscle leads to inadequate perfusion of all organs and tissues.

3. **D:** The patient meets the criteria for hospice admission because her cardiac disease is Class IV of the New York Heart Association (NYHA) for heart failure. That is, she exhibits significant cardiac symptoms even at rest and the inability to carry out minimal activities without dyspnea or angina. The patient also has significant congestive heart failure as documented by an ejection fraction (EF) of ≤20%.

4. **D:** Right heart failure is also called right ventricular failure. Defining characteristics of right heart failure include jugular vein distention, fatigue, ascites, hepatomegaly, splenomegaly, dependent edema, anorexia, gastrointestinal distress, and fluid retention.

5. **D:** The criteria of the New York Heart Association (NYHA) addresses both the functional status of the patient and objective findings of the provider. Consistent with the hospice admission criteria, all hospice patients must meet with NYHA criteria for Class IV heart failure. That is, they exhibit significant cardiac symptoms even at rest and the inability to carry out minimal activities without dyspnea or angina.

6. **C:** New York Heart Association (NYHA) Class III is denoted as marked limitation of physical activity. The patient is comfortable at rest but less than ordinary activity causes fatigue, palpitation, dyspnea, or anginal pain.

7. **A:** Unlike an internal defibrillator, a pacemaker should not be deactivated prior to the patient's death. Deactivation of a pacemaker can result in immediate symptoms related to cardiac disease such as fatigue, dizziness, syncope, dyspnea, and bradycardia.

8. **A:** Sildenafil is a phosphodiesterase 5 (PDE-5) inhibitor. This class of drugs is used in cardiac disease to inhibit the action of PDE-5, thus promoting pulmonary vessel dilation, which combats hypertension.

9. **C:** Patients who have end-stage heart failure are debilitated and experience myriad symptoms such as dyspnea, rales, angina, murmurs, edema, ascites, constipation, orthopnea, nocturia, and paroxysmal nocturnal dyspnea and nocturnal cough. Often the symptoms will be refractory despite traditional interventions. Elevating the patient's head immediately will help to alleviate symptoms. The nurse can then explain that orthopnea is a very common symptom in heart failure patients, check the patient's pulse oximetry, and administer morphine for dyspnea.

10. **B:** Defining characteristics of heart failure include decreased ejection fraction, fatigue with minimal exertion, fluid retention, decreased appetite, dyspnea, arrhythmias, paroxysmal nocturnal dyspnea, cyanosis, tachycardia, orthopnea, pulmonary hypertension, restlessness, and respiratory symptoms such as crackles, wheezing, tachypnea, hemoptysis, and persistent cough.

■ CHAPTER 7

1. **A:** Lung cancer is the most commonly seen pulmonary disease in hospice settings, followed by COPD.

2. **C:** COPD causes dyspnea due to a combination of restricted airways, decreased compliance of alveoli, and air trapping (see Figures 7.1 & 7.2).

3. **B:** Risk factors for COPD include being a current or former smoker, having a history of asthma, age ≥65 years, having American Indian/Alaska Native and multiracial non-Hispanic heritage, female gender, possessing less than a high school education, unemployment, and being divorced, widowed, or separated from spouse. Smoking is the greatest risk factor for COPD.

4. **C:** A definitive diagnosis of COPD can be made only with spirometry. Spirometry reveals the average FEV_1 as well as the FVC. The normal FEV_1/FVC ratio is approximately 70% to 85% and declines

with age due to decreasing lung elasticity. Diagnostic criteria for COPD indicate the diagnosis can be confirmed by the presence of a postbronchodilator FEV_1/FVC <0.70 (GOLD Science Committee, 2017).

5. **D:** Patients who have COPD, particularly end-stage COPD, exhibit a host of symptoms such as increased sputum production, dyspnea, debility due to dyspnea, weight loss due to increased metabolic demands, fatigue due to decreased oxygenation, anxiety and depression, syncope during coughing, rib fractures related to coughing (primarily in frail patients), and cor pulmonale (denoted by ankle edema).

6. **D:** The nurse should assess for signs of abuse because the stem of the question indicates that the patient has multiple caregivers.

7. **C:** All patients who have chronic obstructive pulmonary disease (COPD) should receive education about smoking cessation. Although COPD is incurable, smoking cessation reduces the risk of exacerbation of COPD symptoms. It also reduces the risk of fire due to dropped cigarettes or combustion with supplemental oxygen. Family members should also receive education on reducing the risk of exacerbations of COPD for the patient. The Agency for Healthcare Research and Quality (2012) advises all healthcare professionals to follow the five A's to identify appropriate interventions for smokers. These are Ask, Advise, Assess, Assist, and Arrange.

8. **D:** The nurse should instruct the patient to use albuterol via handheld nebulizer now. It is the only medication listed that will reduce dyspnea, which will then in turn decrease the patient's anxiety. If the patient's anxiety persists after the albuterol is administered, then alprazolam should be taken.

9. **A:** Treatment choices for patients with advanced disease are primarily driven by their goals of care. The other choices may influence their treatment choices but do not provide the overarching framework that goals of care do.

10. **B:** For patients experiencing acute dyspnea, short-acting bronchodilators should be used to rapidly ease symptoms. When symptoms are refractory or severe, opioids should be initiated for dyspnea.

▪ CHAPTER 8

1. **B:** Acute kidney injury (AKI) can manifest in multiple ways, depending on the type and extent of the damage to the renal system, but often includes oliguria, edema, nausea, fatigue, and shortness of breath. AKI can be a consequence of medication toxicity, infection, obstruction of the urinary system, or metabolic diseases.

AKI is often reversible once the cause is identified, although hemodialysis may be necessary for a short period of time. AKI is characterized by the sudden (hours to days) onset of complete lack of kidney function.

2. **D:** Acute kidney injury (AKI) is often reversible once the cause is identified, although hemodialysis may be necessary for a short period of time. AKI is characterized by the sudden (hours to days) onset of complete lack of kidney function. Identification of the cause of AKI requires diagnostic testing, which can be completed in an inpatient setting. Also, AKI can progress quickly. The patient should be transferred to the ED for treatment.

3. **B:** The patient's diagnoses of renal disease and heart failure predispose to fluid volume excess, which can increase blood pressure and cause dyspnea. Because of the potential complications, fluid volume excess is the priority nursing diagnosis.

4. **D:** The kidneys have a significant role in elimination of metabolites. Thus, the dosages of medications should typically be reduced in patients who have renal failure to avoid toxicity.

5. **A:** Albuminuria occurs when albumin, a type of protein normally found in the blood, passes through the kidneys and is identifiable in the urine. Albumin is a large protein molecule that should not be able to pass through the kidneys and into the urine. Therefore, if protein is detected in the urine using a simple urine dipstick test, further investigation using the albumin creatinine ratio (ACR) test may be necessary. The normal result of the ACR is ≤30 mg/g. Results above 30 mg/g may indicate chronic kidney disease (CKD), even if the glomerular filtration rate (GFR) is within normal range (National Kidney Foundation, 2017). Thus, if the patient's ACR results are above normal, consistent follow-up care is recommended. The severity of renal disease can be established using both the GFR and the level of albuminuria (Kidney Disease Improving Global Outcomes, 2013; see Figure 8.2).

6. **D:** Notably, patients may not exhibit signs of chronic kidney disease (CKD) until kidney function "declines to less than 25% of normal when normal adaptive renal reserves have been exhausted" (Doig & Huether, 2014, p. 1364), which corresponds to stage 4 renal failure.

7. **C:** To be eligible for hospice care, patients must decline life-extending or curative interventions such as dialysis or transplantation.

8. **C:** The nurse should make arrangements with the interdisciplinary team to help the patient identify her goals of care. The team can then help the patient choose treatment options that are consistent with her own goals.

9. **A:** The nurse has an obligation to teach the patient about the disease trajectory. Thus the nurse should inform the patient that renal disease typically involves lengthy periods of relative wellness followed by an abrupt change in condition.

10. **C:** Dyspnea is an expected end-of-life symptom that the family should have been taught to expect. Therefore, the nurse should instruct the family on the steps to take to alleviate the patient's dyspnea.

CHAPTER 9

1. **C:** A serious side effect of lactulose is diarrhea, which often causes noncompliance if not addressed. The patient in the question stem is alert and thus it is safe to instruct the patient to hold the next dose of lactulose. The dose of the medication will need to be adjusted so that the patient benefits from the medication without distressing effects.

2. **C:** Pruritus in liver disease often results from "the accumulation of pruritogenic bile acids and bile salts, modulation of itch pathways . . . imbalance between different types of receptors for endogenous opioids, and modulation of the perception of pruritus by serotonin and substance P" (Carrion et al., p. 517).

3. **D:** Chronic liver failure is a sequela of irreversible disease processes such as chronic viral hepatitis (A, B, or C), cancer, nonalcoholic fatty liver disease, or cirrhosis. Without liver transplantation, chronic liver failure (CLF) progresses to end-stage liver disease.

4. **A:** When percussing the abdomen, the nurse expects to hear tympani over most of the abdomen due to the presence of gas in the stomach and intestines. Dullness is heard over solid organs such as the liver, allowing the nurse to approximate the liver borders, which should normally span no more than 10 cm (4 in.) or less.

5. **D:** Ascites indicates a 50% 2-year mortality, with a 6-month median survival rate when it becomes refractory.

CHAPTER 10

1. **A:** Dementia is a form of major neurocognitive disorder, as defined in the *Diagnostic and Statistical Manual of Mental Disorders*, Fifth Edition (*DSM-5*; American Psychiatric Association, 2013). It is most common among those 60 years old or older, with a sharp increase in incidence in those over age 85.

2. **B:** Delirium often has an identifiable cause, such as medication, allergy, pain, dehydration, or infection. When possible, the cause of delirium should be removed and the symptoms will dissipate.

Diagnosis of dementia presumes the exclusion of delirium and other mental disorders as well as the use or abuse of cognition-reducing drugs such as antipsychotics, anticholinergics, opioids, antiepileptics, sedatives, or hypnotics (American Psychological Association, 2013; Brody, 2015).

3. **D:** The criteria for admission to hospice for dementia specify that the patient must be stage 7 or beyond according to the Functional Assessment Staging (FAST) scale **and** have one or more of the following conditions: aspiration pneumonia, septicemia, pyelonephritis, multiple pressure ulcers that are stage 3 or 4, recurrent fever, or other significant condition that suggests limited prognosis. The patient's history should also reflect the inability to maintain sufficient fluid and calorie intake in the past 6 months (10% weight loss or albumin <2.5 gm/dL).

4. **C:** The patient in the question stem is unresponsive to verbal or tactile stimuli and can thus be deemed comatose.

5. **C:** The criteria for admission to hospice for dementia specify that the patient must be stage 7 or beyond according to the Functional Assessment Staging (FAST) scale **and** have one or more of the following conditions: aspiration pneumonia, septicemia, pyelonephritis, multiple pressure ulcers that are stage 3 or 4, recurrent fever, or other significant condition that suggests limited prognosis. The patient's history should also reflect the inability to maintain sufficient fluid and calorie intake in the past 6 months (10% weight loss or albumin <2.5 gm/dL). Weight loss of two pounds over the course of 3 months is not indicative of malnutrition. A stage 1 ulcer on the heel is not part of the criteria for admission to hospice for dementia.

▪ CHAPTER 11

1. **C:** Hypothyroidism can be medically managed with levothyroxine 1 to 2 mg/kg/d. But, when the patient is actively dying, discontinuation of the medication will not harm patient.

2. **A:** Hyperthyroidism results from overproduction of T_4 and/or T_3. Most (60%–80%) of patients who have hyperthyroidism have Graves' disease. Graves' disease is an autoimmune disorder that causes destruction of the thyroid-stimulating hormone (TSH) receptors on thyroid follicular cells.

3. **C:** Hyperthyroidism results from overproduction of T_4 and/or T_3. Most (60%–80%) patients who have hyperthyroidism have Graves' disease. Medical treatment involves antithyroid medications such as methimazole or propylthiouracil. Beta-blockers are used to control adrenergic symptoms such as nervousness, irritability, fine tremor, and muscle weakness.

4. **B:** Type 1 diabetes mellitus occurs most frequently in children and adolescents and has a genetic component. However, genetic predisposition does not account for most cases. In fact, 80% of patients with type 1 diabetes mellitus do not have a family history of the disease.

5. **C:** Wound healing is often delayed in patients who have diabetes due to inflammation and altered glucose levels (Salazar et al., 2016).

CHAPTER 12

1. **D:** The chronicity and incurability of HIV contributes to anxiety and depression. Many antidepressants and anxiolytics are available that can be used in conjunction with antiretroviral therapy. Statements that allude to a desire for death or to thoughts of self-harm are related to depression. The nurse should take immediate action to ensure the patient's safety.

2. **B:** Compliance with the treatment regimen is the highest priority for patients who have HIV. In order to reap the full benefit of pharmacological treatment (see Table 12.1), the patient must strictly adhere to the prescribed treatment regimen or risk viral devastation of the immune system. In fact, adherence to antiviral medications is so important that it is considered the most significant predictor of positive long-term prognosis (Gorman, 2015). Compliance is related to the complexity of the drug regimen, the severity of the patient's symptoms, younger age of the patient, presence of mental illness, and the availability of a support network (Gorman, 2015).

3. **D:** Any patient who reports exposure to HIV should be screened for infection. Screening of at-risk individuals is possible using rapid blood or sputum testing. The results from these tests are available within 5 to 40 minutes. Although rapid testing is useful for screening, positive results from these tests must be confirmed through conventional methods.

4. **C:** The nurse in the question stem overheard a patient stating erroneous information regarding their potential for disease transmission. The nurse must correct the patient's misperception immediately to prevent harm to others.

5. **C:** The hallmark characteristic of HIV, as with other immune deficiency disorders, is the patient's tendency to present with infections that are normally not pathogenic, such as *Pneumocystis jirovecii* (formerly called *Pneumocystis carinii*), widespread and recurrent candida infections, cytomegalovirus, and others. Patients who have not been diagnosed with HIV but test positive for opportunistic pathogens should be screened for HIV.

6. **D:** The nurse should provide teaching on the risk for transmission of HIV through needle sharing.

7. **B:** Because the patient has a compromised immune system, he should avoid exposure to potential infection. The activity that bears the highest risk for exposure to infections is the day-care setting since young children easily transmit colds and other infections to each other.

8. **A:** Compliance with the treatment regimen is the highest priority for patients who have HIV. In order to reap the full benefit of pharmacological treatment (see Table 12.1), the patient must strictly adhere to the prescribed treatment regimen or risk viral devastation of the immune system. In fact, adherence to antiviral medications is so important that it is considered the most significant predictor of positive long-term prognosis (Gorman, 2015). Compliance is related to the complexity of the drug regimen, the severity of the patient's symptoms, younger age of the patient, presence of mental illness, and the availability of a support network (Gorman, 2015).

9. **C:** The symptoms that the patient is experiencing (fatigue and dry mouth) are common in opioid-naïve patients. The side effects will dissipate over time as the patient develops a tolerance to the effects of the medications.

10. **D:** During the dying process, disorientation is common. The patient's family should be assured that no intervention is needed and emotional support should be provided.

▪ CHAPTER 13

1. **C:** Visceral pain is related to injury to an organ or the viscera. It is usually described as achy, dull, or crampy and often radiates away from the site of injury.

2. **D:** The first question that the nurse should ask the patient is whether there are any other symptoms associated with her pain. Associated symptoms lead the nurse to narrow down possible causes of the pain. Then the nurse should ask when the pain began and whether the patient took any actions to decrease the pain. If the assessment questions warrant it, the nurse would then ask if the patient had a cholecystectomy.

3. **C:** The patient is seen in a palliative care clinic for management of symptoms related to COPD. The pain that the patient described may indicate a serious medical problem such as a cardiac event or cholecystitis. The patient should be advised to go to the ED for further evaluation.

4. **C:** Patients who have neuropathies must be provided with teaching to remain safe from cuts, bruises, burns, and falls that could result from sensory impairment. Safety is the highest priority. The

nurse may inquire about the patient's history of diabetes or teach the patient about foot care after a safety plan is in place.

5. **A:** Neuropathic pain originates in the central or peripheral nervous system and is usually described as shooting, burning, stabbing, tingling, or as pins and needles. There are two types of neuropathic pain: peripheral and central. Peripheral neuropathic pain is typically caused by trauma to the peripheral nerves and can result from diabetic neuropathy, nutritional deficiencies, HIV, or carcinoma.

6. **C:** Psychological well-being is inextricably intertwined with pain. Patients who experience pain, particularly on a long-term basis, are more apt to experience anxiety, depression, and hopelessness. Patients who have chronic pain must focus their attention on planning activities around their pain medications and how they feel on a day-to-day basis, which significantly impacts their quality of life. Reliable and valid measures such as the Patient Health Questionnaire (PHQ-9) depression screening tool (Kroenke et al., 2001) and/or the General Anxiety Disorder (GAD-10) tool (Spitzer et al., 2006) should be used to screen patients for depression or anxiety that can result from unrelenting pain.

7. **A:** Pain expression can be influenced by cultural norms and religious beliefs. Acceptance and expression of pain are learned cultural responses. The hospice nurse must be aware of cultural norms related to pain expression, while also avoiding stereotypes.

8. **B:** The patient described in the question stem has end-stage disease that is interfering with his ability to attend religious services. Thus, the most pertinent nursing diagnosis is social isolation since he is no longer able to participate in his faith community.

9. **D:** The Pain Assessment in Advanced Dementia Scale (PAINAD) is the most appropriate tool to assess pain in patients who have dementia.

10. **C:** Roughly 17% of patients who have advanced cancer have alcohol dependence and about 8% have opioid addiction. Patients who have current or past substance abuse disorder (SUD) require special care and attention because they usually have a more severe pain experience and may require a higher dose of opioid medications to manage their pain (Compton & Chang, 2017).

▪ CHAPTER 14

1. **B:** Neuropathic pain is often described as burning or shooting and can be related to nerve damage or pressure on nerves due to tumor growth (Gilron et al., 2014). Neurological pain is caused by injury or disease of the nervous system. It can result from diagnoses such as multiple sclerosis, HIV and AIDS, multiple myeloma, spinal cord surgery or herniated disc, amyotrophic lateral sclerosis, and others.

2. **D:** Treatment of neuropathic pain involves a multimodal approach, which may include "non-opioids, gabapentinoids, tricyclic antidepressants, and serotonin–norepinephrine reuptake inhibitors (all first-line therapies), as well as anticonvulsants and sodium channel blocking antiarrhythmics" (Groninger & Vijayan, 2014, p. 30). The use of opioids for the treatment of neuropathic pain should be considered a second- or even third-line intervention (Smith, 2012). When opioids are used to treat neuropathic pain, methadone is a good choice (Abrahm, 2014). Clinicians should be aware, however, that if opioids are used in the treatment of neuropathic pain, higher doses of opioids are usually needed for effective treatment (Paice, 2015).

3. **A:** The World Health Organization (WHO) developed the WHO pain ladder to help guide interventions for patients experiencing cancer pain (see Figure 14.1). The stepwise approach indicates that the first step in the management of cancer pain is nonopioid medication with or without adjuvant therapies. Adjuvant therapies may include nonsteroidal anti-inflammatory drugs (NSAIDs), COX-2 inhibitors, muscle relaxants, psychotropic medications, antidepressants, antiepileptic drugs, anxiolytics, sedative/hypnotics, amphetamine, antiarrhythmics, calcium channel blockers, ketamine, lidocaine, capsaicin, tramadol, botulinum toxin, and other miscellaneous drugs (Shanti et al., 2012).

4. **C.** Nociceptive pain originates in the peripheral and nociceptive fibers and may involve both physical and psychological dimensions (Zaki et al., 2016). Nociceptive pain is generally categorized as either somatic or visceral. One common source of somatic pain in adults is arthritis pain (Arthritis Foundation, 2018). Other sources of somatic pain in terminally ill patients may include skin or connective tissue damage, such as may occur with a fall or from decubiti. Somatic pain is generally experienced as sharp and localized but can also manifest as dull and diffuse, depending on the source of the pain. Ibuprofen is the best choice for treating the pain described in the question because it decreases inflammation as well as pain. The other options do not have an anti-inflammatory effect.

5. **A:** For most patients, oral administration of an opioid is the most effective and least invasive route. Buccal, transdermal, sublingual, subcutaneous, or rectal routes are possibilities when the oral route is not an option. Administration routes that are invasive or painful, such as intramuscular (IM) or peripheral IV, should be avoided (Paice, 2015). However, if a patient already has a peripherally inserted central catheter (PICC line) or another type of central venous catheter (CVC) in place, it can be used if parenteral medications are needed, such as when pain is severe and/or escalating.

6. **B:** Patients generally develop a tolerance to most side effects of opioids, except constipation. Some patients will experience a

pseudoallergy, which manifests as an allergic reaction to the opioid, such as pruritus (Zhang et al., 2018). However, true allergic reactions to opioids are rare. When pseudoallergy occurs, the nurse should carefully monitor the patient, but intervention is not necessary unless it appears that a true allergic reaction is manifesting.

7. **D:** The conversion guideline for converting an opioid from the oral to route parenteral is roughly 3:1.

8. **C:** When patients are using long-acting pain medications, there is a possibility that they will still experience pain from time to time throughout the day. Therefore, a short-acting (immediate-release) opioid should be prescribed along with the long-acting opioid. When possible, the breakthrough medication should be from the same class of opioid analgesics as the long-acting opioid (Kishner, 2018). To calculate the correct dose of the breakthrough medication, 10% to 20% of the total daily dose of the long-acting opioid should be prescribed for use every 1 to 2 hours for pain (Bodtke & Logon, 2016). The actual amount of the breakthrough dose prescribed will depend on several factors, but as with all opioid prescribing decisions, a lower dose should be used and then titrated upward if necessary.

9. **C:** Patients who require more than three to four breakthrough doses of pain medication while on a long-acting pain medication should have the doses of both medications increased. The number of breakthrough doses needed daily by the patient in the question indicates that the patient's pain is not well controlled. Both the long-acting and short-acting medications should be increased using the appropriate calculation.

10. **D:** Patients who are receiving parenteral opioids for pain management may experience breakthrough pain, just as patients taking oral opioids do. The correct dose of a parenteral breakthrough medication is roughly 50% to 100% of the hourly rate given every 15 minutes as needed (Bodtke & Ligon, 2016). Therefore, the correct breakthrough dose for a patient receiving IV hydromorphone at a rate of 4 mg/hr is 2 mg of hydromorphone q15 minutes PRN.

■ CHAPTER 15

1. **A:** Opioids slow gastric and intestinal motility, which leads to constipation. The body cannot develop a tolerance to this side effect. For some patients, the constipation can be so severe that they discontinue opioid use. Therefore, it is necessary to implement a bowel regimen for every patient taking opioids, which should include both a stool softener (to increase water content of the stool) and a laxative (to increase intestinal motility). In some cases, a prescription medication, such as methylnaltrexone (Relistor), may be necessary

to alleviate opioid-induced constipation. Methylnaltrexone is an opioid receptor agonist, which means that it blocks the effects of opioids in the intestinal tract but not the pain-relieving effects of the opioid. It can be administered orally or subcutaneously.

2. **C:** Patients who are opioid-naïve are at greatest risk for oversedation, especially when the dose is titrated upward. Caution is also required when using opioids with patients who have difficulty clearing the drug, such as geriatric patients or those who have renal dysfunction. Most patients are usually able to develop a tolerance to opioid-induced sedation, but it is a serious concern because it may lead to respiratory depression.

3. **D:** Myoclonus, which is manifested by jerking movements in the patient's arms and legs, is one of the first and most common manifestations of opioid-induced neurotoxicity. Management of opioid-induced neurotoxicity is aimed at reversing the mechanism, so reducing the dose of the opioid or rotating to a different opioid is recommended. Clonazepam, midazolam agents, benzodiazepines, baclofen, or dantrolene can be used for treating myoclonus (Abrahm, 2014; Walker, 2016).

4. **A:** The primary intervention for the reversal of opioid-induced respiratory depression is naloxone.

5. **B:** Each patient's level of pain should be assessed prior to any intervention, and then again approximately 1 hour after the intervention. Even when a patient appears to be relatively comfortable, pain should be evaluated at least every 8 hours using an appropriate pain scale (Song et al., 2015). Each assessment and intervention should be carefully documented in the patient's record.

▪ CHAPTER 16

1. **B:** Dysphagia is difficulty swallowing, which increases the patient's risk for aspiration. Patients who have dysphagia may exhibit choking with eating or drinking, drooling, heartburn, pain behind the sternum, and/or hoarseness (American Speech-Language-Hearing Association, 2018). Nurse-initiated interventions such as proper head and neck positioning, slow introduction of foods and liquids, modification of medication administration, and dysphagia screenings are effective in reducing aspiration pneumonia and other adverse outcomes. The first step that the nurse should take is to conduct a swallowing screen to determine the need for further evaluation. There is no evidence in the stem of the question that indicates that the patient needs to be suctioned. Diet recommendations are not nurse initiated.

2. **B:** A patient's level of consciousness may change due to disease progression, metabolic changes, or structural issues, such as

tumor growth. When a patient's level of consciousness is altered, responses to verbal or tactile stimuli may be delayed or absent. When patients become disoriented, they first become disoriented to time, then to place, and then to person.

3. **B:** Paresthesias are abnormal sensations such as tingling, pins and needles, or burning. Paresthesias can result from nerve impingement or compression, but usually resolve when the pressure is relieved.

4. **A:** Thus, the patient's position should be changed to alleviate the pressure on the nerve.

5. **D:** Nursing interventions for patients experiencing seizures involve protecting the patient's airway, ensuring patient safety throughout the seizure, suctioning as needed, maintaining a calm disposition, and administering lorazepam 2 mg IV. Lorazepam may be repeated up to a total dose of 0.1 mg/kg and infused no faster than 2 mg/min; or phenytoin IV, 15 to 20 mg/kg, may be administered not more than 50 mg/min (following the administration of the lorazepam). As an alternative to phenytoin, valproic acid may be used at a rate of 6 mg/kg/min up to a total dose of 30 mg/kg followed by a maintenance dose of 1 to 2 mg/kg/hr. The highest priority is protecting the patient's airway.

6. **C:** Spinal cord compression (SCC) is a medical emergency that occurs when the thecal sac is compressed by surrounding vertebrae at the level of the spinal cord or cauda equina. The compression causes neurological dysfunction and sometimes irreparable damage (Bobb, 2015). SCC typically manifests as sudden back pain that can be localized, referred, or radicular (Kuriya & Dev, 2016). The pain is worse when the patient is lying down and is relieved when the patients stands. If these symptoms are accompanied by bowel or bladder incontinence, spinal cord compression should be suspected in patients with cancer until proven otherwise (Bobb, 2015). In patients who have cauda equina syndrome, saddle numbness occurs with decreased urethral or rectal tone (Kuriya & Dev, 2016).

7. **C:** Early signs of increased intracranial pressure (ICP) include restlessness, altered consciousness, blurred vision, severe headache, nausea and vomiting, behavioral changes, diminished level of consciousness, fever, and lethargy (Johns Hopkins Medicine, 2018; Weaver, 2015). If interventions are not taken, or are not effective in decreasing increased ICP, hemiplegia or hemiparesis can occur with decorticate and then decerebrate posturing. If the oculomotor nerve becomes compressed, the pupils will stop reacting and will become fixed and dilated. A late sign of increased ICP is Cushing's triad, which involves bradycardia, irregular respirations, and an increase in systolic blood pressure while diastolic blood pressure remains unchanged. If late signs of increased ICP are noted, the patient's prognosis is poor (Weaver, 2015).

8. **A:** For patients who are at risk for bleeding due to esophageal varices, internal hemorrhage, or other conditions, dark-colored towels should be available to reduce the visual impact of the bleeding for the patient and caregivers (Kuriya & Dev, 2016).

9. **C:** The patient in the question stem is actively dying and thus interventions to diagnose or treat a potential DVT are not necessary. The most important interventions would be for the nurse to review the goals of care with the patient's family and to help prepare them for the patient's death.

10. **D:** Treatment choices are primarily dependent on the patient's goals of care. From the question stem, it is not possible to determine whether the patient's symptoms are related to a chronic, or perhaps, terminal condition. Therefore the nurse must clarify the patient's desire for medical intervention before recommending any action.

11. **A:** The patient in the question stem is describing signs of superior vena cava syndrome (SVCS). The signs of SVCS are consistent with obstructed drainage from the head, neck, and upper extremities and include facial swelling, especially after recumbency, jugular vein distension, distention of chest veins, upper extremity edema, and ruddy complexion (facial plethora). Diagnosis of SVCS is confirmed through chest x-ray, CT scan, or magnetic resonance angiography (MRA). The nurse should make arrangements for mobile x-ray in the home to diagnose the SVCS. Once confirmed, treatment options include chemotherapy or radiation, steroid use, diuretics, thrombolytics, and possibly stent placement or bypass. Treatment options offered should be consistent with the patient's goals of care. The head of the bed may be raised 45 to 90 degrees to promote drainage from the head and neck. The prognosis for SVCS is fair to poor and ranges from less than 6 months to 2 years.

12. **D:** The most likely cause of the patient's cough s the angiotensin-converting enzyme (ACE) inhibitor. The nurse should contact the prescriber for a change in medication.

13. **C:** Terminal secretions cause a "rattling" noise with each breath that may be distressing to the family or caregivers. However, neither the accumulation of fluid nor the sound produced is thought to be distressing to the patient (Sharfman & Braun, 2017). Repositioning the patient as needed and suctioning the oropharynx may help to decrease the sound of secretions moving with respirations. However, deep suctioning is not recommended. If the secretions are causing dyspnea or distress to the patient, the following anticholinergic medications may be used: hyoscyamine 0.4 to 0.6 mg subcutaneously every 4 hours as needed, *OR* atropine eye drops 1%, 1 to 2 drops sublingually every 8 hours as needed, *OR* glycopyrrolate 1 mg orally or 0.2 to 0.4 mg subcutaneously

or intravenously every 4 to 8 hours as needed (Dudgeon, 2015; Twomey & Dowling, 2013).

14. **B:** In some cases of fecal impaction only a small amount of liquid stool is able to pass by the impacted stool. The presence of a fecal impaction may be confirmed through digital exam of the rectum. If an impaction is present, a bisacodyl or glycerin suppository may be given. If digital disimpaction is necessary, 2% lidocaine gel should be applied to the rectum prior to the procedure. However, digital disimpaction should be avoided if perforation or bleeding are possible outcomes, especially in patients who have tumors or open areas in the perianal area (Bodtke & Ligon, 2016; Nowicki, 2015).

15. **B:** Pharmacologic interventions for hiccups include simethicone 15 to 30 mL PO every 4 hours to decrease gastric distension, baclofen 5 to 10 mg PO every 6 to 12 hours up to 15 to 37 mg daily or midazolam 5 to 10 mg PO every 4 hours to reduce muscle spasms, gabapentin 300 to 600 mg PO TID for its anticonvulsant effects, amitriptyline 10 to 50 mg PO or sertraline 50 to 150 mg PO QID for central nervous system effects, or haloperidol 2 to 10 mg PO/IV/SQ every 4 to 12 hours to block dopamine and alpha-adrenergic receptors (Dahlin & Cohen, 2015; Walker, 2016).

16. **D:** Benzodiazepines, such as lorazepam 0.5 to 2 mg PO/SC/IV every 8 to 12 hours, are useful for treating nausea and vomiting, especially when anxiety is the cause of or exacerbates the nausea and vomiting. Psychological techniques, such as cognitive behavioral therapy, may have a synergistic effect with lorazepam. Using lorazepam rather than another antiemetic for the patient in the question stem serves the dual purpose of treating the nausea and vomiting as well as the anxiety.

17. **C:** Although urinary catheterization is typically advised when urinary retention occurs, the patient in the question stem has prostate cancer, which complicates placement of a urinary catheter. He needs specialized care to treat his symptoms and to alleviate the retention of urine, if possible. Therefore the patient should be transferred to the inpatient hospice setting for 24-hour symptom management.

18. **D:** Bone metastasis is a common cause of pathological fractures in the hospice and palliative care setting. The most common site of pathological fractures is the femur, of which 75% occur in the proximal end (Willeumier et al., 2016). Other common sites of pathological fractures are the tibia, humerus, ribs, and spine. Symptoms of pathological fractures include localized pain and swelling, and possibly numbness in the affected limb.

19. **B:** The patient in the question stem has reported pruritus and so a thorough skin assessment should be conducted to determine if the

patient has any rashes, jaundice, hives, or infestations. This assessment is particularly important since the patient recently returned from an inpatient setting. Morphine allergies are rare, so the nurse should assess for other causes of the itching first.

20. **A:** Controlling wound odor is an important quality of life issue for patients. Wound odor is often related to the presence of necrotic tissue and/or bacterial overgrowth. Metronidazole gel (0.77%–1.0%) can be applied daily for 1 week to reduce microbial growth. Dressings that contain activated charcoal are useful for absorbing wound odors. In wounds that are not expected to heal, povidone iodine can be used to reduce wound odor.

21. **C:** The highest priority is ensuring safety in the home. If the patient and family cannot remain safe, then other interventions need to be implemented to alleviate danger.

22. **C:** Denial is a state of refusal to believe the truth regarding a present situation. Some patients facing end-of-life situations are not able to accept the reality of their illness. Denial is a protective psychological mechanism that shields the patient from the consequences of their illness until they are psychologically ready to cope. Challenging the patient to face a situation that they are not ready to handle may cause increased emotional distress. Therapeutic communication skills such as reflection, active listening, and therapeutic silence are useful when working with patients who express denial. The patient should be calmly reassured that the interdisciplinary team is available for emotional support as needed.

23. **B:** The first step that the interdisciplinary team should take with the patient in the question stem is to clarify the patient's goals of care. Understanding the patient's goals will help the patient, family, and interdisciplinary team to determine which interventions would be most congruent with the patient's wishes. For example, if the goal is to provide short-term fluid replacement for comfort, then a subcutaneous infusion may be offered. If the goal is to initiate long-term therapy, then a gastric tube might be considered.

24. **B:** Patients who have hypercalcemia may exhibit symptoms such as nausea, vomiting, anorexia, weakness, constipation, thirst, and changes in mentation. Diagnosis of hypercalcemia is confirmed through serum analysis. Patients with a serum calcium level >14 mg/dL require urgent intervention. Even in advanced disease, interventions should be started to reverse hypercalcemia for the patient's comfort. Bisphosphonates such as pamidronate and zoledronate are used most frequently. Intravenous hydration, administration of calcitonin, use of bone reabsorption agents such as gallium nitrate or plicamycin, or dialysis may also be considered (Bobb, 2015; Kuriya & Dev, 2016).

25. **C:** Signs and symptoms of delirium include acute onset, fluctuation in symptoms clearly differentiated from dementia, perceptual changes, sleep–wake cycle alterations, delusions, hallucinations, paranoia, and hyperactivity or lethargy (Bodtke & Ligon, 2016).

▪ CHAPTER 17

1. **D:** Advance care planning is a collaborative effort between healthcare providers, patients, and families through which the patients establish their preferences for future medical treatments (Moore, 2007). Patients may express their advance directives through the development of a living will or by designating a medical power of attorney (Wright, 2017). Advance directives are used to guide care only when patients are unable to speak or make decisions for themselves.

2. **B:** A type of advance directive that is used specifically for patients who have a life expectancy of 1 year or less is a physician (or provider) order for life-sustaining treatment (POLST), also called a medical order for life-sustaining treatment (MOLST). The POLST form specifies which treatments the patient would choose to have in the case of a medical emergency. Unlike an advance directive, the POLST can be followed by emergency care providers because it is a medical order.

3. **D:** When establishing goals, the nurse should ensure that every goal is measurable so that results can be observed and quantified. A goal may be somewhat broad in its scope and thus may have associated objectives. Objectives are more specific than goals and can be seen as steps that need to be achieved to meet the overall goal. Both goals and objectives should be developed according to the patient's preferences and should be specific to the situation, measurable, and realistic.

4. **C:** In the absence of a written advance directive, the decision-makers may have to rely on the previously expressed wishes of the patient when making treatment plans. The nurse and the rest of the interdisciplinary team can help facilitate conversations about the patient's care wishes.

5. **C:** Patients who accept the Medicare hospice benefit agree to forego curative treatments. If a patient later decides to pursue curative therapy, then the Medicare hospice benefit must be revoked.

6. **D:** As a result of the Affordable Care Act, Medicare now requires that hospice patients be seen by the hospice nurse practitioner (who must be employed by the hospice) or the hospice medical director prior to the third benefit period. The purpose of the face-to-face

encounter is to verify continued eligibility for hospice services (Centers for Medicare & Medicaid Services, 2015). The nurse practitioner or medical director should work closely with the hospice nurse to review the patient's status when determining ongoing eligibility.

7. **B:** As a result of the Affordable Care Act, Medicare now requires that hospice patients be seen by the hospice nurse practitioner (who must be employed by the hospice) or the hospice medical director prior to the third benefit period. The purpose of the face-to-face encounter is to verify continued eligibility for hospice services (Centers for Medicare & Medicaid Services, 2015). The nurse practitioner or medical director should work closely with the hospice nurse to review the patient's status when determining ongoing eligibility.

8. **C:** The care needs of terminally ill patients may change frequently. Thus the nurse must update and coordinate the plan of care regularly. To ensure proper coordination of care and interdisciplinary collaboration, the plan of care must be reviewed and revised by the interdisciplinary team at least every 15 days (National Hospice and Palliative Care Organization, 2009).

9. **B:** Hospice care necessarily involves the coordination of services and the development of a plan of care by an interdisciplinary team. Core hospice services that are covered by Medicare and Medicaid include physician services, nursing services with 24 hr/d, 7 d/wk availability, medical social services, and counseling. Non-core services must also be provided according to the patient's unique needs, condition, and living arrangements. These services include physical, occupational, and speech therapy, hospice aide services, homemaker services, volunteers, medical supplies and medications related to the terminal illness, and short-term inpatient care for acute or chronic symptom management in a Medicare/Medicaid participating facility (Centers for Medicare & Medicaid Services, 2015a).

10. **D:** Prior to leaving a patient's home after a death, the nurse must dispose of controlled medications by removing medications from their containers, mixing them with cat litter or used coffee grounds, and placing them in a plastic bag or tub to prevent diversion (Nathan & Deamant, 2015). When disposing of fentanyl patches, each patch should be folded in half with the sticky side inward and flushed down a toilet. Labels on medication bottles should be removed and the bottles should be placed in the trash or recycle container, as appropriate. The nurse should document that medications were properly disposed of, following all agency policies and procedures (Wright, 2017).

CHAPTER 18

1. **A:** The serious illness of one member of the family affects all members of the family and alters normal family processes. Primary caregivers may have multiple domains of their lives affected as they take on the care of the patient and also attempt to balance their other responsibilities (Wittenberg et al., 2014). The hospice and palliative care nurse must identify the family needs, connect the family with needed resources, and provide support as needed. When caregiver burnout is suspected, taking steps such as offering respite care may help to alleviate stress.

2. **C:** The Qur'an is the religious text of Islam.

3. **C:** The most effective therapeutic communication technique to exploring the hopelessness expressed by the patient in the question stem is reflection. Using the technique, the nurse reflects his or her understanding of what the patient has said back for further clarification and discussion.

4. **B:** The patient's spiritual needs should be identified by the hospice and palliative care nurse who is responsible for assessing spiritual suffering, meeting the patient's immediate needs, and working with other members of the health team to develop and implement a plan for ongoing support (Wright, 2017).

5. **D:** When working with patients who are making serious medical decisions, every opportunity for support should be afforded to the patient. Therefore, for the patient in the question stem, a meeting should be arranged at a time when the patient's husband can be present.

CHAPTER 19

1. **A:** Grief reactions for a 4-year-old child include searching for the deceased, dreaming of the deceased, feeling fearful and anxious, wanting to be close with loved ones or social withdrawal, changes in appetite, disturbed sleeping patterns, and regression. Appropriate interventions for a 4-year-old child include maintaining routine, spending as much time as possible with the child, speaking calmly and softly, encouraging the child to express himself or herself through play, explaining death as a change, offering snacks and small meals, and explaining that the deceased will not come back (children of this age do not understand finality so they may ask over and over when the decreased will return).

2. **C:** Kübler-Ross's (1969) work on reactions to one's own impending death indicates that dying patients experience denial that death may actually be near as well anger about their own circumstances.

Patients may engage in bargaining with their higher power or with themselves through "if-then" statements such as "if I recover from this illness, then I will never smoke again."

3. **C:** Complicated grief is a form of grief that involves dysfunctional or maladaptive responses that are prolonged and debilitating and interfere with the person's ability to engage in his or her usual activities on an ongoing basis (Prigerson et al., 1995; Stroebe et al., 2013). The following symptoms are associated with complicated grief: longing, yearning, hallucinations, preoccupation with thoughts of the deceased, intrusive thoughts about the deceased, avoidance of people and places that can trigger grief, altered sleep patterns, and failure to adapt to the loss over time (Horowitz et al., 2003; Prigerson et al., 1996; Shear, 2015; Worden, 1991).

4. **C:** After the patient's death, the hospice or palliative care nurse should help the family break the news to loved ones, as necessary, and remain with the family to offer support. Initial assessment of the family's bereavement reactions should be documented and reassessed as needed. The hospice bereavement coordinator or social worker should develop a bereavement plan of care with the input from the interdisciplinary care team. Bereavement care may include visits, cards, invitations to memorial services, and/or support group attendance. Bereavement care should continue to at least 12 months, as required by Medicare.

5. **B:** Common grief reactions in teens include feeling overwhelmed by emotions, which may lead to risky behaviors, attention deficit, anxiety, distraction, feelings of isolation, and withdrawal from family but drawing nearer to friends. Interventions to support grieving teens include being honest and available, maintaining routine, encouraging involvement in services, and locating teen support groups, if available.

▪ CHAPTER 20

1. **D:** When caregiver stress is noted or when financial burden occurs as a result of caregiving, the resources of the interdisciplinary team are needed to help develop a plan to meet the needs of the family.

2. **C:** Caregiver stress can manifest in myriad ways, especially as death nears. The nurse must provide gentle support to family members, reminding them of the goals of care and the patient's wishes.

3. **A:** Verbal instructions should be supplemented with written instructions and the nurse can use the teach-back method to ensure the caregiver's ability to complete skills. With the teach-back method, the nurse teaches the caregiver the skill, and then the caregiver teaches the skill back to the nurse, demonstrating how to perform the skill.

This method ensures that the caregiver can perform the task and understands the steps involved.

4. **C:** The nurse and other members of the interdisciplinary team must monitor for signs of abuse, such as bruising in unusual places, burns, preventable decubiti, dehydration, evidence of sexual abuse, malnutrition, withheld medications, unexplained fractures, urine burns, or inattention to hygiene. As with any case where abuse is suspected, the caregiver should be asked to leave the room when the patient is interviewed.

5. **B:** Nurses are experts at facilitating communication and advocating for patients. To address the needs of the patient in the question stem, the nurse should first determine if the patient's family is aware of his wishes so that further steps can be taken to shift decision-making ability.

▪ CHAPTER 21

1. **D:** The Centers for Medicare & Medicaid Services (2015) outline the services covered by members of the hospice team, including nursing, medical social services, physician, hospice aide and homemaker, and occupational, physical, or speech therapies.

2. **A:** A nurse practitioner may serve as the attending physician if employed by the hospice and provided that the patient has the option to receive care from a physician. Nurse practitioners cannot certify or recertify terminality or prognosis, but may complete the required face-to-face visits to verify continued eligibility for hospice services, if employed by the hospice.

3. **D:** Prior to delegating a task, the RN should determine whether the task can be delegated according to the state practice act, delegate has the appropriate knowledge and training to perform the task, and whether the patient would benefit from delegation of the task.

4. **B:** Patients and caregivers should be encouraged to join in interdisciplinary team meetings. If a patient is unable to attend due to physical restrictions, alternate arrangements should be made to allow the patient to participate.

5. **C:** When patients express their desire to forego curative treatments, the nurse should open a discussion of types of care that provide comfort and aggressive symptom management without disease-modifying treatments, such as hospice and palliative care.

▪ CHAPTER 22

1. **B:** Ethical principles commonly encountered in end-of-life care include *autonomy*: the right to make decisions for oneself; *beneficence*:

the principle of doing the most good—acting kindly and charitably; *confidentiality*: the expectation that patient's private information not be disclosed to anyone without their consent; *justice*: the promotion of good for all; *nonmaleficence*: doing no harm; *paternalism*: restricting the liberty or rights of another, seemingly for their own good; *truthfulness*: providing information with honesty and integrity.

2. **A:** The ethical principle involved in ensuring that some staff nurses are not overburdened with on-call days is justice, the promotion of good for all.

3. **D:** Hospice and palliative care nurses are expected to develop trusting and therapeutic relationships with their patients while maintaining professional boundaries by avoiding communication with patients outside of work hours, providing only services that are included in one's job description, and openly sharing information about the patient with all members of the team (Perry, 2011).

4. **D:** Avoidance is an appropriate conflict resolution strategy when the issue is not significant.

5. **B:** Professional development (PD) involves voluntary learning and continuing development with the purpose of remaining abreast of the skills, trends, and knowledge development in one's field. Examples of PD include teaching and mentoring, ongoing construction and reconstruction of one's professional identity, participating in informal learning opportunities, maintaining professional competencies and developing new competencies, and embracing and engaging in innovative practice changes (Collin et al., 2012).

■ CHAPTER 23

1. **C:** Routine hospice care may be provided anywhere that a patient lives, such as in their own home, the home of a loved one, a long-term care facility, or an assisted living facility.

2. **C:** Pharmacological interventions commonly used include opioids and anxiolytics such as morphine 2.5 to 5 mg PO, SC, or IV every 4 hours as needed; lorazepam 1 to 2.5 mg sublingually every 4 hours as needed; **OR** midazolam 1 to 2 mg PO or SC (may produce a synergistic effect when used in combination with morphine for severe dyspnea; Dudgeon, 2016; Sharfman & Braun, 2017; Walbert, 2016).

3. **A:** A patient's decisions regarding preferred treatment options are dependent on the patient's values, condition, and concomitant illnesses. Opening a conversation about quality of life encourages the patient to talk about how the treatments are interfering with her daily activities and helps the nurse determine whether any nursing interventions could help improve her quality of life.

4. **B:** Therapeutic interventions for constipation include encouraging a high-fiber diet, recommending 2 to 3 L of fluid per day (if fluid restriction is not in place), exercise as tolerated, and the use of laxatives. Senna laxatives may take up to 72 hours for effect;. thus they should be taken preventatively, not when constipation has occurred.

5. **A:** If hospice care is provided to a patient who resides in a long-term care facility (LTCF), care will be provided according to a written agreement that specifies what services the hospice will provide, the hospice team's role in developing the patient's plan of care, how information will be communicated between the hospice team and the staff of the LTCF, how the staff at the LTCF will immediately notify the hospice team regarding significant changes in the patient's condition, any changes that may warrant modification of the plan of care (i.e., the need to transfer the patient from the LTCF, the patient's death), that the hospice assumes responsibility for determining an appropriate end-of-life plan of care, including the level of care, the LTCF's responsibility in providing room and board and meeting the patient's personal care and nursing needs and for coordinating care with the hospice team, the hospice team's responsibility for providing medical direction and medical management for the patient, nursing care, counseling services, social work, supplies, medical equipment, and medicines related to the terminal illness, all other hospice services that are warranted by the patient's life-limiting condition and related issues that the staff of the LTCF may assist in in the provision of necessary treatments and therapies as allowed by state law and facility policies, that the staff of the LTCF will immediately report any alleged violations including mistreatment, neglect, abuse, or misappropriation of the patient's belongings by hospice staff to the hospice administrator, and designate the responsibilities of the hospice and the LTCF staff to provide bereavement services (National Hospice and Palliative Care Organization, 2013).

6. **D:** The patient in the scenario has reported a significant change in pain level. The physician has stated that the patient might become dependent on the opioid. Although patients may develop dependence to pain medications, as well as many other types of medications, this is not a reason to fail to treat pain. The nurse must advocate for proper pain management immediately and alleviate the patient's suffering. This response is based on the American Society for Pain Management Nursing (ASPMN) "position that nurses and other health care providers must advocate for optimal pain and symptom management to alleviate suffering for every patient receiving end-of-life care" (Reynolds et al., 2013, p.172).

7. **A:** Most patients who have amyotrophic lateral sclerosis (ALS) eventually succumb to respiratory failure, which can ensue quickly and unexpectedly. In the terminal phase of ALS, the hospice team must work with the patient and family to make determinations regarding respiratory support and to provide guidance to the family when symptoms rapidly progress.

8. **C:** Patients, families, and sometimes healthcare providers have beliefs about addiction that prevent proper pain management. However, addiction in terminally ill patients who have no prior history of opioid addiction is rare, but not impossible. Addiction is compulsive use of a substance that occurs when it is used in a way other than intended.

9. **A:** The patient in the scenario is experiencing acute choking and the immediate intervention that is needed is to reposition the patient in an attempt to clear the airway. Interventions for dysphagia must be initiated quickly because dysphagia increases the patient's risk for aspiration. Patients who have dysphagia may exhibit choking with eating or drinking, drooling, heartburn, pain behind the sternum, and/or hoarseness (American Speech-Language-Hearing Association, 2018). Dysphagia may occur together with odynophagia (painful swallowing) and may result from tumor growth, neurological disease, or overall disease progression. Other factors that may affect swallowing in adults include poor dentition or ill-fitting dentures (Son et al., 2013). Nurse-initiated interventions such as proper head and neck positioning, slow introduction of foods and liquids, modification of medication administration, and dysphagia screenings are effective in reducing aspiration pneumonia and other adverse outcomes (Hines et al., 2016).

10. **B:** A family caregiver is a relative, partner, friend, or other significant person in the life of the patient. The caregiver takes responsibility for meeting the daily needs of the patient.

11. **B:** Palliative care can take place in many settings, including in acute care settings. Hospice care is provided only for terminally ill patients who choose to forego curative care. See also, Table 3.1 for the differences between hospice and palliative care.

12. **A:** For nonacute bleeding, the nurse should take measures to stop the bleeding and to alleviate the patient's anxiety. Patients and families should be educated regarding the risks for bleeding, especially in relation to liver disease. Interventions to decrease localized bleeding include packing, compressive dressings, topical hemostatics, positioning to decrease blood flow, and astringents (Kuriya & Dev, 2016). In the scenario, the patient's bleeding must be stemmed. Packing the nostril and remaining with the patient is the most appropriate intervention. Tilting the patient's head back

is no longer recommended due to risk of nausea and vomiting from swallowing blood. Placing the patient in a side-lying position and/or obtaining a red towel will not stop the bleeding.

13. **A:** Cardiac failure–related volume expansion and the buildup of uremic toxins is the leading cause of death in patients with chronic kidney disease (CKD; National Kidney Foundation, 2015).

14. **D:** Kübler-Ross's (1969) work on reactions to one's own impending death indicates that dying patients experience denial that death may actually be near as well anger about their own circumstances. Patients may engage in bargaining with their higher power or with themselves through "if-then" statements such as "if I get well again, then I will never smoke again." Depression may set in as patients take in the inevitability of their death and may feel hopeless at times. Ultimately, the patient accepts that death is near and may take time to resolve past grievances or mend damaged relationships, if possible.

15. **B:** Immobility can be related to numerous end-stage diseases or conditions such as pain, edema, ascites, and others. Immobility increases the risk for skin breakdown, physical deconditioning, activity intolerance, and pathological fractures. When a patient becomes immobile temporarily or permanently, frequent assessment of the condition of the skin and of risk factors for ulceration should be conducted regularly using a reliable tool, such as the Braden scale.

16. **C:** Chronic obstructive pulmonary disease (COPD) causes pulmonary artery hypertension, which predisposes patients to cor pulmonale. If cor pulmonale occurs, the patient is at risk for right ventricular failure. Signs of cor pulmonale include peripheral edema, particularly in the feet and ankles, jugular vein distention, hepatomegaly, and a parasternal lift.

17. **A:** Delirium is an "an acute disorder of attention and cognition" (Inouye et al., 2014, p. 911). Signs and symptoms of delirium include acute onset, fluctuation in symptoms clearly differentiated from dementia, perceptual changes, sleep–wake cycle alterations, delusions, hallucinations, paranoia, and hyperactivity or lethargy (Bodtke & Ligon, 2016). Management of delirium involves determining and reversing the cause, if possible. Safety is a nursing priority, so a one-on-one sitter may be needed or the presence of a family member. The environment should be kept quiet and restful, with minimal disturbance. Although there are no specific treatments for delirium, medications such as haloperidol (2 mg) or risperidone (1 mg) have been used to treat symptoms (Bodtke & Ligon, 2016).

18. **D:** Reiki involves the movement of energy to the patient through the reiki practitioner for the purpose of balancing the patient's

energy and chakras. Reiki is often done with a specific intention tailored to the patient's needs. Palliative care patients who received reiki reported that their self-identified concerns were ameliorated through the session and they felt calmer, more relaxed, and more focused afterward (Nyatanga et al., 2018). It has also been found to be beneficial for improving overall quality of life and perceived well-being at the end of life (Henneghan & Schnyer, 2015). Reiki does not require active participation by the client, as yoga and guided meditation do. Deep tissue massage is not appropriate for actively dying patients.

19. **B:** When a patient's level of consciousness is altered, responses to verbal or tactile stimuli may be delayed or absent. Altered levels of consciousness can be categorized as (Boss & Huether, 2014) *confusion:* the patient is unable to think clearly—judgment and decision-making capacity are impaired; *disorientation:* the patient first becomes disoriented to time, then to place, and then to person; *lethargy:* a decrease in spontaneous speech or movement—the patient responds to verbal or tactile stimuli but may be disoriented; *coma:* there is no verbal response to verbal or tactile stimuli—patient has no motor response to noxious or painful stimuli. Comas can categorized as light coma—the patient exhibits purposeful movement in response to verbal or tactile stimuli; coma—the patient may respond to verbal or tactile stimuli, but response is not purposeful; deep coma: the patient is unresponsive to any stimuli—the patient's level of consciousness can be assessed using the Glasgow Coma Scale. In palliative care settings, the Consciousness Scale for palliative care may be used (Kovach & Reynolds, 2015).

20. **A:** The patient in the scenario has described radicular pain. Radicular pain results from compression of the nerve root(s) in the neck or spine. This type of pain is usually related to sciatica, injury, compression, herniated disk, foraminal stenosis, or inflammation. It is often described as sharp, stabbing, and radiating from the spine or neck to the arms or legs. To determine the type of pain that the patient has and to determine the appropriate treatments, the nurse must ask assessment questions that lead to the identification of the type of pain. Since the patient has already given indications of radicular pain, the most appropriate questions are related to radicular pain assessment.

21. **D:** Routine care involves care in the patient's home setting with regular visits from members of the hospice team. Care is coordinated by the interdisciplinary team and visit schedules may be changed as needed to meet the patient's needs.

22. **C:** Diphenhydramine is not recommended for use in older adults due to its anticholinergic side effects. Topical ointments, creams, or

soaks may be used. Systemic steroids may be used on a short-term basis.

23. **A:** The Centers for Medicare & Medicaid Services (2015) outlined the services covered by members of the hospice team, including nursing care, which "require[s] the skills of a registered nurse (RN), or a licensed practical nurse (LPN) or a licensed vocational nurse (LVN), under the supervision of a Registered Nurse, and must be reasonable and necessary for the palliation and management of the patient's terminal illness and related conditions" (p. 19).

24. **B:** Bladder spasms are sudden, painful contractions of the bladder caused by the action of detrusor muscle against a blocked or partially blocked bladder outlet. Blockage of the bladder outlet may be secondary to tumor, blood clots, or a foreign object such as a urinary catheter or stent. An indwelling urinary catheter that is too large, blocked, or kinked may also block the bladder outlet (Gray & Sims, 2015).

25. **D:** In the scenario, the patient is experiencing signs of deep vein thrombosis (DVT). Signs of DVT generally include edema, pain, localized warmth, venous distention, and tenderness when touched (Blevins, 2015; Powers & Jones, 2012). The "gold standard" for diagnosing DVT is the venogram. However, the test is invasive and may lead to complications. A noninvasive test to detect blood flow is the venous Doppler. The test can be conducted easily and painlessly. Blood flow should be evaluated on both extremities for comparison. Pharmacological treatments for DVT may include heparin, low molecular weight heparin, unfractionated heparin, or fondaparinux. Enoxaparin, a low molecular weight heparin should not be used in patients who have acute renal failure. In the scenario, the nurse needs to gather further assessment data, particularly whether blood flow has been compromised. A venogram is invasive and the patient is approaching death. A Doppler, if available, would be useful, but should be conducted on both legs for comparison. Option D enables the nurse to gather information about blood flow and to compare the blood flow in the affected leg to blood flow in the unaffected leg. With this information, the nurse can then discuss goals of care and possible interventions.

26. **A:** When a family caregiver is unable to fulfill their usual roles, the entire family system is strained, which can lead to disharmony. The nurse must assess the strength and resilience of the family unit in terms of affection and appreciation shown for each other, spiritual well-being, commitment to each other, spending time with each other and sharing positive experiences, and demonstrating

the ability to cope with stressors and deal with crises (Sherman & Cheon, 2015).

27. **B:** Roughly 17% of patients who have advanced cancer have alcohol dependence and about 8% have opioid addiction. Patients who have current or past substance use disorder (SUD) require special care and attention because they usually have a more severe pain experience, and those with a history of opioid abuse may require a higher dose of opioid medications to manage their pain (Compton & Chang, 2017).

28. **A:** The patient in the scenario is experiencing spinal cord compression. Pain medication should be administered immediately. The patient should be transferred to bed, with maximum assistance, because lying down relieves pressure on the spine. The patient's provider should be notified of the change in condition, and the nurse should order appropriate interventions that may include corticosteroids. A discussion should occur with the patient and family regarding transfer to the hospice inpatient setting if the patient's pain is not controllable or for acute management of the new symptom.

29. **C:** The most likely cause of the patient's new-onset incontinence is the newly prescribed temazepam (Restoril). Although the medication may assist with sleep, if used in combination with her other medications, it may cause sedation that would inhibit sensitivity to bladder fullness.

30. **D:** The hospice and palliative care nurse should frequently assess the well-being of the caregiver for signs of role strain, such as feeling tired and overwhelmed, insomnia or increased somnolence, unplanned weight changes, irritability, loss of interest in previously enjoyable activities, somatic complaints, and overuse or reliance on drugs (prescription or nonprescription) or alcohol (Mayo Clinic, 2018). Interventions to help alleviate caregiver burden include offering respite care, encouraging the caregiver to accept help from others, setting realistic goals, connecting with others through classes, support groups, or community services, and maintaining healthy living patterns (Mayo Clinic, 2018; Sherman & Cheon, 2015). In the scenario, the caregiver is so overwhelmed by caregiving that he is overusing prescription drugs. Thus, a respite stay at the hospice inpatient unit for the patient should be arranged.

31. **B:** Patients who must rely on others for repositioning in bed or for transfers are at risk for skin shear injuries or friction abrasions (Bates-Jensen & Petch, 2015). Prevention of pressure ulcers is a priority for patients' ongoing comfort and well-being. Active participation in repositioning should be encouraged through the use of side rails and/or trapeze bars that allow the patient to

use upper body strength to assist with repositioning. Immobile patients should be assisted with repositioning frequently to alleviate pressure on bony surfaces. Pillows, cushions, or antipressure devices or mattresses should be used when possible (Bates-Jensen & Petch, 2015).

32. **D:** Spiritual well-being is impacted by severe or chronic pain as the patient tries to find deeper meaning in their suffering. Besides medicine, spirituality is a common source of solace for patients in pain (Kiser-Larson, 2017). Patients may turn to their faith for strength to get through the difficulties related to pain, or alternatively, may lose faith due to their suffering. The hospice nurse can use a brief screening tool, such as the FICA Spiritual History Tool (Pulchalski & Romer, 2000), to assess for spiritual distress, and should also work closely with the members of the interdisciplinary team, particularly the hospice chaplain, to address the patient's spiritual needs.

33. **C:** Advance care planning is a collaborative effort between healthcare providers, patients, and families through which patients establish their preferences for future medical treatments (Moore, 2007). Patients may express their advance directives through the development of a living will or by designating a medical power of attorney (see Figure 15.1; Wright, 2017). Advance directives are used to guide care only when patients are unable to speak or make decisions for themselves (see also, Chapter 3).

34. **A:** Confusion occurs when a patient is unable to think clearly. When a patient is confused, judgment and decision-making capacity are impaired (Boss & Huether, 2014). Confusion may result from a number of factors, including medical reasons, psychological reasons, or an inability to keep track of time and dates due to illness, hospitalization, or altered sleep cycles. The patient in the scenario may be admitted to hospice with the consent of his proxy but he may not sign the consent himself due to his confusion.

35. **B:** Hallmark motor symptoms that occur in patients who have Parkinson's disease are bradykinesia, muscle rigidity, postural instability or unbalance, and resting tremor. Tremor, rigidity, and movement disorder are the three components of the "classic triad" of Parkinson's disease (PD) symptoms.

36. **B:** The World Health Organization (WHO) developed the WHO pain ladder to help guide interventions for patients experiencing cancer pain. The stepwise approach indicates that the first step in the management of cancer pain is nonopioid medication with or without adjuvant therapies. Adjuvant therapies may include nonsteroidal anti-inflammatory drugs (NSAIDs), COX-2 inhibitors, muscle relaxants, psychotropic medications,

antidepressants, antiepileptic drugs, anxiolytics, sedative/hypnotics, amphetamine, antiarrhythmics, calcium channel blockers, ketamine, lidocaine, capsaicin, tramadol, botulinum toxin, and other miscellaneous drugs (Shanti et al., 2012). If the patient's pain is not responsive to the interventions initiated in step 1, then step 2 involves the use of opioid medications with or without adjuvants. Nonopioids may also be used with opioids, if indicated. If the pain persists or worsens, then step 3 involves the use of opioids for moderate to severe pain, which may involve the use of both long-acting and short-acting pain medications as well as adjuvants.

37. **B:** When establishing goals, it is important to ensure that they are measurable so that results can be observed and quantified. A goal may be somewhat broad in its scope and thus may have associated objectives. Objectives are more specific than goals and can be seen as steps that need to be achieved to meet the overall goal. Both goals and objectives should be developed according to the patient's preferences and should be specific to the situation, measurable, and realistic. A commonly used mnemonic used to describe the necessary components of goals and objectives is the SMART model, which stands for specific, measureable, achievable, relevant, and timely.

38. **B:** Inhaled corticosteroids can cause overgrowth of candida. The risk of thrush is decreased by thoroughly rinsing the mouth after use of inhalers. Addition of a spacer may also help.

39. **B:** In patients who have cancer, the disease trajectory involves a period of stability followed by a period of decline. The expected time from terminal diagnosis to death is approximately 6 months without intervention. During the period of decline, the patient may experience symptoms of weight loss, gradual decreased ability to engage in activities of daily living, and a progressive decline in overall condition.

40. **C:** In order to provide proper care for the patient, the family must be well-informed regarding the illness, disease progression, medication use, and use of equipment. The nurse must identify barriers to family education such as low English proficiency, low literacy, caregiver confidence, family dynamics, and cultural beliefs regarding care during illness. Verbal instruction should be supplemented with written instructions, and the nurse can use the teach-back method to ensure the caregiver's ability to complete skills. There is no evidence that the caregiver is unable to complete to the skill, thus the skill does not need to be completed by someone else. Also, allowing the caregiver to practice with water is not contraindicated. But the teach-back method ensures that the caregiver understands the skills well enough to explain it step by step.

41. **D:** The patient in the scenario is experiencing opioid-induced constipation. A senna/docusate combination will take up to 72 hours to be effective. Methylnaltrexone may be an option for the patient, but first the nurse should rule out impaction. Methylnaltrexone will not remove an impaction. Although the nurse should auscultate the patient's bowel sounds, ascultating does not meet the patient's needs. The intervention that most effectively meets the patient's need at this time is determining whether an impaction exists. If so, the nurse can attempt digital impaction and alleviate the patient's pain immediately.

42. **B:** Selective serotonin reuptake inhibitors such as citalopram, 20 to 60 mg daily, escitalopram 10 to 20 mg daily, paroxetine 20 to 50 mg daily, fluoxetine 20 to 60 mg daily, fluvoxamine 50 to 100 mg twice daily, or sertraline 50 to 200 mg daily are useful for decreasing symptoms of depression but may take several weeks to achieve therapeutic effect. If the patient's life expectancy is thought to be less than 2 weeks, methylphenidate (Concerta, Ritalin) may be used to treat symptoms of depression (Periyakoil, 2016). Benzodiazepines are not recommended for depression.

43. **A:** As with any open wound, partial or full-thickness pressure ulcers incur risk for infection. The wound, combined with the patient's compromised immunity, increases the risk of sepsis.

44. **B:** For patients who have been diagnosed with a terminal illness and have a life expectancy of approximately 6 months, hospice services may be an option. Patients who are eligible for Medicare Part A may receive services provided that they accept hospice care instead of curative treatments, sign a statement choosing hospice care and revoking Medicare benefits for curative treatment of the terminal condition, and receive certification of terminality (life expectancy of 6 months or less) from *both* the primary care physician *and* the hospice medical director (Centers for Medicare & Medicaid Services, 2015a). Other criteria used to support terminality and eligibility for services, such as local coverage determinations (LCDs), determine eligibility for hospice care.

45. **B:** Artificial nutrition can be considered when it is consistent with the patient's wishes. However, the hospice nurse should explain that artificial nutrition does little good at the end of life and may actually increase distressing symptoms (Heidrich, 2007). When patients have artificial nutrition orders in place, a decrease in the amount administered or discontinuation should be considered if the patient experiences untoward effects such as vomiting, aspiration, edema, congestive heart failure, pulmonary edema, or other signs of fluid overload.

46. **B:** The patient is exhibiting symptoms of pulmonary embolism. Pharmacological interventions center on intravenous (IV) resuscitation and vascular stabilization. If aggressive or curative treatments are not in alignment with the goals of care, steps should be taken to alleviate dyspnea and anxiety. Sedation may be required if the patient is severely distressed and symptomatic. Family education is needed throughout the process, as a pleural effusion (PE) can occur suddenly and the prognosis is poor if interventions are not initiated quickly.

47. **C:** A pain scale that was developed specifically for patients who have dementia is the Pain Assessment in Advanced Dementia (PAINAD) scale (Warden et al., 2003). In addition to dementia, the patients who were part of the original validation study for this tool were aphasic or otherwise lacked the ability to communicate their level of pain verbally. The PAINAD includes only five items, so it is a quick assessment for nonverbal patients that is easy to use in the clinical setting (Ware et al., 2006).

48. **D:** The hospice and palliative nurse should frequently assess the well-being of the caregiver for signs of role strain such as feeling tired and overwhelmed, insomnia or increased somnolence, unplanned weight changes, irritability, loss of interest in previously enjoyable activities, somatic complaints, and overuse or reliance on drugs (prescription or nonprescription) or alcohol (Mayo Clinic, 2018).

49. **A:** A foam dressing is most appropriate for a stage 2 ulcer with exudate. Thin film dressings are used only to protect skin; hydrocolloid and hydrogel dressings are used for wounds without exudate.

50. **C:** When patients are cared for at home, caregiver stress, lack of support, resentment, or other issues may sometimes lead to aggressive behavior toward the patient. Thus, the nurse and other members of the interdisciplinary team must monitor for signs of abuse such as bruising in unusual places, burns, preventable decubiti, dehydration, evidence of sexual abuse, malnutrition, withheld medications, unexplained fractures, urine burns, or inattention to hygiene (Hoover & Polson, 2014).

51. **C:** According to the National Hospice and Palliative Care Organization, all hospice members should be invited to the interdisciplinary team meetings. Because hospice care is holistic and family-centered, it is critical that the patient and/or family be invited to participate in interdisciplinary team meetings. During team meetings, the nurse offers input regarding nursing assessments, changes in the patient's condition, responses to medication or treatment changes, and the types of supportive care needed. It is not necessary to invite outside support persons, such as personal spiritual advisors.

52. **A:** Spiritual issues, such as loss of faith or feelings of meaninglessness, may arise at the end of life as patients face the unknown and question what might happen after they take their last breaths. The ability to recognize and address patients' spiritual concerns is central to end-of-life care because "patients' learn to cope and understand their suffering through their spiritual beliefs, or the spiritual dimension of their lives" (Pulchalski & Roma, 2000, p. 129). The patient's spiritual needs should be identified by the hospice and palliative care nurse who is responsible for assessing spiritual suffering, meeting the patients' immediate needs, and working with other members of the health team to develop and implement a plan for ongoing support (Wright, 2017). The hospice and palliative care chaplain or social worker are key members of the interdisciplinary team whose expertise is invaluable in supporting patients through spiritual distress.

53. **D:** Grief is the manifestation of physical and emotional responses to an impending or actual loss. Grief involves deep sorrow and emotions such as sadness, guilt, anger, despair, and shame (Potter & Wynne, 2015). Typically, the intensity of grief symptoms slowly lessen over time. As the intensity of grief decreases, the person is more and more able to reengage in their usual activities.

54. **A:** Visceral pain is related to pain in the organs or viscera. It is experienced as gnawing and achy and usually requires a multimodal approach to pain management. Visceral pain is also common at the end of life and is often related to "metastases, biliary obstruction, and pancreatitis, as well as pancreatic tumors and small bowel or colon obstruction" (Groninger & Vijayan, 2014, p. 30).

55. **A:** Diagnosis of bladder spasm is primarily based on the patient's report of symptoms such as stabbing, cramping, or colicky pain in the suprapubic area. The pain may be associated with urinary urgency or leakage. Management of bladder spasm involves addressing the underlying etiology, if possible. If a urinary catheter is in place, it should be changed to a smaller size. The balloon should be inflated to the appropriate size. Patients who experience bladder spasm should be taught to drink sufficient fluids and avoid bladder irritants such as caffeine and alcohol. Anticholinergic medications may also be used to inhibit contractions.

56. **B:** The FICA tool can be used to assess spiritual beliefs and needs. FICA stands for **F:** faith or beliefs; **I:** importance and influence of one's faith in life; **C:** community of faith (if any); **A:** address the patient's spiritual concerns (Pulchalski & Roma, 2000).

57. **D:** Although pain clearly has a physiologic basis, McCaffery's (1968) well-accepted definition of pain emphasizes the primacy of the patient's experience and personal description of his or her pain. McCaffery's definition states that "pain is whatever the experiencing person says it is, existing whenever he says it does"

(p. 95). Thus, the cornerstone of good pain management is masterful assessment, which is predicated on gathering both subjective and objective data. Subjective data includes the patient's perception of the pain in terms of intensity, temporality, radiating nature, and character. Objective data that lends clarity to the pain assessment includes the patient's medical history.

58. **C:** There is a direct correlation between pressure ulcer risk and severity and nutritional deficiencies, particularly low protein, and albumin.

59. **D:** Incomplete cross-tolerance occurs when the newly introduced drug causes unexpected hyperalgesia. When changing opioids, incomplete cross-tolerance is thought to be due to the individual's response to the new opioid or the molecular differences between opioids (Botke & Ligon, 2016). To account for cross-tolerance, the equianalgesic dose of the newly introduced drug should be reduced by 50% to avoid overdose and/or hyperalgesia (Prescriber's Letter, 2012). The newly introduced drug can be slowly titrated upward to achieve effective pain management. Throughout the titration process, the patient should be carefully monitored and breakthrough medication should be available (Kishner, 2018).

60. **C:** Complicated grief responses are more common among those who have a history of mental illness or have experienced disenfranchised grief. Disenfranchised grief results when a significant loss is not openly or publicly recognized, such as in the case of suicide, pregnancy loss, or loss at war (Doka, 2008). The social recognition of loss and grief are critical to garnering support and sharing grief with others.

61. **B:** The patient is experiencing pruritus as a side effect of morphine. Pruritus is common with morphine use, but is also associated with the use of other opioids. In palliative care settings, opioid-induced pruritus may necessitate opioid rotation, dose reduction, discontinuance of the opioid, or the addition of other medications (Rashid et al., 2018). Patients usually develop a tolerance to pruritus within a few days of beginning to use an opioid medication. Therefore, in this case, the opioid should be rotated for the comfort of the patient.

62. **A:** The patient is experiencing symptoms consistent with infection; thus, the fever should be treated with acetaminophen. Antidiarrheals, such as loperamide, should be used cautiously when fever is present. Oral liquids are not appropriate as the patient is vomiting. Antibiotics are not indicated by the scenario.

63. **D:** The following symptoms are associated with complicated grief: longing, yearning, hallucinations, preoccupation with thoughts of the deceased, intrusive thoughts about the deceased, avoidance of people and places that can trigger grief, altered sleep patterns,

and failure to adapt to the loss over time (Horowitz et al., 2003; Prigerson et al., 1996; Shear, 2015; Worden, 1991).

64. **C:** The patient in the scenario is exhibiting early signs of increased intracranial pressure (ICP). Signs of ICP include restlessness, altered consciousness, blurred vision, severe headache, nausea and vomiting, behavioral changes, diminished level of consciousness, fever, and lethargy (Johns Hopkins Medicine, 2018; Weaver, 2015). Hyperosmolar therapy, such as mannitol, may be used intravenously at a rate of 0.25 to 1 mg/kg body weight. If mannitol is used, arterial hypotension, defined as a systolic blood pressure of <90 mmHg, should be avoided. Side effects of mannitol include headache, blurred vision, dry mouth, dizziness, and nausea, among others. Because headache is a sign of increased ICP and a possible sideeffects of mannitol, the nurse would not be surprised if the patient reported severe headache.

65. **C:** According to Maslow's hierarchy of needs, safety is a more basic priority than psychological needs, which include family processes. There is no evidence in the stem of the question to indicate that the patient is bedbound or otherwise at risk for infection or skin breakdown. However, all neurological disorders affect movement, which increases the risk for falls.

66. **A:** During patient transitions, such as transfer of the patient to an inpatient setting from home, or at the time of a patient's death, the use of a standard communication tool, such as the SBAR (Pope et al., 2008), has been recommended to facilitate smooth transitions (The Joint Commission, 2012). SBAR is used in healthcare settings to convey the *situation:* identify yourself, identify the patient, and succinctly explain what the issue is—in hospice settings this may also entail information about the patient's home situation and family dynamics; *background:* provide information that helps to situate the current problem such as pertinent medical history, lab results, and any recent changes in condition; *assessment:* describe what you think the problem is and the severity of the problem; *recommendation:* provide a recommendation for what should happen next. Recommendation may be the need to prescribe a different prescription drug or change the dosage of currently used medications. Other recommendations may include a change in the level of care, such as, a transfer from home to the inpatient unit for symptom management.

67. **D:** According to the World Health Organization, "to maintain freedom from pain, drugs should be given 'by the clock' or 'around the clock' rather than only 'on demand' (i.e., PRN). This means they are given on a regularly scheduled basis. The frequency will depend on whether it is a long- or short-acting preparation"

(WHO, 2018). Therefore, in the scenario presented in the question, the patient's pain medication should be converted to a long-acting opioid given on a schedule.

68. **B:** In the scenario, the patient is expressing fears related to faith and spiritual beliefs. The nurse has taken a position near the patient and sat down, indicating that there is no rush and the nurse is fully available and focused on the patient. This is an example of providing active listening and presence. Providing spiritual support may also entail upholding the patient's dignity throughout the course of her or his illness; providing a compassionate and caring environment; providing active listening, presence, respect, and support; being available to listen to the patient's concerns; encouraging attendance at religious services or a visit from the patient's faith leader; facilitating the use of meditation, prayer, or other religious practices; encouraging life review; helping patients clarify their beliefs and values, as appropriate; providing spiritual music, literature, radio, or television programs for the patient; praying with the patient, as appropriate (Kisvetrová et al., 2013).

69. **C:** Anorexia is loss of appetite that can occur from illness, emotional stress, or medications. Severe or prolonged anorexia can lead to cachexia, but these conditions are actually two separate medical issues that can occur independently of each other. Cachexia is manifested by weight loss, fluid retention, muscle wasting, and metabolic changes. When these two conditions occur together, particularly at the end stage of a disease process, the condition is referred to as anorexia/cachexia syndrome (ACS; Wholihan, 2015).

70. **B:** Family disagreements can occur regarding the plan of care, especially when the patient's condition is deteriorating. The nurse should determine who is the primary decision-maker and discuss how other members of the family can offer input and feel heard. In the scenario, there is no indication that the patient is unable to make her own decisions, so the patient is the primary decision-maker. There is no indication that security or a patient advocate are needed at this time.

71. **A:** Angina, also called angina pectoris, is chest pain caused by increased oxygen demands on the cardiac muscle. It can result from exercise, strenuous activity, an obstruction within a cardiac vessel, or myocardial infarction. Angina can be classified as either stable or unstable. Typical manifestations of angina include sudden chest pain, heaviness, tightness, or a squeezing sensation. The pain can sometimes radiate to the jaw, arms, or back. Associated symptoms can include shortness of breath, fatigue, and nausea

(McDonald, 2015). When angina occurs, the patient should discontinue precipitating activities. Nitroglycerin should be administered sublingually, orally, transdermally, intravenously, or as a lingual spray.

72. **C:** Appropriate grief responses for teenagers may include feeling overwhelmed by emotions and engaging in risky behaviors. The teen may exhibit attention deficit, anxiety, and distraction; feelings of isolation; and withdrawal from family. The teen may draw nearer to friends.

73. **B:** The use of acetaminophen has been effective for the patient and there is no indication of increased pain. The medication does not need to change, but the route needs to change due to the patient's new-onset dysphagia. Thus, the acetaminophen should be administered rectally.

74. **D:** Ascites is the accumulation of fluid in the abdominal cavity due to portal hypertension and hypoalbuminemia. Other causes include malignancy and heart failure. Regardless of the cause, ascites is an indication of end-stage disease. It causes abdominal discomfort, altered body image, decreased mobility, and dyspnea as the fluid increases pressure on the diaphragm.

75. **A:** Most branches of Abrahamic faith traditions, such as Judaism, Christianity, and Islam, teach that there is some form of an afterlife. Some believe that the soul continues on, some believe that there will be a resurrection of the body, and others believe that the afterlife is a new life in the presence of God (Sherman & Free, 2015). Eastern faith traditions, such as Hinduism and Buddhism, teach that when the current life ends, a new life may begin through reincarnation. The circumstances of death may influence the next reincarnation, so the nurse must take steps to ensure that a calm and peaceful environment is maintained.

76. **B:** The patient in the scenario is experiencing symptoms of hypercalcemia as a result of bone deterioration secondary to metastasis. Patients who have hypercalcemia may exhibit symptoms such as nausea, vomiting, anorexia, weakness, constipation, thirst, and changes in mentation. Diagnosis of hypercalcemia is confirmed through serum analysis. Patients with a serum calcium level >14 mg/dL require urgent intervention. Even in advanced disease, interventions should be started to reverse hypercalcemia for the patient's comfort. Bisphosphonates such as pamidronate and zoledronate are used most frequently. Intravenous hydration, administration of calcitonin, use of bone reabsorption agents such as gallium nitrate or plicamycin, or dialysis may also be considered (Bobb, 2015; Kuriya & Dev, 2016).

77. **D:** All nursing practice is governed by the board of nursing in each state or territory. Every nurse is responsible for adhering to the rules and regulations set forth by the board of nursing.

78. **B:** Hospice and palliative care nurses must develop cultural awareness, which is the ability to identify and appreciate cultural differences between themselves and their patients. In healthcare settings, cultural preferences influence medical decisions, family decision-making, and the types of nonmedical interventions the patient might choose.

79. **C:** In the allopathic medical model, illness is viewed as a "disruption in physical or biochemical processes that can be manipulated by health care" (Sherman & Free, 2015, p. 93). In holistic or naturopathic health models, illness is viewed as an imbalance in energy, or in yin and yang, the vital life forces. Moreover, some cultures associate illness with evil, sin, or curses (Sherman & Free, 2015). The patient in the scenario is viewing her illness through the lens of a holistic healthcare model. In order to convey understanding of the patient's perspective, the nurse should determine if there are any interventions that would help the patient feel more comfortable or "balanced" at this time.

80. **B:** Causes of urinary retention can include mechanical obstruction, neurological issues, infection, or medications. In particular, opioids when used in combination with anticholinergics are more likely to cause urinary retention.

81. **C:** The patient is describing gastric symptoms that could be the result of excessive doses of ibuprofen. The maximum daily dose of ibuprofen is 2,400 mg/d. Side effects are similar to other NSAIDs and may include bleeding and exacerbation of peptic ulcer disease. Therefore, the most appropriate teaching intervention focuses on the maximum daily dose of ibuprofen.

82. **B:** Patients may not exhibit signs of chronic kidney disease (CKD) until kidney function "declines to less than 25% of normal when normal adaptive renal reserves have been exhausted" (Doig & Huether, 2014, p. 1364). This percentage correlates with stage 4 renal disease, characterized by a GFR between 15 and 29 or 15% to 29% of normal kidney function (National Kidney Foundation, 2017).

83. **D:** The report from the National Consensus Project (NCP) provided the first coherent account of what quality end-of-life care entailed. The Clinical Practice Guidelines were endorsed by the National Quality Forum (NQF) in 2006, lending further credence to this excellent work. The Clinical Practice Guidelines underpin the provision of high-quality, uniform end-of-life care across multiple practice settings and serves as the foundation for many other

hospice and palliative care initiatives and guidelines (Dahlin, 2015).

84. **C:** In providing care for patients who have language barriers, the priority intervention is accessing translation services to ensure that the patient has an accurate understanding of the care provided. Overall, nondominant cultural groups are at risk for poor access to healthcare services, provider bias, gender inequity, and language barriers. In addition to cultural groups, nurses must be aware that healthcare disparities also affect several other disenfranchised groups, such as older adults, patients who have disabilities, veterans, those who have low English proficiency, and those of lower socioeconomic status. Specifically, vulnerable populations may have poor access to transportation, steady healthcare providers, insurance coverage, or needed medications (Ritter & Graham, 2017; Wright & Hanson, 2016).

85. **A:** Respiratory depression is a decrease in respiratory function that can occur after the administration of an opioid. It may be mild, with the patient fully conscious, or it may lead to respiratory arrest. Opioid-induced respiratory depression is most common among opioid-naïve patients, but other risk factors include history of sleep apnea, older age, anatomic anomalies, comorbid conditions, psychological state, functional status, drug–drug interactions, cardiac or respiratory disorders, obesity (Jarzyna et al., 2011).

86. **D:** Patients must strictly adhere to the treatment regimen or risk viral devastation of the immune system. In fact, adherence to antiviral medications is so important that it is considered the most significant predictor of positive long-term prognosis (Gorman, 2015). Compliance is related to the complexity of the drug regimen, the severity of the patient's symptoms, younger age of the patient, presence of mental illness, and the availability of a support network (Gorman, 2015). Goals of care in the early stages of HIV should center on maximizing function and longevity within the limits of the disease process and preventing transmission of the virus (Centers for Disease Control and Prevention, 2017).

87. **A:** The serious illness of one member of the family affects all members of the family and alters normal family processes. The primary caregivers may have multiple domains of their lives affected as they take on the care of the patient and also attempt to balance their other responsibilities (Wittenberg et al., 2014). The hospice and palliative care nurse must identify the family needs, connect the family with needed resources, and provide support as needed. Further, the nurse should work with the interdisciplinary care team to help manage manifestations of family disputes and/or dysfunction.

88. **B:** Without curative treatment, the life expectancy for colon cancer is 6 months or less. The disease trajectory of COPD and dementia is less certain. Therefore, the diagnosis of cancer should be used as the terminal diagnosis for the purposes of hospice care.

89. **C:** T1, T2, T3, and T4 refer to the size and/or extent of the main tumor. The higher the number after the T, the larger the tumor or the more it has grown into nearby tissues. T's may be further divided to provide more detail, such as T3a and T3b. N1, N2, and N3 refer to the number and location of lymph nodes that contain cancer. The higher the number after the N, the more lymph nodes that contain cancer. M0 means there is no evidence that cancer has spread to other parts of the body.

90. **A:** A RN may delegate certain tasks to licensed practical nurses/licensed vocational nurses (LPNs/LVNs) and to unlicensed assistive personnel (UAP). "Delegation is the act of empowering another person to act. Delegation occurs in a downward manner" (Williams et al., 2015, p. 24). The nurse who chooses to delegate tasks must be aware of the state laws and regulations related to delegation because the delegator remains responsible for the outcomes of the delegate's tasks (National Council of the State Boards of Nursing, 2018).

91. **C:** The patient has end-stage dementia and is, therefore, nonverbal. The patient is exhibiting physical manifestations of pain such as grimacing, jaw clenching, and calling out. The patient's pain should be addressed immediately.

92. **D:** When opioid-naïve patients begin using opioids, common side effects include sedation, dry mouth, nausea, lightheadedness, drowsiness, loss of appetite, diaphoresis, restlessness, euphoria, and constipation, among others. Patients will develop a tolerance to all side effects except constipation because opioids slow motility of the gastrointestinal tract.

93. **B:** Delegation involves excellent communication between the delegator and the delegate. Before the delegate carries out delegated tasks, the RN should check the five rights of delegation: (a) the right task, (b) under the right circumstances, (c) to the right person, (d) with the right directions and communication, and (e) under the right supervision and evaluation (American Nurses Association/National Council of State Boards of Nursing, 2005).

94. **A:** Anxiety is a very common end-of-life symptom and should be addressed by teaching and coaching the patient in deep breathing and relaxation techniques, visualization, meditation, and the use of essential oil (topically or diffused; Buckle, 2015; Martinez-Kratz, 2015). For patients with persistent anxiety with or without depressive features, escitalopram 10 to 20 mg daily may

be effective. For patients who have intermittent or situational anxiety, or a life expectancy of less than 2 weeks, a benzodiazepine such as lorazepam (0.5–1 mg PO/IM/IV/SC BID or TID) is recommended. Short-acting anxiolytics are less useful than a long-acting medication such as escitalopram for patients such as the one described in the scenario.

95. **D:** Bereavement is the condition of being separated from someone, usually through death. It is often seen as a period of mourning.

96. **C:** In collaboration with the other members of the interdisciplinary team, the nurse can take the following steps to provide spiritual support: uphold the patient's dignity throughout the course of their illness; provide a compassionate and caring environment; provide active listening, presence, respect, and support; be available to listen to the patient's concerns; encourage attendance at religious services or a visit from the patient's faith leader; facilitate the use of meditation, prayer, or other religious practices; encourage life review; help the patient clarify personal beliefs and values, as appropriate; provide spiritual music, literature, radio, or television programs for the patient; and pray with the patient, as appropriate (Kisvetrová et al., 2013).

97. **B:** Family disagreements can occur regarding the plan of care, especially when the patient's condition is deteriorating. The nurse must collaborate with the interdisciplinary team to plan family discussions and to mediate conflict. Family meetings are structured by setting an agenda, inviting family members to share their feelings about the current circumstances, discussing the patient's daily care needs, determining who is the primary decision-maker, discussing how other members of the family can offer input and feel heard, and problem-solving regarding how to honor the patient's wishes, ensure comfort, and promote dignity (Family Caregiver Alliance, 2018). When a meeting takes place, the first step is to set the agenda so that everyone knows the focus of the meeting.

98. **C:** Early diagnosis of dementia is crucial because, although it is incurable, several interventions are available to slow disease progression and maintain quality of life for as long as possible. Physical, occupational, and speech therapies should be initiated early in the disease process to maintain physical integrity and preserve speech and swallowing ability.

99. **C:** A RN may delegate certain tasks to icensed practical nurses/licensed vocational nurses (LPNs/LVNs) and to unlicensed assistive personnel (UAP). "Delegation is the act of empowering another person to act. Delegation occurs in a downward manner" (Williams et al., p. 24). The nurse who chooses to delegate tasks

must be aware of the state laws and regulations related to delegation because the delegator remains responsible for the outcomes of
the delegate's tasks (National Council of the State Boards of Nursing, 2018).

100. **B:** Confidentiality is the expectation that the patient's private
information not be disclosed to anyone without consent.

101. **A:** To effectively advocate for the patient, the nurse must rely on
written documents, conversations with the patient, and the documentation in the medical record to ascertain the patient's stated
wishes.

102. **D:** Neuropathy, which means nerve damage or disease, can
result from high glucose levels, nerve injury, tumor growth, and
ischemia (National Institute of Neurological Disorders and Stroke,
2018c). Peripheral neuropathy is particularly common in the lower
extremities and can lead to undetected foot infection, injury, or
ulceration.

103. **D:** The patient has described pain that is dull and crampy. More
assessment information is needed. Thus the nurse should determine when the patient's last bowel movement was, and also ask
assessment questions related to the P-Q-R-S-T tool. Assessment of
a patient is structured in the following order: assessment, auscultation, percussion, palpation.

104. **B:** Patients generally develop a tolerance to most side effects
of opioids, except constipation. Constipation must, therefore, be
aggressively managed using both pharmacological and nonpharmacologic interventions (Rogers et al., 2013).

105. **D:** Regardless of cancer type, the greatest risk for cancer is advancing age. Risk for specific types of cancers are related to gender,
diet, genetic predisposition, and other factors.

106. **B:** Ethical dilemmas occur in clinical practice when treatment
options or other aspects of the patient's care, including the
patient's treatment preferences, conflict with one or more ethical
principles.

107. **A:** True allergic reactions to opioids are rare. If an allergic reaction
does occur, it is usually to a morphine derivative. In such cases, a
test dose of a synthetic opioid, such as fentanyl, may be attempted
(Paice, 2015; Wahler et al., 2017). If the patient has a true allergy to
morphine drugs as well as to fentanyl and meperidine, methadone
may be used (Abrahm, 2014).

108. **B:** According to the Centers for Disease Control and Prevention
(2017), heart disease is the leading cause of death for American
men and women.

109. **C:** Around the time of the patient's death, family members may draw near to spend the last days or hours with the patient. Often this time is referred to as the "death vigil." Hospice and palliative care nurses can provide support for families by providing teaching them about the process of dying (see Chapter 10, Dementia). The nurse should also encourage the family and caregivers to say their goodbyes and seek closure, as appropriate.

110. **D:** Moral distress, grieving, frequent exposure to death and dying, workload pressure, lack of support, existential issues, and intrateam conflicts can lead to occupational stress for hospice nurses. Other factors that can contribute to occupational stress include workplace bullying, generational differences, personality types, and work values. Serious consequences of workplace stress include disengagement, increased absenteeism, decreased job satisfaction, decreased productivity, low morale, and compassion fatigue (Wright, 2017).

111. **A:** A definitive diagnosis of chronic obstructive pulmonary disease (COPD) can be made only with spirometry.

112. **D:** When a patient is no longer eligible for hospice due to an improvement in health, the patient will be discharged from the service. Patients who choose curative treatment rather than palliative and end-of-life care may also initiate discharge by revoking the hospice benefit. When a patient is discharged, a discharge order must be written by the hospice medical director and the hospice team must include the patient and family in the discharge planning process (National Hospice & Palliative Care Organization, 2016).

113. **A:** Grief reactions may include avoidance of places, people, and things associated with the loss of a loved one. This mechanism is a way to suppress grief responses for a short time. When avoidance becomes routine and interferes with daily activities, it may be a sign of complicated grief.

114. **C:** Nursing management of pathological fractures centers on determining risks and providing teaching regarding proper positioning and patient safety. If a pathological fracture occurs, pain management and joint stabilization are priorities. The interdisciplinary team should collaborate with the patient and family to develop a plan of care that promotes quality of life and is consistent with the goals of care.

115. **C:** The assessment findings indicate left-sided heart failure. The most common cause of right-sided heart failure is left-sided heart failure. Thus, since the patient already has left-sided heart failure, they are at risk for right-sided heart failure.

116. **D:** Superior vena cava syndrome (SVCS) is a condition caused by obstruction of the superior vena cava and/or nearby lymph nodes or vessels. Most commonly, the obstruction occurs from a

primary tumor or metastasis from lung or breast cancer or lymphoma (Abrahm, 2014; Manthey & Ellis, 2016).

117. **D:** After the patient's death, the hospice or palliative care nurse should help the family break the news to loved ones, as necessary, and remain with the family to offer support. Initial assessment of the family's bereavement reactions should be documented and reassessed as needed. The hospice bereavement coordinator or social worker should develop a bereavement plan of care with the input from the interdisciplinary care team. Bereavement care may include visits, cards, invitations to memorial services, and/or support group attendance.

118. **B:** Neuropathic pain originates in the central or peripheral nervous system and is usually described as shooting, burning, stabbing, tingling, or as pins and needles. There are two types of neuropathic pain: peripheral and central.

119. **A:** When an eligible patient chooses hospice services, the first benefit period is for 6 months (two 90-day periods). After two 90-day periods, recertification of the terminal illness is required every 60 days for as long as the patient continues to meet the eligibility requirements (see Figure 15.3).

120. **C:** Palliative care is team-based care. The team's goal is to reduce the burden of disease through effective symptom management. The patient has stage 4 cardiac disease, which is a requirement for hospice care. However, the patient is inquiring about further intervention, not hospice care. Therefore the palliative care nurse should arrange for a team meeting, including the cardiologist, to discuss whether an LVAD is an option for the patient. If so, the team should discuss how symptoms will be managed and goals of care.

121. **B:** For patients who are unable to speak, such as those very near death, or those who have dysarthria or dysphasia due to medical issues, an appropriate scale should, such as the FLACC scale, be used to routinely and uniformly assess and document the patient's level of comfort. Each category is scored on the 0 to 2 scale, which results in a total score of 0 to 10. The FLACC scale includes five categories rated on a 0 to 2 scale. The total score is interpreted as 0: relaxed and comfortable; 4 to 6: moderate pain; 1 to 3: mild discomfort; 7 to 10: severe discomfort or pain, or both.

122. **B:** Every 60 days after the initial two 90-day periods, a face-to-face visit must be made to the patient by the hospice physician or nurse practitioner to verify ongoing eligibility for hospice services.

123. **A:** In 2016, reimbursement regulations were changed to take into account the intense care that is provided for patients during their

final week of life. According to the Centers for Medicare & Medicaid Services (2015b), in order to receive the additional reimbursement, the following criteria must be met: the patient's level of care must be "routine home care," the billing dates of care occur within the last 7 days of the patient's life, and direct patient care is provided by a RN or licensed social worker.

124. **D:** The patient has end-stage Parkinson's disease with dementia. The patient is nonverbal and is, therefore, unable to rate his pain. The nurse needs more assessment information to determine the best course of action. Response D allows the nurse to affirm the daughter's assessment of her father and allows the nurse to gather the needed assessment data that will determine the next steps.

125. **D:** Diabetes-related complications include retinopathy, neuropathy, and macrovascular problems that increase the risk of stroke and cardiac events (Centers for Disease Control & Prevention, 2018a; Leontis & Hess-Fischl, 2019). Weight loss is an early sign of diabetes, especially in the presence of increased appetite. Thus it is more likely related to the diagnosis of pancreatic cancer. Poor appetite is not usually related to diabetes, except in the presence of uncontrolled blood glucose. Thus loss of appetite is likely related to the diagnosis of pancreatic cancer. Insulinomas are insulin-producing tumors that a consequence of pancreatic cancer.

126. **D:** The patient in the scenario is exhibiting signs of an opioid overdose. Signs of opioid overdose include confusion and/or delirium, vomiting, pinpoint pupils, lethargy and/or unresponsiveness, loss of consciousness, cyanosis, and/or respiratory distress or respiratory failure (American Addiction Centers, 2018).Hospice and palliative care nurses must be skilled at recognizing risk for and symptoms of opioid overdose and responding appropriately. Treating opioid overdose involves administration of naloxone intranasally, sublingually, intravenously, or intramuscularly. The onset of action is 1 to 2 minutes.

127. **A:** Physical symptoms associated with grief include nausea, fatigue, and myalgias. Grief support should begin with therapeutic listening, empathetic support, and assurance that the experience is normal. The team social worker and chaplain can provide expertise in facilitating life review, teaching cognitive behavioral therapy techniques, and providing spiritual support and guidance.

128. **B:** The patient has chronic pain and has set a pain goal that is in the range of moderate pain. The patient's reason for setting this goal is to promote safety, which is a misconception. The patient should be taught that unlike acute pain, chronic pain serves no useful purpose (Huether et al., 2014).

129. **C:** Adverse effects of opioids are sometimes related to the accumulation of toxic metabolites. This situation is especially concerning in patients whose drug metabolism and elimination are impaired due to hepatic or renal disease; so close monitoring of patients with organ failure is warranted (Paice, 2015). When toxicity occurs, opioid rotation becomes necessary. Other reasons for opioid rotation include lack of analgesic efficacy, drug–drug interactions, change in the patient's clinical status, and practical issues such as cost or lack of availability of a drug (Smith & Peppin, 2014).

130. **A:** When patients lose hope or face their own death, they may become fearful or depressed, which can lead to suicidal thoughts or thoughts of self-harm. Some warning signs of suicidal ideation are changes in behavior, giving away prized possessions, talking about suicide, withdrawing from friends or activities, or increasing use of alcohol or drugs (American Psychological Association, 2018). The key assessment questions for the nurse to ask are *Are you considering harming yourself?* and *Do you have a plan to harm yourself?* If the answer is *yes* to either of these questions, the patient is considered to be at risk for suicide and steps must be taken urgently to assure the patient's safety.

131. **D:** Immediate-release morphine is given for pain. Pain should be assessed prior to the intervention and then approximately 1 hour after the intervention. All assessments and interventions should be carefully documented in the patient's chart.

132. **A:** A Jewish religious leader is called a rabbi.

133. **A:** According to the Centers for Disease Control and Prevention (2017), the following are risk factors for chronic obstructive pulmonary disease (COPD): unemployment; being divorced, widowed, or separated from spouse; having less than a high school education; being a current or former smoker; history of asthma; age ≥65 years; American Indian/Alaska Native and multiracial non-Hispanic heritage; and female gender. In the United States, smoking is a key factor in the development and progression of COPD.

134. **D:** Hospice care involves four levels of care. The appropriate level of care is determined through conversations between the patient, the patient's family, and the interdisciplinary team. *Routine home care* is provided in the patient's home, which may be a long-term care facility. Visits from members of the hospice team are scheduled regularly as indicated by the patient's needs. *Continuous home care* is provided in the patient's home, predominantly by nurses, but also by hospice nurses' aides. The goal of continuous home care is to provide support for patients and families during a short-term crisis, such as a pain crisis. *Inpatient respite care* may be provided in an approved facility for a short period of time to allow respite for the caregiver(s). *General inpatient (GIP) care* takes place

in an inpatient facility with the goal of addressing acute pain or other symptoms (Centers for Medicare & Medicaid Services, 2015a).

135. **C:** The conversion guideline for converting an opioid from the oral to parenteral route is roughly 3:1

136. **B:** When a patient who has an AICD is actively dying, the device should be deactivated to prevent defibrillation. Placing a medical magnet over the AICD temporarily deactivates the device, but it must be permanently deactivated by a trained professional. The pacemaker function of the device should remain functional to prevent shortness of breath and irregular heart rhythm.

137. **C:** A Kennedy ulcer, also called a Kennedy terminal ulcer, is a form of decubiti that develops suddenly in patients who are near death. The ulcer may begin as a discoloration or a blister and then quickly deteriorates to a full-thickness ulcer. The ulcer usually appears on the sacral area and is often pear or butterfly shaped.

138. **D:** Hospice care necessarily involves the coordination of services and the development of a plan of care by an interdisciplinary team. Core hospice services that are covered by Medicare and Medicaid include physician services, nursing services with 24 hr/d, 7 d/wk availability, medical social services, and counseling. Noncare services must also be provided according to the patient's unique needs, condition, and living arrangements. These services include physical, occupational, and speech therapy, hospice aide services, homemaker services, volunteers, medical supplies and medications related to the terminal illness, and short-term inpatient care for acute or chronic symptom management in a Medicare/Medicaid participating facility (Centers for Medicare & Medicaid Services, 2015a).

139. **A:** 5 mg of oxycodone × 12 doses in 24 hours = 5 mg × 12 doses = 60 mg (total daily dose), then the long-acting dose would be calculated as 60 mg divided into two doses to be given every 12 hours = 30 mg of long-acting oxycodone every 12 hours.

140. **C:** During the last 72 hours of life, the symptoms most frequently experienced by patients with end-stage renal disease (ESRD) are dyspnea, fatigue, edema, pain (including angina), and anorexia. Most patients have more than one of these symptoms concomitantly (Kwok et al., 2016). Because of the unusual disease trajectory, patients may report feeling fairly well and may decline hospice admission until very late in the disease process.

141. **A:** The patient in the question scenario has signs and symptoms of thyroid storm. Thyroid storm is an acute manifestation of thyrotoxicosis. It can result from undertreatment of hyperthyroidism, noncompliance with the treatment regimen, or an inability to

take the medication. Thyroid storm is a medical emergency that is associated with hyperthyroidism. Symptoms include sweating, fever, tachycardia, hypertension, agitation, confusion, and diarrhea. It must be promptly treated with antithyroid drugs, inorganic iodine, bile acid sequestrants, beta-blockers, and glucocorticoids (De Leo et al., 2016; Levesque, 2012). Therefore, the most important question for the nurse to ask at this time is whether the patient has been able to take her prescribed medications, including the medications for hyperthyroidism. This piece of information would confirm the nurse's suspicion that the patient is in thyroid crisis, which in turn, would lead to proper decision-making regarding how to handle this medical emergency.

142. **B:** In patients who have advanced disease, palliation of symptoms is the primary goal. The least invasive approach to reducing a pulmonary embolism (PE) is pleuroscopy and placement of an indwelling pleural catheter (see Figure 14.3), which should be initiated when the benefits of the intervention outweigh the risks (Engleka, 2016).

143. **D:** The most common sites of lung cancer metastasis, in order, are the opposite lung, adrenal gland, bone, brain, liver.

144. **D:** Opioid-induced neurotoxicity (OIN) is a syndrome that results from an accumulation of opioid metabolites. Any opioid drug can induce OIN, but it is most commonly associated with morphine. Myoclonus is one of the first and most common manifestations of OIN. Management of OIN is aimed at reversing the mechanism; so reducing the dose of the opioid or rotating to a different opioid is recommended. Clonazepam, midazolam agents, benzodiazepines, baclofen, or dantrolene can be used for treating myoclonus (Abrahm, 2014; Walker, 2016).

145. **B:** Seizures may be of two sorts: focal or generalized. Focal seizures are characterized by an altered level of consciousness during which the patient may have uncontrollable repetitive movements, called automatisms. Focal seizures result from abnormal electrical activity in only one part of the brain. Focal seizures do not cause the same widespread symptoms as generalized symptoms, so the patient in the scenario should be taught to ambulate with assistance. The other interventions are more appropriate precautions for generalized seizures.

146. **A:** Consistent engagement in self-care activities can help nurses to avoid burnout, build resilience, and reduce stress. Self-care activities are important because "clinicians meeting the criteria for burnout deliver poorer quality of care, make more medial errors, and display low empathy" (Back et al., 2016, p. 285). Thus nurses must engage in self-care as part of their professional responsibilities.

147. **B:** Nausea and vomiting related to the use of opioids may occur due to the effects of opioids on gastric motility and stimulation of the chemoreceptor trigger zones (CTZ).

148. **C:** A patient who states that he can smoke in his home while wearing oxygen requires teaching about safety risks, especially risk of fire. The other statements are true and do not need to be corrected.

149. **C:** Ondansetron is specifically indicated for preventing chemotherapy-induced nausea and vomiting. Dronabinol is useful if other treatments fail. Scopolamine is not indicated for nausea caused by chemotherapy treatments. Octreotide is recommended for nausea and vomiting associated with bowel obstruction.

150. **C:** The primary cause of liver disease is hepatitis C, followed by alcohol abuse-related cirrhosis (American Liver Foundation, 2017).

Index

CPSIA information can be obtained
at www.ICGtesting.com
Printed in the USA
BVHW082131020621
608674BV00004B/12